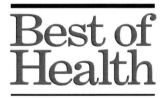

Best of Health

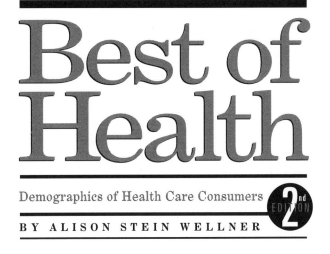

Best of Health

Demographics of Health Care Consumers **2**nd EDITION

BY ALISON STEIN WELLNER

New Strategist Publications, Inc.
Ithaca, New York

New Strategist Publications, Inc.
P.O. Box 242, Ithaca, New York 14851
800-848-0842
<www.newstrategist.com>

ISBN 1-885070-32-2

Printed in the United States of America

Table of Contents

List of Tables

Chapter 3. Changing Medical Relationships

Chapter 4. Growing Diversity in Health Care

Chapter 5. Making Sense of Health Information

Chapter 6. The Emerging Self-Care Industry

Chapter 7. Staying Fit and Eating Right

Chapter 8. Managing Diseases

Chapter 9. Living with Disability

Chapter 10. Mental Health Care Needs

Chapter 11. Treating Addictions

Chapter 12. Birth, Aging, and Death

List of Charts

INTRODUCTION

The consumers of health care drive one of the nation's largest and most important industries. Understanding who those consumers are, what they want, and how their wants and needs are changing is vital to health insurance companies, hospitals, doctors, pharmaceutical companies, government policy makers, and many others. Fortunately, there are enough statistics about health care consumers to answer almost any question researchers may pose. The problem is not whether the data exist, but finding them and making sense of them.

The second edition of *Best of Health: Demographics of Health Care Consumers* brings together in one volume the many sources of data on health care consumers, providing a comprehensive look at the demand for health care. More than a reference book, *Best of Health* goes beyond the numbers—the demographics—to examine how demographic change is influencing health care wants and needs now and in the future. New to the second edition is additional information about Americans' attitudes towards doctors, HMOs, death, and dying.

How to use this book

Best of Health is divided into 12 chapters, each of which explores the intersection between an important facet of the health care industry and the consumers of health care. Topics examined include the rapid rise of health care spending, the diversity of health care consumers, the changing relationship between medical providers and patients, the Internet's growing importance to health care, the deinstitutionalization of medical care, and changing attitudes towards disability, mental health, and even death. Each chapter includes explanatory text and charts which describe the most important trends. Detailed tables complete each chapter, revealing the characteristics of the consumers behind the trends.

Most of the tables in *Best of Health* draw on data collected by the federal government, in particular the National Center for Health Statistics. The federal government continues to be the best source of up-to-date, reliable information on the changing characteristics of Americans. Despite the volume of data produced by the federal government, finding relevant health care information and compiling it in a meaningful way is time-consuming—and often frustrating—because the government publishes its health care information in a mind-boggling variety of separate reports. The National Center for Health Statistics attempts to collate its information in the annual publication, *Health, United States*, but because the purpose of *Health, United States* is to provide an overview of health care, it focuses only briefly on health care consumers. *Best of Health* goes further by giving readers a comprehensive look at health care from the customer's perspective.

A great deal of information about health care lies inside the world's most authoritative medical journals. The author of *Best of Health* sifted through those journals for the latest data on health care consumers. From how to reach underserved minority markets to the emerging disability culture, *Best of Health* brings you leading-edge ideas from a variety of health care specialists.

To explore the attitudes of Americans toward health care, New Strategist extracted data from the nationally representative General Social Survey of the University of Chicago's National Opinion Research Center. NORC conducts the GSS as a biennial survey through face-to-face interviews with an independently drawn, representative sample of 1,500 to 3,000 noninstitutionalized English-speaking people aged 18 or older who live in the United States. The GSS is one of the best sources of attitudinal data available today.

While most of the data in *Best of Health* were collected by the government, the majority of the tables published here are not just reprints of the government's tabulations. Instead, New Strategist's editors individually compiled and created most of the tables to reveal the trends—the story behind the statistics. If you need more information than a table provides, explore the data source cited at its bottom.

Best of Health includes a list of tables to help you locate the information you need. For a more detailed search, use the index at the back of the book. At the end of each chapter and at the back of the book is a bibliography of data sources. Also at the back of the book is a comprehensive glossary defining the terms used in tables and text.

With *Best of Health* in hand, you will discover the changes that lie ahead for the health care industry. Because health care is one of the largest industries in the U.S., the ever-changing demands of its customers will shape the future of every American alive today—and those yet to be born.

1

The New Health Care Consumer

In 1900, life expectancy in the United States was just 47 years. Today, it is 77 years—or 30 years longer. During the past century, we've bought ourselves (literally) almost one additional lifetime.

Health care has come a long way in 100 years. At the beginning of the 20th century, drugs consisted of aspirin, opium, morphine, codeine, and heroin—or the doctor's own blend of ingredients. A physician's prescription was most often bed rest, a special diet, or quarantine. Millions of older Americans can remember a time when today's basic medical tools, such as penicillin, insulin, and the polio vaccine, were unavailable.

The rapid acceleration of medical technology has created a new health care consumer. One hundred years ago, a physician could hold all medical knowledge in his head. Today, the sheer volume of data about every aspect of human physiology has created innumerable

Life expectancy is up sharply since 1900

(years of life remaining at birth, 1900–98)

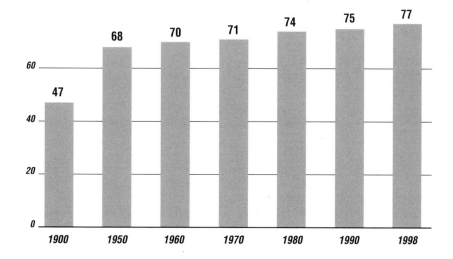

specialists. When we get sick today, treatment is no simple matter. We must coordinate all those specialists.

The role of medical care coordinator is a new one for consumers. The very word "patient"—which means submissive and calm—conflicts with the coordinator role. The new health care consumer is not patient at all. These less-than-patient "patients" enter the medical arena with the same concerns as people had a century ago. We have jumped from aspirin to lasers, but the basic goal of health care—prolonging life—is the same. Everything else has changed, however.

Although health care has become exceedingly complex, trends in the health care industry are not so difficult to foretell. The aging of the population, coupled with the changing attitudes of older Americans as the baby-boom generation becomes the nation's elders, will reshape the health care industry and affect the well-being of everyone alive today. Three major trends will determine the future of health care in the U.S.: rising expectations, growing consumer power, and the shift from disease treatment to lifestyle management.

Most Americans feel good or excellent

(percent of people reporting good or excellent health, by age, 1998)

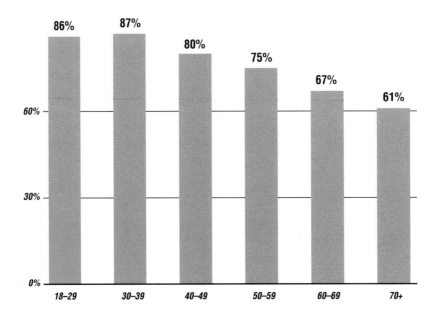

TREND 1: RISING EXPECTATIONS

The bar dividing good health from bad has been raised. "We have a culture that emphasizes youth, vigor, and good health, which in turn leads individuals to think they should feel well continuously," says Dr. Benjamin H. Natelson in his book, *Tomorrow's Doctors: The Path to Successful Practice in the 1990's.*[1]

Americans are feeling better than they once did. Between 1974 and 1998, despite the aging of the population, the percentage of people reporting "fair" or "poor" health fell from 27 to 21 percent. Even more telling, the percentage of the oldest Americans—people aged 70 or older—who report "fair" or "poor" health fell from 51 to 39 percent during those years.

In the past, feeling poorly was an accepted part of the aging process. Today we know better. We have discovered that many aging-related health problems are not only treatable, but preventable. This knowledge gives us more control over our physical well-being through diet, exercise, and other lifestyle decisions. It also makes us more demanding health care consumers.

TREND 2: CONSUMER POWER

Today, machines scan our insides and light beams are replacing scalpels. We have mapped the human genome, and the possibility of cloning humans has leapt from sci-fi movies to the front page of newspapers. It is all the more frustrating and bewildering when the medical community, armed with so much knowledge and technology, cannot save a life, particularly that of someone we love.

Americans have less confidence in the medical system

(percent of people aged 18 or older having "a great deal" of confidence in the people running medicine, 1974 and 1998)

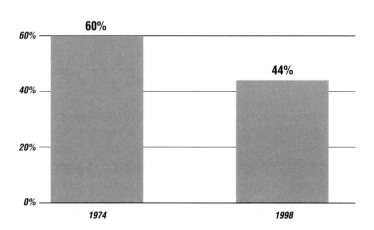

Despite a century of medical advances, we are more disillusioned with health care today than ever before. The percentage of Americans who have a "great deal" of confidence in the people running medicine fell from 60 percent in 1974 to 44 percent in 1998, according to the General Social Surveys of the University of Chicago's National Opinion Research Center. Perhaps it's our heightened expectations that have caused this disillusionment, or the contradictory opinions in the medical community regarding key health issues. Most likely, it's that consumers have learned to question authority. Whatever the reason, the result is that health care is no longer a physician-directed experience. It is now controlled by the consumer.

One factor driving the public to question medical authority is the deluge of information about health care in the popular media. This information may come from sources that are reputable or disreputable, paid or unpaid. Pharmaceutical companies, for example, spend more than $1 billion a year on consumer advertising, up from $50 million just ten years ago, according to *Advertising Age*.[2] Today's patients march into doctors' offices demanding brand name medications, a practice that would have shocked physicians of yesteryear.

Celebrities now publicize diseases and promote research into cures. Health information—both good and bad—is growing exponentially on the Internet. And as always, friends and family are important sources of medical information and advice. Armed with this jumble of information, consumers are questioning the medical care they receive, searching for the best doctor, demanding leading-edge procedures, and evaluating medical facilities. They are no longer willing to settle for second best. The growing power of consumers in the health care industry is turning the traditional practice of medicine upside down.

One of the demands of new health care consumers is recognition of their diversity. As the population has become more diverse, medical research and practice have been forced to broaden. In the past, most medical studies were limited to how a disease or course of treatment affected white men, ignoring differences by sex or race. Those studies are no longer acceptable to the public or to the medical community. Within medicine itself, diversity is also an issue. Health care providers are changing. In 1999, 25 percent of the nation's physicians were women, up from 16 percent in 1983. Asians accounted for 18 percent of medical students in 1997-98, up from 3 percent in 1980-81.

TREND 3: FROM DISEASE TREATMENT TO LIFESTYLE MANAGEMENT

"Remember natural causes? Now they're treatable conditions," writes Janice Castro in *The American Way of Health*.[3] Many diseases that were once fatal, like whooping cough, polio, and measles, have been virtually eliminated.

With some exceptions, we've come a long way in reducing the physical dangers of the world around us. Today the greater dangers lie within. Although survival rates have improved, cancer is not yet conquered—in fact, the incidence rate has grown by double digits over the past two decades. And we still battle a host of lifestyle-related health problems, from drug use to sexually transmitted diseases. Chronic conditions trouble a growing number of people. Americans with arthritis or high blood pressure now far outnumber those with tuberculosis. The most common serious health problems of today cannot be fixed in one office visit. They require preventive efforts beginning years before the first manifestation of disease. They require lifestyle changes to lessen the impact of disease. And they require long-term monitoring to improve the quality of life for those with disease.

The aging of the baby-boom generation will accelerate the trend away from disease treatment toward lifestyle management. In a few years, most boomers will be older than 50. The rise in chronic conditions accompanying the aging of this educated and demanding generation will change medical care. It will force the nation to confront out-of-control health care spending. It will pressure policy makers to set priorities for the delivery of health care. It will focus attention on healthy living. And it may lead to even faster advances in medical technology and treatment.

There has never been a better time to grow old.

Notes

1.   Benjamin H. Natelson, *Tomorrow's Doctors: The Path to Successful Practice in the 1990's* (New York: Plenum Press, 1990): 2.

2.   "DTC drug ads should hit $1 bil for 1998," *Advertising Age* (January 4, 1999): 1.

3.   Janice Castro, *The American Way of Health: How Medicine is Changing and What it Means to You* (Boston: Little, Brown, 1994): 108.

Confidence in Medicine, 1974 and 1998

"As far as people running medicine are concerned, would you say
you have a great deal of confidence, only some confidence,
or hardly any confidence at all in them?"

*(percent of people aged 18 or older responding "a great deal of confidence," 1974 and 1998;
percentage point change, 1974–98)*

	1998	1974	percentage point change
Total	**44%**	**60%**	**–16**
Men	49	59	–10
Women	40	61	–21
Black	44	58	–14
White	44	61	–17
Aged 18 to 29	49	71	–22
Aged 30 to 39	46	62	–16
Aged 40 to 49	40	59	–19
Aged 50 to 59	41	55	–14
Aged 60 to 69	41	52	–11
Aged 70 or older	46	52	–6
Not a high school graduate	49	57	–8
High school graduate	41	63	–22
Bachelor's degree	52	58	–6
Graduate degree	45	60	–15

*Source: 1974 and 1998 General Social Surveys, National Opinion Research Center, University of Chicago;
calculations by New Strategist*

Health Status, 1974 and 1998

"Would you say your own health, in general,
is excellent, good, fair, or poor?"

(percent of people aged 18 or older responding "excellent/good" or "fair/poor," 1974 and 1998; percentage point change, 1974–98)

	excellent/good			fair/poor		
	1998	*1974*	*percentage point change*	*1998*	*1974*	*percentage point change*
Total	**79%**	**73%**	**6**	**21%**	**27%**	**−6**
Men	78	77	1	22	24	−2
Women	79	69	10	21	31	−10
Black	72	57	15	28	42	−14
White	80	74	6	20	25	−5
Aged 18 to 29	86	88	−2	14	12	2
Aged 30 to 39	87	82	5	12	18	−6
Aged 40 to 49	80	74	6	20	26	−6
Aged 50 to 59	75	63	12	25	38	−13
Aged 60 to 69	67	58	9	33	42	−9
Aged 70 or older	61	48	13	39	51	−12
Not a high school graduate	56	56	0	44	43	1
High school graduate	79	80	−1	21	20	1
Bachelor's degree	91	90	1	9	10	−1
Graduate degree	86	81	5	14	19	−5

Source: 1974 and 1998 General Social Surveys, National Opinion Research Center, University of Chicago; calculations by New Strategist

Life Expectancy by Age and Sex, 1900 to 1998

(years of life remaining at birth and age 65 by sex, selected years 1900–98)

	total	men	women
At birth			
1998	76.7	73.8	79.5
1990	75.4	71.8	78.8
1980	73.7	70.0	77.4
1970	70.8	67.1	74.7
1960	69.7	66.6	73.1
1950	68.2	65.6	71.1
1900	47.3	46.3	48.3
At age 65			
1998	17.8	16.0	19.2
1990	17.2	15.1	18.9
1980	16.4	14.1	18.3
1970	15.2	13.1	17.0
1960	14.3	12.8	15.8
1950	13.9	12.8	15.0
1900	11.9	11.5	12.2

Source: National Center for Health Statistics, Health, United States, 2000; *and* Deaths: Final Data for 1998, *National Vital Statistics Report, Vol. 48, No. 11, 2000; calculations by New Strategist*

2

The Rapid Rise of Health Care Spending

It is no secret that Americans spend an enormous amount of money on health care—$4,094 per capita in 1998, including out-of-pocket expenses and the contributions of private employers and governments. For that tidy sum, we get the lowest rates of stomach cancer and cerebrovascular disease in the world. The Swiss spend much less per capita, yet have lower rates of infant mortality, lung cancer, ischemic heart disease, and chronic liver disease.

Switzerland is not the only country that fares better than the United States while spending less. Most other industrialized nations get more for their money than the U.S.— although we devote 13.5 percent of our gross domestic product to health care. After Social Security, health care consumes more of the federal budget than any other spending item.

But the news isn't all bleak. The United States has relatively low death rates not only from stomach cancer and cerebrovascular disease, but also from bronchitis, emphysema, asthma, chronic liver disease, and cirrhosis. Americans are less likely to die from a motor vehicle accident or by suicide than adults in many other industrialized nations. And for the well-off or well-insured, the United States offers the highest quality health care in the world, attracting the affluent ailing from around the globe.

For decades, health care costs in the U.S. have been spiraling upwards. Government projections of health care spending show no end to the upward trajectory. A look at the history of health care spending tells us what we can expect in the future.

The history of health care spending

Between 1965 and 1990, U.S. health care expenditures rose at double-digit annual rates, peaking at a 13.6 percent average annual gain between 1975 and 1980. To understand the future of health care spending, it's important to know why expenditures have grown so rapidly. Behind the double-digit increases have been spiraling costs in almost every facet of health care with little to slow the climb.

The distribution of blame for rising costs depends on who does the analysis. Experts have blamed dozens of factors including poor government management, a surplus of medical specialists, too many unnecessary medical procedures, futile medical intervention, defensive medicine as protection against malpractice suits, too much paperwork, theft and fraud, physicians' salaries, social factors such as violence, teen pregnancy, and AIDS, and an aging population. It is interesting to note, however, that the rapid escalation of health care costs occurred after the bulk of health care spending shifted from out-of-pocket expenditures by individuals to employer-provided health insurance and government health care programs.

National health care expenditures soared from $27 billion in 1960 to $699 billion in 1990. Whatever the cause of this increase, a solution was needed. Enter managed care. This was a business revolt against the high cost of health care, says George Anders in *Health Against Wealth: HMOs and the Breakdown of Medical Trust*. Put bluntly, managed care amounted to a power grab by employers and insurance companies, says Anders.[1]

Seeing their profits eroded by health care costs, employers—who typically bear most of the expense of health insurance—wanted to reverse the trend. Anders points out that this resolve coincided with the erosion of trust between the public and the medical community. These two factors—the need to cut costs and increasing scrutiny of the health care industry by the public—created a climate ripe for managed care.

Spending on health care keeps rising

(total annual health care expenditures, 1960 to 1998; in billions of dollars)

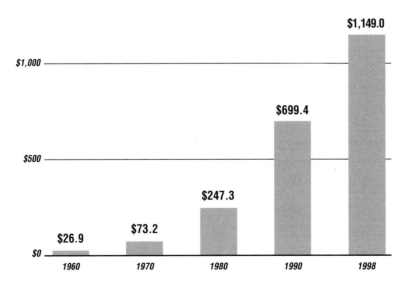

Since 1990, the rate of increase in health care spending has slowed, falling into the single digits. But spending rose 5.6 percent between 1997 and 1998, higher than the 4.7 percent increase between 1996 and 1997. The 1997-98 gain was the biggest since a 7.4 percent jump between 1992 and 1993.

It is not clear whether managed care is entirely responsible for the slowdown in health care spending during the 1990s—although it does deserve some credit, according to Eli Ginzberg of Columbia University writing in the *Journal of the American Medical Association*.[2] Managed care programs have been able to negotiate lower prices due to surpluses of hospital beds and health care personnel. Other factors are also at work, however. The emergence of home health care, which is less expensive than institutionalization, and the decline in the length of hospital stays have also reduced costs.

Another factor that has slowed spending growth is the increased use of part-time and temporary employees, say Alan Krueger and Helen Levy in a *National Bureau of Economic Research Working Paper*.[3] They argue that managed care is not directly responsible for significant cost savings because the average managed care premium is now almost as high as the average fee-for-service plan.

Whatever capped the growth rate of health care spending during the 1990s, the slowdown did not prevent spending from topping the $1 trillion mark in 1996 and continuing to rise in 1997 and 1998. And annual spending increases are likely to return to double digits as the population ages.

Out-of-pocket spending on health care is falling

(percent of personal health care expenditures paid for out-of-pocket, 1960 to 1998)

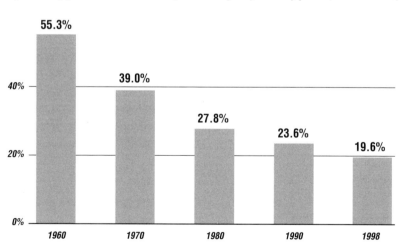

Year	Percent
1960	55.3%
1970	39.0%
1980	27.8%
1990	23.6%
1998	19.6%

Who spends what?

What comprises the more than $1 trillion health care market? Local, state, and federal governments account for 44 percent of total spending on personal health care. Private funds—most of it employer-provided health insurance—account for the rest.

Among consumers, the biggest spenders on health care are the oldest Americans. Householders aged 75 or older spend much more out-of-pocket on health care than the average household—$2,938 versus $1,903 in 1998. The oldest age group spends more per capita than any other on health insurance, medical services, drugs, and medical supplies. Combine the high out-of-pocket spending of the elderly with the government's spending on the older population through Medicare, and it becomes apparent that older Americans are by far the dominant consumers of health care.

Older Americans are not the only consumers of health care, however. The middle aged spend lavishly on medical services, in part because many have children requiring doctor visits, dental checkups, eyeglasses, and so on. Householders aged 45 to 54 spend as much as 36 percent more than average on physician services. Those aged 55 to 64, many of whom are just becoming aware of health problems, spend the most out-of-pocket on lab tests, X-rays, and hospital services other than rooms.

The culprits are many

In 1998, the nation spent a total of $1.1 trillion on health care. The figure is projected to grow at a rate of 6.5 percent a year for the next ten years, according to the Health Care Financing Administration, which tracks health costs for the nation. Although this seems like rapid growth, it's slower than the rate previously projected by HCFA. Still, even with a slower rate of growth, health care spending will double by 2008, to $2.2 trillion, or 16.6 percent of GDP.

There are many factors behind the rise in health care spending. Insurance premiums are one. The cost of health insurance rose 14.9 percent in 1998 following three years of declines.

Drug costs are another factor behind the increase in health care costs. Spending on prescription drugs grew more than any other category in 1998, climbing 15.4 percent to $90.6 billion. This growth is due to a record-setting number of new drug introductions between 1994 and 1996, following new FDA fast-approval procedures and a drop in out-of-pocket costs to consumers as prescription drug coverage became more widespread. The number of drug introductions has slowed since its 1994–1996 peak.

The rise in health care spending could have been worse. Spending on Medicare rose only 2.4 percent between 1997 and 1998. This lull is just temporary, however, since Medicare costs are expected to jump sharply when the baby-boom generation becomes eligible for coverage after 2010. Other factors keeping costs down are the growing ranks of the uninsured, the increased use of cost containing measures by health insurers, and the shift by hospitals from inpatient to outpatient procedures.

The proportion of hospital surgical procedures performed on outpatients rather than inpatients has grown from just 16 percent in 1980 to 62 percent in 1998. This development has helped to keep the lid on health care spending since outpatient services are much less expensive than inpatient care. According to the government's Healthcare Cost and Utilization Project, a study that measures the cost of typical hospital services, the five most expensive hospital diagnoses are spinal cord injury, infant respiratory distress syndrome, low birth weight, leukemia, and heart valve disorders.

The HCUP has found that different treatments for the same illness result in radically different costs. For uterine cancer, for example, abdominal hysterectomy is nearly 20 percent more expensive than vaginal hysterectomy. Such financial analyses help insurers decide on the procedures they will cover—and how they can keep costs down.

Health insurance

Insurance has emerged as a central issue in the health care spending debate. In the early 1990s, when the Clinton administration was attempting to reform the health care system, horror stories about families facing bankruptcy because of medical bills abounded. Although the debate has quieted some, it is certain to rise again.

Health insurance first emerged in the 1930s when a group of school teachers asked Baylor University Hospital to guarantee them a certain number of days each year in the hospital in exchange for a set monthly fee of 55 cents per person. Eventually, this modest plan became the behemoth Blue Cross. By 1952, one-half of Americans had health insurance, primarily to cover hospitalization, and the concept of third-party payment was firmly established.[4]

Today, 82 percent of Americans under age 65 have some kind of health insurance, either public or private. Nearly 90 percent of those with private insurance are covered through an employer. Virtually all Americans aged 65 or older have health insurance through Medicare.

The rise of the health insurance industry and government-subsidized health care has shifted the payment burden from individuals to employers and governments. Until a few decades ago, out-of-pocket spending by individuals accounted for most of the nation's personal health care expenditures. Between 1960 and 1998, the share of personal health care expenditures paid for by individual Americans fell from 55 to just 20 percent. The share accounted for by private health insurance rose from 21 to 32 percent, while government's share doubled from 22 to 44 percent. Interestingly, as individual control over health care spending eroded, health care costs soared. Today, as employers and governments try to shift more of the spending burden back to individuals, we are returning to what was once the norm. The difference, of course, is that doctor visits, medical procedures, and disease treatments are much more complex and expensive than they once were.

While 84 percent of all Americans had health insurance in 1998, that left 16 percent (or 44 million) uninsured. Whites are more likely to have health insurance than blacks. Non-Hispanics are more likely to have coverage than Hispanics. Among people aged 18 to 64 who are not poor, workers are more likely to have health insurance than nonworkers. But among the poor, workers are less likely to have health insurance than nonworkers because the nonworking poor are eligible for public insurance programs. More than half the nation's immigrants are without health insurance.

Older people are well insured thanks to Medicare. Children and young adults are not. Thirty percent of people aged 18 to 24 lack health insurance. Because young adults tend to

Older Americans spend the most out-of-pocket on health care

(average out-of-pocket spending on health care by age of householder, 1998

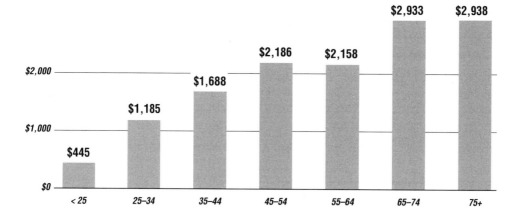

be healthier than older people, they may not regard health insurance as a necessity. On the other hand, since young adults are so healthy, it is baffling that insurers ignore this low-risk market.

Most Americans without insurance (87 percent) have a working adult in the family. Employees of small businesses, low-wage workers, and the self-employed are disproportionately represented among the uninsured, according to a study by the Agency for Health Care Policy Research. Young workers and minorities—especially Hispanic men—are also a disproportionate share of the uninsured. A Bureau of the Census study has shown that over a 28-month period, the 52 percent majority of 18-to-24-year-olds lacked insurance for at least one month. Among Americans of all ages, only 27 percent were uninsured for one or more months during the same time period.

Health insurance status can determine access to health care, reports the Agency for Health Care Policy Research. People who lack health insurance are much less likely to receive regular medical care. Thirty-eight percent of those without insurance do not have a usual source of medical care, compared with 15 percent of those with private insurance and 13 percent of the publicly insured.

Health insurance status also determines how much a household spends on health care overall. According to G. D. Paulin and W. D. Weber writing in *Family Economics and Nutrition*

Americans aged 18 to 24 are most likely to be uninsured

(percent of persons not covered by health insurance, by age, 1998)

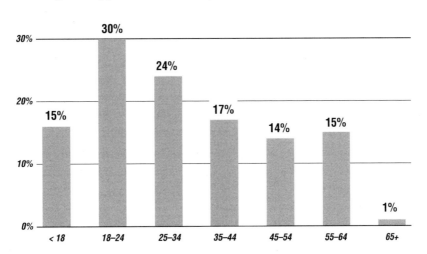

Review, fully insured households devote 7 percent of their total expenditures to health care, partially insured households devote 5 percent, and the uninsured spend only 3 percent of their budgets on health care.[5] One explanation for the lower spending of the uninsured is that they are younger, healthier, and may not need medical care. But in fact, the uninsured are the ones most likely to rate their health as only fair, according to the 1996 Medical Expenditure Panel Survey. Clearly, there is a market for medical products and services for the uninsured if the price is right.

Medicare's growing importance

Medicare is a federal program that provides health insurance to people aged 65 or older. Since the oldest baby boomers are only about 10 years away from qualifying for coverage, the long-term outlook for Medicare will be of concern to a growing number of Americans.

One area of brewing controversy is the idea of bringing managed care into Medicare. Traditionally, Medicare operates as a fee-for-service plan, with the great majority of Medicare's 39 million beneficiaries still receiving care in that way. But more than 6 million Medicare beneficiaries are enrolled in managed care plans, known as Medicare+Choice. the hope that managed care would cut the cost of Medicare was dashed when a number of private-sector managed care organizations discovered they could not make enough from their Medicare patients to stay afloat. In 1999, 41 Medicare+Choice plans did not renew their contracts, and 58 reduced their service areas, affecting a total of 327,000 enrollees. The General Accounting Office determined that Medicare's managed care plans weren't working because they could not compete effectively in their local areas and had difficulty establishing provider networks, while Medicare enrollees were dissatisfied with what they had to pay. Many managed care organizations that remain in the Medicare program are raising their rates—to the tune of about 5 percent in 1999. Twenty-five percent of counties enrolled in managed care programs saw increases as large as 7.5 percent, according to the Health Care Financing Administration.

As the number of Medicare beneficiaries rises with the aging population, scrutiny of the Medicare system—providers, patients, and suppliers—has increased. In 1995, Department of Health and Human Services secretary Donna Shalala initiated Operation Restore Trust, coordinating federal, state, local, and private resources in anti-fraud efforts. In 1998, the HCFA doubled its audits of home health care agencies and increased its claim reviews by 25 percent. In 1999, it began contracting its fraud-fighting work to outside organizations that specialize in this type of investigation.

The future of health care spending

Considering the changing characteristics of health care consumers, it becomes frightfully obvious that health care spending is going to be difficult to contain. Although most analysts agree that the growth in spending will remain in single digits for the next few years, it won't be much below the double-digit level.

Health care spending is destined to continue its rapid rise not only because demand for health care will increase, but also because the nation lacks the political will to force individual Americans to shoulder much of the health care bill. This responsibility would soon put the brakes on spending, although not without dire consequences for the health and well-being of many.

Several important trends will have the most influence on health care spending in the decades ahead.

TREND 1: AGING BABY BOOMERS

Boomers are certain to boost health care spending as they age, but their full impact remains decades away. Because the oldest Americans are the biggest consumers of health care, it will be at least another two decades before boomers enter the peak-spending age group.

TREND 2: CHANGES IN MANAGED CARE

Consumers are tired of being "managed" by their health care plans. The public's dissatisfaction with managed care is evident in responses to questions about HMOs asked in the 1998 General Social Survey of the University of Chicago's National Opinion Research Center. While 48 percent of people aged 18 or older believe HMOs help control costs, only 23 percent agree that they improve the quality of care. A 40 percent plurality believe HMOs prevent people from getting the care they need, and a 46 percent plurality believe HMOs take important medical decisions out of the hands of doctors.

Americans are demanding more options and flexibility from their health care plans. In an economy with only 4 percent unemployment, employers have little choice but to give them what they want. Consequently, if the economy were to remain robust, expect faster growth in health care spending. On the other hand, if unemployment were to rise, employers would be able to shift health care costs back to their employees. Restrictive managed care plans would become the only affordable choice.

No matter how hot the economy, the managed care model will not disappear entirely. It's more likely to be modified by keeping the best of it and eliminating the worst. The Preferred Provider Organization is one step in that direction. It allows consumers more choice if they spend more money.

Managed care reform comes down to the issue of cost. Health care is expensive, and the only way to control that expense is to reduce services. The Internet may offer a relatively painless way to do this, allowing medical providers to transmit information and eliminate the expense of paperwork. Today, some companies are building business models around administering health benefits online. Within a few years, those models should be in operation.

Trend 3: More state and federal cooperation

As the ranks of the uninsured and the elderly grow, public health care programs will feel the pressure. Inevitably, there must be more cooperation between federal and state governments to handle the growing demand. Each state must be allowed to meet its unique population needs, while at the same time assuring the federal government that its dollars are well spent. A good example of this kind of cooperation is the State Children's Health Insurance Program, commonly known as SCHIP. This federal program provides health insurance for children whose family income is too high to qualify for Medicaid but too low to purchase private health insurance. In 1999, SCHIP covered nearly 2 million children. States have the flexibility to determine eligibility for the program but they must meet guidelines provided by the federal government.

Notes

1. George Anders, *Health against Wealth: HMOs and the Breakdown of Medical Trust* (New York: Houghton Mifflin, 1996): 18–25.

2. Eli Ginzberg, "Managed Care and the Competitive Market: What They Can and Cannot Do," *Journal of the American Medical Association* 277, no. 22 (June 11, 1997): 1812–1814.

3. Alan Krueger and Helen Levy, "Accounting for the Slowdown in Employer Health Care Costs," *National Bureau of Economic Research Working Paper* 589 (January 20, 1998).

4. Victoria Sherrow, *The U.S. Health Care Crisis* (Brookfield, Connecticut: Millbrook Press, 1994): 33.

5. G.D. Paulin and W.D. Weber, "The Effects of Health Insurance on Consumer Spending," *Family Economics and Nutrition Review* 9 (Winter 1996): 42–47.

Health Care Spending by Country, 1997

(per capita and indexed per capita health care expenditures in selected countries, 1997; ranked by per capita expenditures)

	per capita expenditures	indexed per capita expenditures
United States	$3,912	100
Switzerland	2,611	67
Germany	2,364	60
Luxembourg	2,303	59
Canada	2,175	56
France	2,047	52
Denmark	2,042	52
Norway	2,017	52
Iceland	1,981	51
Netherlands	1,933	49
Australia	1,909	49
Austria	1,905	49
Belgium	1,768	45
Sweden	1,762	45
Japan	1,760	45
Italy	1,613	41
Finland	1,525	39
United Kingdom	1,391	36
New Zealand	1,357	35
Ireland	1,293	33
Greece	1,196	31
Spain	1,183	30
Portugal	1,148	29
Czech Republic	943	24
Korea	870	22
Hungary	642	16
Poland	386	10
Mexico	363	9
Turkey	259	7

Note: Per capita health expenditures for each country have been adjusted to U.S. dollars using gross domestic product purchasing power parities.
Source: National Center for Health Statistics, Health, United States, 2000; *calculations by New Strategist*

National Health Care Expenditures, 1960 to 1998

(total national health care expenditures and average annual percent change in expenditures, 1960 to 1998)

	total (billions of dollars)	average annual percent change from previous year shown
1998	$1,149.10	5.6%
1997	1,088.2	4.7
1996	1,039.4	4.6
1995	993.3	4.8
1994	947.7	5.5
1993	898.5	7.4
1992	836.5	9.1
1991	766.8	9.6
1990	699.4	11.0
1985	428.7	11.6
1980	247.3	13.6
1975	130.7	12.3
1970	73.2	12.2
1965	41.1	8.9
1960	26.9	–

Source: Health Care Financing Administration, Office of the Actuary, National Health Statistics Group; and National Center for Health Statistics, Health, United States, 2000

National Health Care Expenditures by Type of Expenditure, 1998

(national health care expenditures and percent distribution by type of expenditure, 1998)

	total (billions of dollars)	percent distribution
Total national health care spending	**$1,149.1**	**100.0%**
Health services and supplies	**1,113.7**	**96.9**
Personal health care	1,019.3	88.7
Hospital care	382.8	33.3
Physician services	229.5	20.0
Dental services	53.8	4.7
Other professional services	66.6	5.8
Home health care	29.3	2.5
Drugs and other medical nondurables	121.9	10.6
Prescription drugs	90.6	7.9
Vision products and other medical durables	15.5	1.3
Nursing home care	87.8	7.6
Other personal health care	32.1	2.8
Program administration and net cost of health insurance	57.7	5.0
Government public health activities	36.6	3.2
Research and construction	**35.3**	**3.1**
Research	19.9	1.7
Construction	15.5	1.3

Source: Health Care Financing Administration, Office of the Actuary, National Health Statistics Group

Personal Health Care Expenditures, 1960 to 1998

(total personal health care expenditures and percent distribution by source of funds, 1960 to 1998)

	total (billions of dollars)	percent	out-of-pocket payments	private health insurance	government federal	government state and local
1998	$1,019.3	100.0%	19.6%	33.1%	33.7%	9.9%
1997	968.6	100.0	19.5	32.3	34.4	10.1
1996	924.0	100.0	19.3	32.3	34.5	10.3
1995	879.1	100.0	19.4	32.6	34.0	10.5
1990	614.7	100.0	23.6	33.8	28.8	10.4
1985	376.4	100.0	26.7	30.3	29.5	9.7
1980	217.0	100.0	27.8	28.6	29.2	10.9
1975	114.5	100.0	33.3	24.8	27.0	12.5
1970	63.8	100.0	39.0	23.2	23.0	12.2
1965	35.2	100.0	52.7	24.7	8.4	12.2
1960	23.6	100.0	55.3	21.2	9.0	12.6

Note: Numbers will not add to total because "other" is not shown.
Source: Health Care Financing Administration, Office of the Actuary, National Health Statistics Group; and National Center for Health Statistics, Health, United States, 2000; *calculations by New Strategist*

Out-of-Pocket Payments for Personal Health Care Expenditures, 1960 to 1998

(total personal health care expenditures and percent paid out-of-pocket by type of expenditure, 1960 to 1998)

	total		hospital care		physician services		nursing home care		other	
	amount (billions)	percent paid out-of-pocket	amount (billions)	percent paid out-of-pocket	amount (billions)	percent paid out-of-pocket	amount (billions)	percent paid out-of-pocket	amount (billions)	percent paid out-of-pocket
1998	$1,019.3	19.6%	$382.8	3.4%	$229.5	15.6%	$87.8	32.5%	$319.2	38.4%
1997	968.6	19.5	370.2	3.3	217.8	15.5	84.7	32.8	296.0	39.0
1996	924.0	19.3	359.4	3.2	208.5	14.9	80.2	33.6	275.9	39.3
1995	879.1	19.4	347.0	3.3	201.9	15.0	75.5	35.2	254.8	40.1
1990	614.7	23.6	256.4	4.3	146.3	22.0	50.9	43.1	161.0	49.6
1985	376.4	26.7	168.3	5.2	83.6	29.2	30.7	44.3	93.9	57.3
1980	217.0	27.8	102.7	5.2	45.2	32.4	17.6	41.8	51.5	63.9
1975	114.5	33.3	52.6	8.3	23.9	36.7	8.7	42.6	29.4	72.4
1970	63.8	39.0	28.0	9.0	13.6	42.2	4.2	53.5	18.0	79.9
1965	35.2	52.7	14.0	19.6	8.2	60.6	1.5	60.1	11.5	86.7
1960	23.6	55.3	9.3	20.7	5.3	62.7	0.8	77.9	8.2	87.4

Source: Health Care Financing Administration, Office of the Actuary, National Health Statistics Group; and National Center for Health Statistics, Health, United States, 2000

Whose Responsibility Are Health Care Costs? 1975 and 1998

"In general, some people think it is the responsibility of the government in Washington to see to it that people have help in paying for doctor and hospital bills. Others think these matters are not the responsibility of the federal government and that people should take care of these things themselves. Where would you place yourself on a scale of 1 to 5?"

(percent of people aged 18 or older responding by sex, race, age, and education, 1975–98)

	government (1 and 2)		both (3)		individual (4 and 5)	
	1998	*1975*	*1998*	*1975*	*1998*	*1975*
Total	47%	49%	32%	29%	18%	21%
Men	44	51	32	26	22	21
Women	49	46	32	30	15	21
Black	59	69	28	22	10	7
White	44	46	33	29	20	23
Aged 18 to 29	54	56	29	25	13	16
Aged 30 to 39	50	52	31	25	16	22
Aged 40 to 49	49	40	28	34	21	23
Aged 50 to 59	47	39	31	33	18	26
Aged 60 to 69	35	48	41	28	23	23
Aged 70 or older	37	51	40	29	20	16
Not a high school graduate	48	53	33	28	13	15
High school graduate	47	44	32	29	19	25
Bachelor's degree	46	46	32	29	20	24
Graduate degree	50	52	28	20	21	24

Note: Numbers may not add to 100 because "don't know" and no answer are not shown.
Source: General Social Surveys, National Opinion Research Center, University of Chicago; calculations by New Strategist

Out-of-Pocket Spending on Health Care by Age of Householder, 1998: Average Spending

(average annual out-of-pocket spending of consumer units on health care, by age of consumer unit reference person, 1998)

	total consumer units	under 25	25 to 34	35 to 44	45 to 54	55 to 64	65 to 74	75+
Number of consumer units (in thousands)	107,182	8,255	19,969	24,241	20,058	12,829	11,874	9,957
Average number of persons per consumer unit	2.5	1.8	2.8	3.3	2.7	2.2	1.9	1.5
Average out-of-pocket health care spending	$1,902.76	$445.31	$1,185.31	$1,688.40	$2,186.11	$2,158.29	$2,933.41	$2,938.27
HEALTH INSURANCE	**$913.20**	**$206.41**	**$604.04**	**$790.47**	**$940.47**	**$991.15**	**$1,549.35**	**$1,502.98**
Commercial health insurance	**198.36**	**53.23**	**168.99**	**229.54**	**273.90**	**254.39**	**164.81**	**117.28**
Traditional fee for service health plan (not BCBS)	94.97	20.15	71.06	101.88	118.79	123.02	96.79	101.79
Preferred provider health plan (not BCBS)	103.39	33.08	97.94	127.66	155.12	131.36	68.03	15.50
Blue Cross, Blue Shield	**224.82**	**44.98**	**123.39**	**189.45**	**278.71**	**306.26**	**323.43**	**332.36**
Traditional fee for service health plan	77.42	8.59	36.34	50.41	107.93	123.94	105.62	127.62
Preferred provider health plan	54.53	18.96	37.82	54.58	79.85	97.28	43.73	24.20
Health maintenance organization	56.26	16.85	46.32	77.82	77.69	62.47	42.01	22.23
Commercial Medicare supplement	30.42	0.44	0.15	3.98	2.80	10.47	120.88	153.89
Other BCBS health insurance	6.18	0.15	2.76	2.65	10.44	12.11	11.20	4.42
Health maintenance organization (not BCBS)	**240.44**	**91.97**	**277.36**	**311.19**	**316.40**	**254.10**	**132.26**	**75.67**
Medicare payments	**157.87**	**5.82**	**10.21**	**22.45**	**32.41**	**100.53**	**640.97**	**660.22**
Commercial Medicare supplements/other health insurance	**91.71**	**10.41**	**24.08**	**37.85**	**39.55**	**75.88**	**287.87**	**317.44**
Commercial Medicare supplement (not BCBS)	56.97	1.94	2.13	6.18	8.17	25.12	236.41	261.62
Other health insurance (not BCBS)	34.74	8.47	21.95	31.67	31.37	50.76	51.46	55.82

(continued)

(continued from previous page)

	total consumer units	under 25	25 to 34	35 to 44	45 to 54	55 to 64	65 to 74	75+
MEDICAL SERVICES	**$542.15**	**$136.20**	**$372.63**	**$556.93**	**$737.78**	**$641.62**	**$591.95**	**$601.08**
Physician's services	137.82	36.70	118.18	155.97	187.85	174.24	108.60	103.98
Dental services	212.95	40.09	104.77	223.44	312.40	230.62	325.34	190.57
Eye care services	29.70	8.00	15.77	29.37	58.47	29.88	25.91	22.77
Service by professionals other than physician	30.51	13.91	21.15	30.37	52.00	33.98	25.14	21.98
Lab tests, X-rays	21.09	7.56	10.54	21.25	32.00	36.28	21.88	10.60
Hospital room	38.47	3.29	27.68	33.49	45.36	69.11	29.73	58.42
Hospital service other than room	44.73	20.86	42.62	54.29	42.49	56.17	41.18	39.46
Care in convalescent or nursing home	15.60	–	0.29	3.36	1.12	3.02	6.76	144.93
Repair of medical equipment	0.36	–	–	–	1.44	0.76	–	–
Other medical services	10.93	5.80	31.63	5.39	4.65	7.56	7.41	8.37
DRUGS	**345.71**	**79.34**	**142.96**	**240.34**	**376.97**	**429.41**	**664.24**	**675.69**
Nonprescription drugs	71.21	24.39	40.44	69.84	94.36	80.58	92.84	88.31
Nonprescription vitamins	43.19	16.42	15.83	39.34	68.72	45.35	63.26	50.36
Prescription drugs	231.31	38.54	86.69	131.16	213.89	303.48	508.14	537.02
MEDICAL SUPPLIES	**101.70**	**23.36**	**65.68**	**100.66**	**130.39**	**96.11**	**127.88**	**158.52**
Eyeglasses and contact lenses	55.71	18.46	40.55	59.90	83.83	60.67	53.55	46.35
Hearing aids	12.46	0.06	1.45	1.33	9.74	7.34	25.36	68.65
Topicals and dressings	25.78	4.45	20.41	31.50	28.92	23.12	32.67	28.10
Medical equipment for general use	2.74	–	0.62	4.03	2.43	2.59	5.32	3.84
Supportive/convalescent medical equipment	2.67	0.42	1.65	1.15	3.62	0.88	5.73	7.00
Rental of medical equipment	1.08	0.07	0.28	2.54	1.00	0.32	0.45	1.83
Rental of supportive, convalescent medical equipment	1.26	–	0.71	0.20	0.85	1.19	4.80	2.74

Note: (–) means sample is too small to make a reliable estimate.
Source: Bureau of Labor Statistics, unpublished data from the 1998 Consumer Expenditure Survey

Out-of-Pocket Spending on Health Care by Age of Householder, 1998: Indexed Spending

(indexed average annual out-of-pocket spending of consumer units on health care, by age of consumer unit reference person, 1998; index definition: an index of 100 is the average for all consumer units; an index of 125 means spending by consumer units in the age group is 25 percent above the average for all consumer units; an index of 75 means spending by the age group is 25 percent below the average for all consumer units)

	total consumer units	under 25	25 to 34	35 to 44	45 to 54	55 to 64	65 to 74	75+
Health care, spending index	**100**	**23**	**62**	**89**	**115**	**113**	**154**	**154**
HEALTH INSURANCE	**100**	**23**	**66**	**87**	**103**	**109**	**170**	**165**
Commercial health insurance	**100**	**27**	**85**	**116**	**138**	**128**	**83**	**59**
Traditional fee-for-service health plan (not BCBS)	100	21	75	107	125	130	102	107
Preferred provider health plan (not BCBS)	100	32	95	123	150	127	66	15
Blue Cross, Blue Shield	**100**	**20**	**55**	**84**	**124**	**136**	**144**	**148**
Traditional fee-for-service health plan	100	11	47	65	139	160	136	165
Preferred provider health plan	100	35	69	100	146	178	80	44
Health maintenance organization	100	30	82	138	138	111	75	40
Commercial Medicare supplement	100	1	0	13	9	34	397	506
Other BCBS health insurance	100	2	45	43	169	196	181	72
Health maintenance organization (not BCBS)	**100**	**38**	**115**	**129**	**132**	**106**	**55**	**31**
Medicare payments	**100**	**4**	**6**	**14**	**21**	**64**	**406**	**418**
Commercial Medicare supplements/ other health insurance	**100**	**11**	**26**	**41**	**43**	**83**	**314**	**346**
Commercial Medicare supplement (not BCBS)	100	3	4	11	14	44	415	459
Other health insurance (not BCBS)	100	24	63	91	90	146	148	161

(continued)

(continued from previous page)

	total consumer units	under 25	25 to 34	35 to 44	45 to 54	55 to 64	65 to 74	75+
MEDICAL SERVICES	**100**	**25**	**69**	**103**	**136**	**118**	**109**	**111**
Physician's services	100	27	86	113	136	126	79	75
Dental services	100	19	49	105	147	108	153	89
Eye care services	100	27	53	99	197	101	87	77
Service by professionals other than physician	100	46	69	100	170	111	82	72
Lab tests, X-rays	100	36	50	101	152	172	104	50
Hospital room	100	9	72	87	118	180	77	152
Hospital service other than room	100	47	95	121	95	126	92	88
Care in convalescent or nursing home	100	–	2	22	7	19	43	929
Repair of medical equipment	100	–	–	–	400	211	–	–
Other medical services	100	53	289	49	43	69	68	77
DRUGS	**100**	**23**	**41**	**70**	**109**	**124**	**192**	**195**
Nonprescription drugs	100	34	57	98	133	113	130	124
Nonprescription vitamins	100	38	37	91	159	105	146	117
Prescription drugs	100	17	37	57	92	131	220	232
MEDICAL SUPPLIES	**100**	**23**	**65**	**99**	**128**	**95**	**126**	**156**
Eyeglasses and contact lenses	100	33	73	108	150	109	96	83
Hearing aids	100	0	12	11	78	59	204	551
Topicals and dressings	100	17	79	122	112	90	127	109
Medical equipment for general use	100	–	23	147	89	95	194	140
Supportive/convalescent medical equipment	100	16	62	43	136	33	215	262
Rental of medical equipment	100	6	26	235	93	30	42	169
Rental of supportive, convalescent medical equipment	100	–	56	16	67	94	381	217

Note: (–) means sample is too small to make a reliable estimate.
Source: Calculations by New Strategist based on unpublished data from the Bureau of Labor Statistics 1998 Consumer Expenditure Survey

Out-of-Pocket Spending on Health Care by Age of Householder, 1998: Total Spending

(total annual out-of-pocket spending on health care by consumer unit age groups, 1998; numbers in thousands)

	total consumer units	under 25	25 to 34	35 to 44	45 to 54	55 to 64	65 to 74	75+
Health care, total spending	$203,941,622	$3,676,034	$23,669,455	$40,928,504	$43,848,994	$27,688,702	$34,831,310	$29,256,354
HEALTH INSURANCE	97,878,602	1,703,915	12,062,075	19,161,783	18,863,947	12,715,463	18,396,982	14,965,172
Commercial health insurance	21,260,622	439,414	3,374,561	5,564,279	5,493,886	3,263,569	1,956,954	1,167,757
Traditional fee-for-service health plan (not BCBS)	10,179,075	166,338	1,418,997	2,469,673	2,382,690	1,578,224	1,149,284	1,013,523
Preferred provider health plan (not BCBS)	11,081,547	273,075	1,955,764	3,094,606	3,111,397	1,685,217	807,788	154,334
Blue Cross, Blue Shield	24,096,657	371,310	2,463,975	4,592,457	5,590,365	3,929,010	3,840,408	3,309,309
Traditional fee-for-service health plan	8,298,030	70,910	725,673	1,221,989	2,164,860	1,590,026	1,254,132	1,270,712
Preferred provider health plan	5,844,634	156,515	755,228	1,323,074	1,601,631	1,248,005	519,250	240,959
Health maintenance organization	6,030,059	139,097	924,964	1,886,435	1,558,306	801,428	498,827	221,344
Commercial Medicare supplement	3,260,476	3,632	2,995	96,479	56,162	134,320	1,435,329	1,532,283
Other BCBS health insurance	662,385	1,238	55,114	64,239	209,406	155,359	132,989	44,010
Health maintenance organization (not BCBS)	25,770,840	759,212	5,538,602	7,543,557	6,346,351	3,259,849	1,570,455	753,446
Medicare payments	16,920,822	48,044	203,883	544,210	650,080	1,289,699	7,610,878	6,573,811
Commercial Medicare supplements/ other health insurance	9,829,661	85,935	480,854	917,522	793,294	973,465	3,418,168	3,160,750
Commercial Medicare supplement (not BCBS)	6,106,159	16,015	42,534	149,809	163,874	322,264	2,807,132	2,604,950
Other health insurance (not BCBS)	3,723,503	69,920	438,320	767,712	629,219	651,200	611,036	555,800

(continued)

(continued from previous page)

	total consumer units	under 25	25 to 34	35 to 44	45 to 54	55 to 64	65 to 74	75+
MEDICAL SERVICES	**$58,108,721**	**$1,124,331**	**$7,441,048**	**$13,500,540**	**$14,798,391**	**$8,231,343**	**$7,028,814**	**$5,984,954**
Physician's services	14,771,823	302,959	2,359,936	3,780,869	3,767,895	2,235,325	1,289,516	1,035,329
Dental services	22,824,407	330,943	2,092,152	5,416,409	6,266,119	2,958,624	3,863,087	1,897,505
Eye care services	3,183,305	66,040	314,911	711,958	1,172,791	383,331	307,655	226,721
Service by professionals other than physician	3,270,123	114,827	422,344	736,199	1,043,016	435,929	298,512	218,855
Lab tests, X-rays	2,260,468	62,408	210,473	515,121	641,856	465,436	259,803	105,544
Hospital room	4,123,292	27,159	552,742	811,831	909,831	886,612	353,014	581,688
Hospital service other than room	4,794,251	172,199	851,079	1,316,044	852,264	720,605	488,971	392,903
Care in convalescent or nursing home	1,672,039	–	5,791	81,450	22,465	38,744	80,268	1,443,068
Repair of medical equipment	38,586	–	–	–	28,884	9,750	–	–
Other medical services	1,171,499	47,879	631,619	130,659	93,270	96,987	87,986	83,340
DRUGS	37,053,889	654,952	2,854,768	5,826,082	7,561,264	5,508,901	7,887,186	6,727,845
Nonprescription drugs	7,632,430	201,339	807,546	1,692,991	1,892,673	1,033,761	1,102,382	879,303
Nonprescription vitamins	4,629,191	135,547	316,109	953,641	1,378,386	581,795	751,149	501,435
Prescription drugs	24,792,268	318,148	1,731,113	3,179,450	4,290,206	3,893,345	6,033,654	5,347,108
MEDICAL SUPPLIES	10,900,409	192,837	1,311,564	2,440,099	2,615,363	1,232,995	1,518,447	1,578,384
Eyeglasses and contact lenses	5,971,109	152,387	809,743	1,452,036	1,681,462	778,335	635,853	461,507
Hearing aids	1,335,488	495	28,955	32,241	195,365	94,165	301,125	683,548
Topicals and dressings	2,763,152	36,735	407,567	763,592	580,077	296,606	387,924	279,792
Medical equipment for general use	293,679	–	12,381	97,691	48,741	33,227	63,170	38,235
Supportive/convalescent medical equipment	286,176	3,467	32,949	27,877	72,610	11,290	68,038	69,699
Rental of medical equipment	115,757	578	5,591	61,572	20,058	4,105	5,343	18,221
Rental of supportive, convalescent medical equipment	135,049	–	14,178	4,848	17,049	15,267	56,995	27,282

Note: (–) means sample is too small to make a reliable estimate.
Source: Calculations by New Strategist based on unpublished data from the Bureau of Labor Statistics 1998 Consumer Expenditure Survey

Out-of-Pocket Spending on Health Care by Age of Householder, 1998: Market Shares

(percent of total annual out-of-pocket spending on health care accounted for by consumer unit age groups, 1998)

	total consumer units	under 25	25 to 34	35 to 44	45 to 54	55 to 64	65 to 74	75+
Share of health care spending	**100.0%**	**1.8%**	**11.6%**	**20.1%**	**21.5%**	**13.6%**	**17.1%**	**14.3%**
HEALTH INSURANCE	**100.0**	**1.7**	**12.3**	**19.6**	**19.3**	**13.0**	**18.8**	**15.3**
Commercial health insurance	**100.0**	**2.1**	**15.9**	**26.2**	**25.8**	**15.4**	**9.2**	**5.5**
Traditional fee-for-service health plan (not BCBS)	100.0	1.6	13.9	24.3	23.4	15.5	11.3	10.0
Preferred provider health plan (not BCBS)	100.0	2.5	17.6	27.9	28.1	15.2	7.3	1.4
Blue Cross, Blue Shield	**100.0**	**1.5**	**10.2**	**19.1**	**23.2**	**16.3**	**15.9**	**13.7**
Traditional fee-for-service health plan	100.0	0.9	8.7	14.7	26.1	19.2	15.1	15.3
Preferred provider health plan	100.0	2.7	12.9	22.6	27.4	21.4	8.9	4.1
Health maintenance organization	100.0	2.3	15.3	31.3	25.8	13.3	8.3	3.7
Commercial Medicare supplement	100.0	0.1	0.1	3.0	1.7	4.1	44.0	47.0
Other BCBS health insurance	100.0	0.2	8.3	9.7	31.6	23.5	20.1	6.6
Health maintenance organization (not BCBS)	**100.0**	**2.9**	**21.5**	**29.3**	**24.6**	**12.6**	**6.1**	**2.9**
Medicare payments	**100.0**	**0.3**	**1.2**	**3.2**	**3.8**	**7.6**	**45.0**	**38.9**
Commercial Medicare supplements/ other health insurance	**100.0**	**0.9**	**4.9**	**9.3**	**8.1**	**9.9**	**34.8**	**32.2**
Commercial Medicare supplement (not BCBS)	100.0	0.3	0.7	2.5	2.7	5.3	46.0	42.7
Other health insurance (not BCBS)	100.0	1.9	11.8	20.6	16.9	17.5	16.4	14.9

(continued)

(continued from previous page)

	total consumer units	under 25	25 to 34	35 to 44	45 to 54	55 to 64	65 to 74	75+
MEDICAL SERVICES	**100.0%**	**1.9%**	**12.8%**	**23.2%**	**25.5%**	**14.2%**	**12.1%**	**10.3%**
Physician's services	100.0	2.1	16.0	25.6	25.5	15.1	8.7	7.0
Dental services	100.0	1.4	9.2	23.7	27.5	13.0	16.9	8.3
Eye care services	100.0	2.1	9.9	22.4	36.8	12.0	9.7	7.1
Service by professionals other than physician	100.0	3.5	12.9	22.5	31.9	13.3	9.1	6.7
Lab tests, X-rays	100.0	2.8	9.3	22.8	28.4	20.6	11.5	4.7
Hospital room	100.0	0.7	13.4	19.7	22.1	21.5	8.6	14.1
Hospital service other than room	100.0	3.6	17.8	27.5	17.8	15.0	10.2	8.2
Care in convalescent or nursing home	100.0	–	0.3	4.9	1.3	2.3	4.8	86.3
Repair of medical equipment	100.0	–	–	–	74.9	25.3	–	–
Other medical services	100.0	4.1	53.9	11.2	8.0	8.3	7.5	7.1
DRUGS	**100.0**	**1.8**	**7.7**	**15.7**	**20.4**	**14.9**	**21.3**	**18.2**
Nonprescription drugs	100.0	2.6	10.6	22.2	24.8	13.5	14.4	11.5
Nonprescription vitamins	100.0	2.9	6.8	20.6	29.8	12.6	16.2	10.8
Prescription drugs	100.0	1.3	7.0	12.8	17.3	15.7	24.3	21.6
MEDICAL SUPPLIES	**100.0**	**1.8**	**12.0**	**22.4**	**24.0**	**11.3**	**13.9**	**14.5**
Eyeglasses and contact lenses	100.0	2.6	13.6	24.3	28.2	13.0	10.6	7.7
Hearing aids	100.0	0.0	2.2	2.4	14.6	7.1	22.5	51.2
Topicals and dressings	100.0	1.3	14.8	27.6	21.0	10.7	14.0	10.1
Medical equipment for general use	100.0	–	4.2	33.3	16.6	11.3	21.5	13.0
Supportive/convalescent medical equipment	100.0	1.2	11.5	9.7	25.4	3.9	23.8	24.4
Rental of medical equipment	100.0	0.5	4.8	53.2	17.3	3.5	4.6	15.7
Rental of supportive, convalescent medical equipment	100.0	–	10.5	3.6	12.6	11.3	42.2	20.2

Note: (–) means sample is too small to make a reliable estimate.
Source: Calculations by New Strategist based on unpublished data from the Bureau of Labor Statistics 1998 Consumer Expenditure Survey

Health Insurance Coverage by Age, 1998

(number and percent distribution of people by age and health insurance coverage status, 1998; numbers in thousands)

| | | covered by private or government health insurance | | | | | | | not covered |
| | | | private health insurance | | government health insurance | | | | |
	total	total	total	employment based	total	Medicaid	Medicare	military	
Total people	**271,743**	**227,462**	**190,861**	**168,575**	**66,087**	**27,854**	**35,887**	**8,747**	**44,281**
Under age 18	72,021	60,949	48,627	45,593	16,400	14,274	325	2,241	11,073
Aged 18 to 24	25,968	18,191	15,872	13,107	3,347	2,538	149	795	7,776
Aged 25 to 34	38,474	29,347	26,726	25,096	3,616	2,476	423	991	9,127
Aged 35 to 44	44,744	37,036	34,134	32,019	4,190	2,579	749	1,232	7,708
Aged 45 to 54	35,232	30,427	28,153	26,401	3,522	1,610	1,139	1,225	4,805
Aged 55 to 64	22,910	19,476	17,179	15,210	3,845	1,415	2,016	1,077	3,434
Aged 65 or older	32,394	32,037	20,171	11,150	31,167	2,961	31,085	1,186	358
Percent distribution by age									
Total people	**100.0%**	**100.0%**	**100.0%**	**100.0%**	**100.0%**	**100.0%**	**100.0%**	**100.0%**	**100.0%**
Under age 18	26.5	26.8	25.5	27.0	24.8	51.2	0.9	25.6	25.0
Aged 18 to 24	9.6	8.0	8.3	7.8	5.1	9.1	0.4	9.1	17.6
Aged 25 to 34	14.2	12.9	14.0	14.9	5.5	8.9	1.2	11.3	20.6
Aged 35 to 44	16.5	16.3	17.9	19.0	6.3	9.3	2.1	14.1	17.4
Aged 45 to 54	13.0	13.4	14.8	15.7	5.3	5.8	3.2	14.0	10.9
Aged 55 to 64	8.4	8.6	9.0	9.0	5.8	5.1	5.6	12.3	7.8
Aged 65 or older	11.9	14.1	10.6	6.6	47.2	10.6	86.6	13.6	0.8

(continued)

(continued from previous page)

Percent distribution of type of coverage

| | total | covered by private or government health insurance | | | | | | | not covered |
| | | private health insurance | | government health insurance | | | | |
		total	employment based	total	Medicaid	Medicare	military	
Total people	**100.0%**	**83.7%**	**70.2%**	**62.0%**	**24.3%**	**10.3%**	**13.2%**	**3.2%**	**16.3%**
Under age 18	100.0	84.6	67.5	63.3	22.8	19.8	0.5	3.1	15.4
Aged 18 to 24	100.0	70.1	61.1	50.5	12.9	9.8	0.6	3.1	29.9
Aged 25 to 34	100.0	76.3	69.5	65.2	9.4	6.4	1.1	2.6	23.7
Aged 35 to 44	100.0	82.8	76.3	71.6	9.4	5.8	1.7	2.8	17.2
Aged 45 to 54	100.0	86.4	79.9	74.9	10.0	4.6	3.2	3.5	13.6
Aged 55 to 64	100.0	85.0	75.0	66.4	16.8	6.2	8.8	4.7	15.0
Aged 65 or older	100.0	98.9	62.3	34.4	96.2	9.1	96.0	3.7	1.1

Note: Numbers will not add to total because people may have more than one type of health insurance coverage.
Source: Bureau of the Census, Internet site <http://www.census.gov/hhes/lthins/historic/hihist2.html>; calculations by New Strategist

People without Health Insurance by Age, 1987 and 1998

(number and percent of people without health insurance coverge by age 1987 and 1998; percent change in number and percentage point change in share, 1987–98; numbers in thousands)

	1998	1987	percent change 1987–98
Total without coverage	**44,280**	**31,026**	**42.7%**
Under age 18	11,073	8,193	35.2
Aged 18 to 24	7,776	6,108	27.3
Aged 25 to 34	9,127	7,308	24.9
Aged 35 to 44	7,708	4,135	86.4
Aged 45 to 54	4,805	2,695	78.3
Aged 55 to 64	3,434	2,281	50.5
Aged 65 or older	358	306	17.0

	1998	1987	percentage point change, 1987–98
Percent without coverage	**16.3%**	**12.9%**	**3.4**
Under age 18	15.4	12.9	2.5
Aged 18 to 24	29.9	23.4	6.5
Aged 25 to 34	23.7	17.0	6.7
Aged 35 to 44	17.2	11.9	5.3
Aged 45 to 54	13.6	11.3	2.3
Aged 55 to 64	15.0	10.5	4.4
Aged 65 or older	1.1	1.1	0.0

Source: Bureau of the Census, Internet site <http://www.census.gov/hhes/hlthins/historic/hihist2.html>; calculations by New Strategist

Health Care Benefits in Private Establishments, 1996 and 1997

(health care benefits provided to full-time employees in small private nonfarm establishments, 1996; and health care benefits provided to full-time employees in medium and large private non-farm establishments, 1997)

	small firms	medium and large firms
Percent receiving		
Medical care	64%	76%
Dental care	31	59
Vision care	12	26
Prescription drug coverage	57	73
Type of coverage		
Total with medical care benefits	**100**	**100**
Traditional fee-for-service	36	27
Preferred provider organization	35	40
Prepaid health maintenance organization	27	33
Retiree coverage available	16	43
Average flat monthly contribution for individual coverage (dollars)	**$43**	**$39**
Average flat monthly contribution for family coverage (dollars)	**182**	**130**

Note: Small establishments have fewer than 100 employees; medium and large establisments have 100 or more employees.
Source: National Center for Health Statistics, Employee Benefits in Small Private Establishments, 1996, *Bulletin 2507, 1999; and* Employee Benefits in Medium and Large Private Establishments, 1997, *Bulletin 2517, 1999*

Employers' Costs for Health Insurance, 1999

(amount employers pay for health insurance per employee-hour worked, and health insurance as a percent of total compensation, by type of employer, 1999)

	amount per hour (dollars)	percent of compensation
State and local government	**$2.12**	**7.6%**
Private industry	**1.03**	**5.4**
Industry		
Goods producing	1.52	6.6
Service producing	0.88	4.9
Manufacturing	1.58	6.9
Nonmanufacturing	0.91	5.0
Occupation		
White collar	1.15	5.0
Blue collar	1.20	6.7
Service	0.40	4.2
Region		
Northeast	1.19	5.7
Midwest	1.07	5.8
South	0.89	5.2
West	1.00	4.8
Union status		
Union	2.02	8.2
Nonunion	0.89	4.9
Establishment employment size		
Under 100 employees	0.77	4.7
100 or more employes	1.30	5.9
100 to 499 employees	1.01	5.6
500 or more employees	1.64	6.2

Source: National Center for Health Statistics, Health, United States, 2000

Health Insurance Coverage by HMO Status, 1997

(percent of employees with health insurance by type of service covered and HMO status, for full-time workers in private nonfarm establishments with 100 or more employees, 1997)

	total	non-HMO plans	HMO plans
Percent of insured with coverage for:			
Hospital room and board	100%	100%	100%
Inpatient surgery	100	100	100
Outpatient surgery	100	100	100
Inpatient physician visits	100	100	100
Office physician visits	100	100	100
Diagnostic X-ray and laboratory	99	99	100
Extended care	78	76	84
Home health care	85	81	93
Hospice care	60	69	43
Inpatient mental health	96	97	95
Outpatient mental health	95	93	99
Inpatient alcohol detoxification	98	97	99
Inpatient alcohol rehabilitation	80	84	72
Outpatient alcohol rehabilitation	84	85	82
Inpatient drug detoxification	97	96	98
Inpatient drug rehabilitation	80	84	72
Outpatient drug rehabilitation	83	84	81
Hearing care	35	12	84
Physical exam	63	47	97
Well-baby care	66	51	96
Immunization and inoculation	52	34	90

Source: National Center for Health Statistics, Employee Benefits in Medium and Large Private Establishments, 1997, *Bulletin 2517, 2000*

People Covered by Health Maintenance Organizations, 1989 and 1997

(number and percent of people with private health insurance provided by health maintenance organizations by age, sex, race, Hispanic origin, region, and metropolitan status, 1989 and 1997; percentage point change in HMO coverage, 1989–97)

	1997	1989	percentage point change
Number (in millions)	**76.5**	**45.0**	–
Percent	**28.7%**	**18.5%**	**10.2**
Age			
Under age 18	29.9	20.1	9.8
Aged 18 to 24	24.9	16.6	8.3
Aged 25 to 34	32.4	21.2	11.2
Aged 35 to 44	34.1	21.7	12.4
Aged 45 to 54	33.6	19.6	14.0
Aged 55 to 64	27.9	15.3	12.6
Aged 65 or older	12.5	10.4	2.1
Sex			
Male	29.0	18.9	10.1
Female	29.1	18.6	10.5
Race			
White	29.3	18.2	11.1
Black	27.9	20.3	7.6
Asian or Pacific Islander	35.2	24.6	10.6
Hispanic origin and race			
Hispanic	25.4	18.8	6.6
Mexican	23.6	16.8	6.8
Puerto Rican	23.9	16.1	7.8
Cuban	37.7	25.6	12.1
Other Hispanic	27.4	22.2	5.2
White, non-Hispanic	30.0	18.6	11.4
Black, non-Hispanic	27.9	20.0	7.9
Region			
Northeast	37.7	20.6	17.1
Midwest	25.6	20.8	4.8
South	23.6	11.9	11.7
West	34.9	26.0	8.9
Metropolitan status			
Within metropolitan area	32.1	21.7	10.4
Outside metropolitan area	17.0	8.4	8.6

Source: National Center for Health Statistics, Health United States, 2000; *calculations by New Strategist*

HMOs Help Control Costs, 1998

"Health Maintenance Organizations (HMOs) help to
control costs. Do you agree or disagree?"

(percent of people aged 18 or older responding by sex, race, age, and education, 1998)

	agree	neither agree nor disagree	disagree	don't know
Total	**48%**	**15%**	**22%**	**15%**
Men	52	14	22	12
Women	46	15	22	17
Black	45	19	19	17
White	49	14	23	14
Other	49	10	16	24
Aged 18 to 29	49	18	17	16
Aged 30 to 39	49	19	21	11
Aged 40 to 49	56	11	25	8
Aged 50 to 59	51	15	22	12
Aged 60 to 69	43	13	22	20
Aged 70 or older	34	8	26	31
Not a high school graduate	37	12	19	32
High school graduate	46	15	25	15
Bachelor's degree	60	16	19	6
Graduate degree	63	16	15	5

Source: General Social Survey, National Opinion Research Center, University of Chicago; calculations by New Strategist

HMOs Improve Quality of Care, 1998

"Health Maintenance Organizations (HMOs) improve
the quality of care. Do you agree or disagree?"

(percent of people aged 18 or older responding by sex, race, age, and education, 1998)

	agree	neither agree nor disagree	disagree	don't know
Total	23%	23%	41%	13%
Men	24	26	37	12
Women	20	22	44	14
Black	31	24	27	18
White	20	23	45	12
Other	26	29	24	21
Aged 18 to 29	33	29	23	14
Aged 30 to 39	20	26	43	10
Aged 40 to 49	25	21	46	7
Aged 50 to 59	15	18	56	11
Aged 60 to 69	22	24	38	16
Aged 70 or older	15	20	38	28
Not a high school graduate	27	17	28	29
High school graduate	22	24	39	14
Bachelor's degree	21	25	48	6
Graduate degree	12	29	56	3

Source: General Social Survey, National Opinion Research Center, University of Chicago; calculations by New Strategist

HMOs Deny Needed Care, 1998

"Health Maintenance Organizations (HMOs) prevent people from getting the care they need. Do you agree or disagree?"

(percent of people aged 18 or older responding by sex, race, age, and education, 1998)

	agree	neither agree nor disagree	disagree	don't know
Total	**40%**	**17%**	**29%**	**14%**
Men	34	21	33	12
Women	43	15	27	15
Black	27	21	34	18
White	42	16	29	12
Other	29	20	30	22
Aged 18 to 29	28	25	34	15
Aged 30 to 39	41	20	29	10
Aged 40 to 49	44	15	34	7
Aged 50 to 59	48	16	25	11
Aged 60 to 69	43	15	24	18
Aged 70 or older	34	9	28	29
Not a high school graduate	29	12	29	30
High school graduate	39	17	31	13
Bachelor's degree	43	20	30	7
Graduate degree	49	24	23	4

Source: General Social Survey, National Opinion Research Center, University of Chicago; calculations by New Strategist

HMOs Limit Doctors' Decision Making, 1998

"Health Maintenance Organizations (HMOs) take important medical decisions out of the hands of physicians. Do you agree or disagree?"

(percent of people aged 18 or older responding by sex, race, age, and education, 1998)

	agree	neither agree nor disagree	disagree	don't know
Total	**46%**	**16%**	**22%**	**15%**
Men	43	18	26	14
Women	48	14	21	17
Black	34	16	29	20
White	49	15	21	14
Other	37	20	19	24
Aged 18 to 29	38	20	26	16
Aged 30 to 39	45	20	23	12
Aged 40 to 49	54	14	24	8
Aged 50 to 59	54	12	23	12
Aged 60 to 69	47	18	15	20
Aged 70 or older	40	7	20	33
Not a high school graduate	33	13	22	33
High school graduate	47	15	23	16
Bachelor's degree	49	20	25	7
Graduate degree	61	18	19	3

Source: General Social Survey, National Opinion Research Center, University of Chicago; calculations by New Strategist

HMOs Damage Doctor-Patient Trust, 1998

"Health Maintenance Organizations (HMOs) damage the trust between doctors and patients. Do you agree or disagree?"

(percent of people aged 18 or older responding by sex, race, age, and education, 1998)

	agree	neither agree nor disagree	disagree	don't know
Total	**36%**	**19%**	**30%**	**13%**
Men	34	21	33	12
Women	38	18	28	15
Black	26	20	35	17
White	39	20	29	12
Other	25	17	36	22
Aged 18 to 29	24	24	37	15
Aged 30 to 39	33	22	33	11
Aged 40 to 49	43	19	31	7
Aged 50 to 59	46	18	28	8
Aged 60 to 69	47	17	18	18
Aged 70 or older	33	12	26	29
Not a high school graduate	29	13	29	30
High school graduate	38	20	29	14
Bachelor's degree	37	23	34	6
Graduate degree	42	29	25	4

Source: General Social Survey, National Opinion Research Center, University of Chicago; calculations by New Strategist

HMOs Limit Necessary Tests, 1998

"Health Maintenance Organizations (HMOs) prevent doctors from prescribing tests necessary for treatment. Do you agree or disagree?"

(percent of people aged 18 or older responding by sex, race, age, and education, 1998)

	agree	neither agree nor disagree	disagree	don't know
Total	**42%**	**18%**	**24%**	**16%**
Men	39	21	26	15
Women	44	15	24	17
Black	29	18	32	21
White	45	17	23	15
Other	33	26	15	25
Aged 18 to 29	33	25	25	16
Aged 30 to 39	43	19	25	13
Aged 40 to 49	47	16	28	9
Aged 50 to 59	56	13	19	13
Aged 60 to 69	45	18	16	22
Aged 70 or older	31	11	25	32
Not a high school graduate	29	17	23	32
High school graduate	40	18	24	17
Bachelor's degree	50	20	22	8
Graduate degree	59	16	22	4

Source: General Social Survey, National Opinion Research Center, University of Chicago; calculations by New Strategist

HMOs Limit Mental-Health Care, 1998

"HMOs make it more difficult to see a specialist for problems like emotional, nervous, and mental health problems. Do you agree or disagree?"

(percent of people aged 18 or older responding by sex, race, age, and education, 1998)

	agree	neither agree nor disagree	disagree	don't know
Total	**48%**	**14%**	**19%**	**18%**
Men	43	17	22	18
Women	51	13	17	19
Black	41	15	24	19
White	50	14	18	18
Other	41	15	19	25
Aged 18 to 29	41	20	22	18
Aged 30 to 39	47	16	21	16
Aged 40 to 49	60	11	17	12
Aged 50 to 59	53	12	20	14
Aged 60 to 69	47	16	13	25
Aged 70 or older	35	10	19	35
Not a high school graduate	33	13	20	34
High school graduate	47	14	19	20
Bachelor's degree	56	15	19	10
Graduate degree	62	16	15	6

Source: General Social Survey, National Opinion Research Center, University of Chicago; calculations by New Strategist

3

Changing Medical Relationships

A health care system is a network of experiences. Although analysts attempt to turn those experiences into statistics, health care remains a place where two people—provider and patient—meet.

Americans contact a doctor more than 1 billion times a year. They visit doctors hundreds of millions of times a year. In 1997 alone, the public logged 959 million trips to a doctor's office, emergency room, or hospital outpatient department. These medical consumers are not who they used to be. No longer passive, obedient, and eager to follow the doctor's orders, they have become critical, questioning, and willing to chart their own course of medical treatment. They regard a doctor's advice as just one piece of the puzzle. The new health care consumer has gained more control over the medical relationship, as have health insurers and administrators. With patients, third-party payers, and accountants questioning their authority, doctors have less power than they once did.

"The discretion that the profession once enjoyed has been increasingly circumscribed by an almost bewildering number of parties and procedures participating in medical decision making," writes David J. Rothman in his book, *Strangers at the Bedside: A History of How Law and Bioethics Transformed Medical Decision Making.*[1] That discretion once meant the physician was king. The physician alone made life-and-death decisions, without the scrutiny of the media, the courts, or even the patient's family.

Critical change occurred between 1966 and 1976, according to Rothman, when medical decisions were formalized, often to be made by committees with third party intervention. Now doctors must cope with insurers, lawyers, and demanding customers. All these layers put greater distance between patient and doctor and erode trust.

The transformation of the doctor-patient relationship has arguably hurt the medical profession, and it has done little to boost consumer satisfaction. The proportion of Americans who have a "great deal" of confidence in the people running medicine dropped from the 60 percent majority in 1974 to just 44 percent in 1998, according to the General Social Survey of the University of Chicago's National Opinion Research Center. The public is increasingly wary of the health care establishment.

Visiting the doctor

Americans contacted physicians fully 1.6 billion times in 1996—including telephone calls, visits to doctor's offices, and seeing doctors in hospitals and clinics. In 1997, the American public walked into the nation's health care establishments (including physician's offices, hospital outpatient departments, and emergency rooms) an average of 3.6 times per person. During 95 percent of those visits, the patient saw a physician—making the doctor-patient interaction one of the most pervasive relationships in modern life. It is a relationship that is increasingly troubled as the complexity and cost of health care grow.

Age determines how frequently people visit a doctor. Not surprisingly, the oldest Americans need medical care most often. People aged 75 or older visit health care providers an average of 7.5 times a year. This number compares with just 2.3 visits per year for people aged 15 to 24. People aged 45 or older account for nearly half of visits to physician's offices. They account for only 32 percent of trips to emergency rooms. Older Americans are a smaller share of emergency-room patients because they are less likely to be injured than children or young adults.

Doctor visits increase with age

(average annual number of physician's office visits per person, by age, 1998)

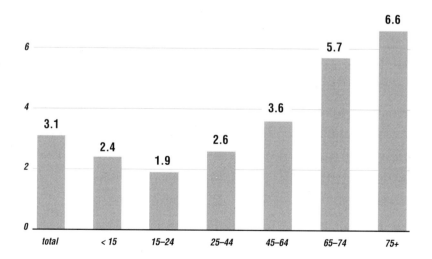

Gender and race also determine how often people seek health care. Women visit health care providers more frequently than men (4.2 visits per year for females versus 3.0 for males). For women, many doctor visits are pregnancy related.

Whites contact health care providers an average of 3.7 times a year, while blacks do so 3.4 times. Health care visits by whites are more likely than those of blacks to occur at a physician's office, while blacks are more likely than whites to visit hospital outpatient departments and emergency rooms. People of other races (Asians and Native Americans) visit health care providers less frequently than whites or blacks, averaging 2.6 visits per person in 1997.

New providers

The pressure to keep medical costs down is changing the type of provider seen by consumers during health care visits. While physicians attend 95 percent of all health care visits, they are present at a smaller 80 percent of visits to hospital outpatient departments. In 40 percent of outpatient department visits, the provider is a registered nurse.

The downshifting of medical care to lesser-trained providers is occurring in health care facilities across the nation. While this development once meant shifting the provision of medical care from physicians to nurses, it's now going beyond that. As registered nurses become overloaded, care is shifting to providers with less training—such as licensed practical nurses. Because hospitals can pay LPNs 20 to 40 percent less than RNs, many hospitals replace RNs with LPNs when downsizing.

"To make sure workers are productive, hospitals may also cross train janitors, house-keepers, transport workers and security guards to do nursing work," writes Suzanne Gordon in *The American Prospect*.[2] "The consequences of cuts in nursing care are extremely serious. Patients who could recover, don't. Preventable complications escalate. Some patients die. Moreover as nurses are stretched too thin in the hospital and as patients are denied expert nursing care at home, the burden of care is shifted to ill-prepared family caregivers." While the American Hospital Association claims that the number of RNs employed in hospitals has increased slightly over the past few years, Gordon contends that the number includes all RNs regardless of whether they provide direct care or are administrators.

Cost is not the only factor that can limit the presence of physicians during health care visits. Another limiting factor is a pending shortage of doctors. The number of applicants to medical school fell to 66,489 in 1998-99, 4.7 percent less than one year earlier.[3] It is an ominous sign that the number of physicians-in-training is falling just as we face a surge in demand for health care because of the aging of the baby-boom generation.

One positive trend is that physicians are slowly becoming more diverse. In 1998, 44 percent of enrolled first-year students were women, while 35 percent were members of a minority group. For minorities, progress has not been steady. Although the number of minority medical students was 6.2 percent greater in 1998 than in 1997, it was 2.8 percent less than in 1996.[4]

The need for doctors to represent the diversity of the U.S. population is important. Female doctors, for example, are a wanted commodity. Many consumers—especially women—request female doctors. A Northeastern University study found that female doctors spend more time with patients. A *JAMA* study found that female doctors were more likely to involve patients in decision making and spent more time listening rather than talking than male doctors. A Robert Wood Johnson Medical Center study found that female doctors were less likely than male doctors to be sued for malpractice. The news is not all good, however. The Northeastern study found that patient satisfaction scores were lower for female than male doctors. The study authors speculate that this may be due to societal prejudice.[5]

The erosion of trust

With the percentage of people having a great deal of confidence in the leaders of medicine falling over the past quarter-century, it is no surprise that the public's trust in their own medical doctors also shows signs of erosion. While 81 percent of Americans aged 18 or older say they trust their doctor's judgment about their medical care, one in five agree that their doctor "does not do everything he should for my medical care," according to the 1998 General Social Survey of the University of Chicago's National Opinion Research Center. One in four worries that his or her doctor puts cost considerations above care. Nearly half disagree that doctors are very careful to check everything when examining patients. And fully 50 percent agree that doctors aren't as thorough as they should be.

The cause of this distrust does not seem to be the factor sometimes blamed for the breakdown in the doctor-patient relationship—that patients see a different doctor each time they visit a medical establishment. Only 19 percent of Americans say they "hardly ever see the same doctor" when they go for medical care. Seventy-five percent disagree with that statement. Instead, the big problem between doctors and patients appears to be a lack of communication. When asked whether doctors always do their best to keep their patients from worrying, a substantial 28 percent disagree. Forty-one percent say that doctors cause people to worry because they don't explain their medical problems. One-third do not believe doctors treat patients with respect.

The distrust runs even deeper. The fifty-five percent majority of Americans do not believe that doctors always avoid unnecessary patient expenses. Thirty-four percent think doctors take unnecessary risks when treating their patients. One in five does not think doctors would tell them if they made a mistake in their treatment.

One reason for the public's growing distrust of the medical establishment is the fear that privacy could be violated by the deliberate or inadvertent release of confidential medical information. Privacy has become an increasingly important issue now that employers are storing personnel files on the Internet and health care providers are considering using the Internet to distribute medical records to all doctors working with a particular patient.

Sixty-five percent of Americans say protecting the privacy of consumer information is very important, according to a 1996 Equifax/Harris Consumer Privacy Survey. Medical information is what Americans are most concerned about protecting.[6]

A nationally representative survey by the California Health Care Foundation, fielded in 1999, found 54 percent of the public believing that computerization was the most serious threat to medical privacy. Fifty-five percent worried about hackers breaking into computer-

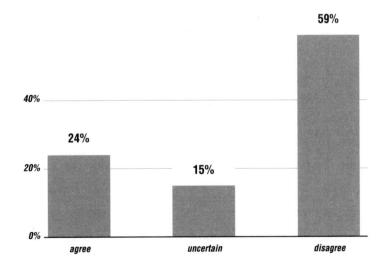

Many worry that doctors consider cost over care

(percent distribution of people aged 18 or older responding to the question, "I worry that my doctor will put cost considerations above the care I need. Do you agree or disagree?")

ized medical records system.[7] Fully 60 percent do not want potential employers to see their medical records, and the same percentage do not want hospitals with preventive care programs to be able to access their records.[8]

Following up on a study of medical privacy by the Health Privacy Project at Georgetown University and the California Healthcare Foundation, the Federal Trade Commission is currently investigating how commercial health web sites protect privacy. After investigating the privacy practices of high profile web sites like medscape.com, drkoop.com, and others, Health Privacy Project researchers reported disturbing findings. Health web sites are constantly gathering information about consumers through devices such as cookies—often without a consumer's knowledge or consent, the researchers found. Many web sites with stated privacy policies are violating those policies. Even when companies intend to protect privacy, many do not have adequate computer security to fight hackers.[9]

The Internet is not the only arena where the battle for privacy is being waged. Smart card technology—which links consumers' medical records with physicians and insurance companies—also threatens to expose personal medical information to unauthorized parties. Real Med Corporation of Indianapolis, for example, has developed smart card technology for reducing the cost and increasing the speed of health claims processing. Working with companies such as MCI and Digital Equipment, Real Med plans to link patients, physicians,

Many think doctors don't explain enough

(percent distribution of people aged 18 or older responding to the question, "Doctors cause people to worry a lot because they don't explain medical problems to patients. Do you agree or disagree?")

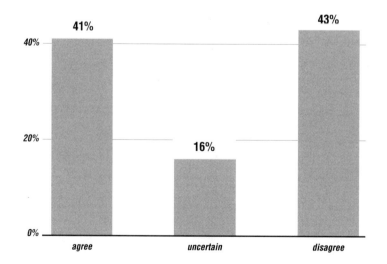

and insurance companies through a single claims resolution network. Similar systems tested in Europe have reduced costs by as much as 30 percent, according to *Industry Week*.[10] But for such a system to gain acceptance, it will have to guarantee privacy to consumers.

The future of medical relationships

The public's growing distrust of doctors and the health care system overall will shape future relationships between health care providers and patients. Several trends will influence how the relationship will evolve.

TREND 1: REBUILDING CREDIBILITY

Americans' negative feelings toward the health care system—particularly health insurance companies—are held in check today because most haven't personally experienced problems with the system yet. But over time, particularly as the population ages, insurers and providers will pay the price for the erosion of public trust. They will face increasing consumer anger and government regulation, leaving them vulnerable to competition from alternative health care providers and delivery systems.

Traditional medical providers are concerned, publicly distancing themselves from insurers. An example of this occurred in the fall of 1997, when the Ad Hoc Committee to Defend Health Care, a group of more than 2,000 doctors and nurses in Massachusetts, wrote an open letter to the *Journal of the American Medical Association* protesting the shift to profit-driven care.[11] Efforts such as these will not entirely deflect consumer anger away from physicians. Instead, physicians must be ever vigilant in their attempts to improve the doctor-patient relationship.

TREND 2: LOOKING FOR ALTERNATIVES

As Americans become increasingly distrustful of the current health care system, many hunger for alternative providers and delivery systems. Technological and economic change will speed the acceptance of alternatives—even among consumers reluctant to use them. New medical technologies are creating specialists to whom the public must relate. Economics is pushing more consumers into the hands of physician assistants, nurse practitioners, chiropractors, and other nonphysicians.

Many consumers welcome this shift. One sign of acceptance is the growing popularity of alternative medicine. In 1997, 42 percent of adults with health insurance used some form of alternative therapy to treat a health problem, according to a survey by Landmark Healthcare, Inc., a managed alternative care company based in Sacramento, California. The search for alternatives promises to boost competition in the already turbulent health care industry.

Trend 3: Better communication

Regardless of who provides health care, communication skills will be more important in the future than they are today. Already valued highly by patients, physicians who are good communicators are less likely to be sued by their patients, according to an article in *Hippocrates*, a magazine for physicians.[12] Because malpractice suits are costly in terms of money, morale, and reputation, physicians are likely to sit up and take notice of this finding. Many medical schools offer courses in communication skills. For practicing physicians, several organizations offer training in effective communication.

To communicate effectively with patients, medical providers must ask the right questions, probing topics patients may be hesitant to discuss, such as sex or healthy aging. For a population aging as rapidly as ours, too few doctors have sufficient knowledge of the aging process or how to age well. To solve this problem, the Department of Health and Human Services is funding more than two dozen geriatric education centers across the nation, training medical professionals in caring for the needs of older patients.

Accommodating the spiritual beliefs of patients is another area likely to receive more attention. Eighty percent of Americans believe in the power of God or prayer to affect the course of an illness, according to a 1996 Time/CNN poll.[13] Nearly 70 percent of physicians say patients with terminal illnesses have asked them about religious counseling, but only 10 percent of physicians ever ask about a patient's beliefs or practices. Physicians of the future will have to connect with the spiritual needs of patients or lose this important role to alternative medical providers.

Encouraging good communication may help the medical community avoid embarrassing mistakes that hurt credibility. Of 461 pharmacists surveyed by the Department of Health and Human Services, for example, 45 percent said they sometimes or often saw inappropriate drugs prescribed to nursing home patients. Poor communication is blamed for these mistakes.[14]

The public has little tolerance for such errors. Books like *When Your Doctor Doesn't Know Best* and *How to Get Out of the Hospital Alive* are drawing attention to the mistakes doctors make.[15,16] This hostile climate guarantees an important place for quality comparisons of health care providers and facilities in the future. Comparative reports are likely to focus on the experience of patients—such as the number of complaints about a doctor or health care plan or the percentage of members who change plans. Patient satisfaction surveys will also add to the knowledge base. Americans already find such surveys influential if they are available. In the increasingly competitive health care market of the future, such surveys could build a word-of-mouth network that will bring patients in the door.

TREND 4: PROTECTING PRIVACY

The battle over privacy has become one of the most important health issues of the new century. A survey of Fortune 500 companies found one-third used health records when making job-related decisions—with or without an applicant's knowledge, according to *Atlantic Monthly*.[17] Although Congress passed the Health Insurance Portability and Account-ability Act of 1996, government is moving more slowly than technology in this area. Both the Department of Health and Human Services and Congress are considering the best ways to protect the privacy of medical records, but both organizations missed their deadlines for creating standards. They are finding it difficult to protect privacy without hamstringing health care providers.[18]

Any implementation of government privacy protection rules is likely to be delayed—possibly until 2006. It's important to remember, however, that although consumers say they worry about the privacy of health records, most do not think their privacy has been violated, according to the California Health Care Foundation survey. Only 18 percent of adults think their health care provider, insurance plan, government agency, or employer has ever improperly disclosed personal medical information. For the most part, Americans have not changed the way they interact with the health care industry because of privacy concerns. Only 15 percent say they have done something out of the ordinary to keep their medical information confidential.

TREND 5: CUSTOMIZING CARE

Thanks to the Internet, patients are taking a more active role in their health care. But social mores about doctor-patient communication don't change overnight. Although many pa-tients are eager to speak up, many are rightfully nervous about assuming responsibility for their own health. A study of patients with breast cancer found that only 22 percent wanted to select their own treatment, compared with one-third who wanted to delegate the choice of cancer treatment to their physician and 44 percent who wanted to select their treatment collaboratively. On the physician's side, attitudes are also slow to change. One study found that 30 percent of requests to physicians for specific medical interventions caused the physician to object or become angry. An additional 20 percent of physicians simply showed no interest in the patient's request.[19]

In an *Archives of Family Medicine* article, Forest Lang, M.D., points out, "Such diversity of expectation suggest that a 'one size fits all' model will lead to frustrations and problems on both sides . . . A patient centered approach does not insist on patient decision making. An approach that is truly patient centered explores the patients' preference for involvement and decision making and respects that preference."[20] In other words, there needs to be a sliding scale of involvement in medical decisions, and it should be up to the patient to determine how involved he or she wants to be.

Trend 6: The Internet

The number of consumers who feel comfortable making health care decisions will grow because of the Internet. According to a Harris Poll, 70 million consumers, or "cyberchondriacs" in the poll's terminology, have logged on at some point to learn more about their health. That's nearly three-quarters of the entire online population. These consumers are most often researching serious conditions requiring prescription treatment. The top conditions or diseases of interest to consumers online include depression, cancer, bipolar disorder, and hypertension.[21]

Today, the search online is for information. Tomorrow, full care could be received via computer. At least that's the hope of Virtual Clinic, a collaboration of Overlake Hospital near Seattle and Microsoft Corporation. Using Virtual Clinic, Microsoft employees can seek advice from doctors via the Internet and the software company's intranet. If an employee suffers from back pain, for example, a doctor at Virtual Clinic can call up an anatomical image of a back and ask the patient to point to where it hurts, *The Lancet* reports. "If a prescription is needed, it can be e-mailed to an online pharmacy for delivery to the patient. Thus, the physician will be able to provide all the services of a doctor's visit except that of touching the patient," writes author Jon Ferry.[22] This system is not without controversy, of course. But if medical care can be provided as easily as buying a book online, then it's obvious the relationship between patient and doctor is going to change dramatically. And it's likely that costs will decrease.

Even before virtual clinics become widespread, many physicians will use e-mail to stay in touch with patients. E-mail is especially helpful to patients seeking information on sensitive subjects. A Harris Interactive study found that one-third of physicians worked in practices with web sites—a figure likely to grow to 50 percent within the next 18 months.[23]

Many doctors have yet to develop the technological skills to fully participate in the Internet revolution. The computer industry is investing to help with the training effort. Intel, for example, has developed the Internet Health Road Show in partnership with the American Medical Association, intended to show doctors the potential of technology. Intel has also developed "digital credentials" to help doctors and other health care professionals feel more secure about transmitting confidential medical information online.[24]

Notes

1. David J. Rothman, *Strangers at the Bedside: A History of How Law and Bioethics Transformed Medical Decision Making* (New York: Basic Books, 1991): 1.

2. Suzanne Gordon, "Nurse, Interrupted," *The American Prospect* (February 14, 2000): 26.

3. Barbara Baransky, Harry S. Jonas, and Sylvia I. Etzel, "Educational Programs in U.S. Medical Schools, 1998-1999," *Journal of the American Medical Association* 282, no. 9 (September 1, 1999): 840–846.

4. Ibid.

5. Jim Ritter, "Women Redefining Art of Being a Doctor; Gender a Factor in Patient Choices," *Sunday News, Chicago Sun-Times* (February 13, 2000): 6.

6. The Equifax/Harris Consumer Privacy Survey, 1996. <www.equifax.com>.

7. Janlori Goldman, and Zoe Hudson, "Promoting Health/Protecting Privacy: A Primer," Health Privacy Project, Georgetown University, written for the California HealthCare Foundation and Consumers Union, January 1999. <www.chcf.org>.

8. Ibid.

9. Janlori Goldman, Zoe Hudson, and Richard M. Smith, "Report on the Privacy Policies and Practices of Health Web Sites," Health Privacy Project, Georgetown University, January 2000. <www.chcf.org>.

10. Industry Week Online Editor (January 7, 1998). <www.industryweek.com>.

11. Open Letter from the Ad Hoc Committee to Defend Health Care, *Journal of the American Medical Association* 278, no. 21 (December 3, 1997): 1733–1739.

12. Jane Goldman, "Preventing Malpractice," *Hippocrates* 11, no. 10 (1997): 27–33.

13. Claudia Wells, "Faith and Healing," *Time* (June 24, 1996): 58.

14. Associated Press report via America Online News, "Report: Elderly Get Wrong Drugs" (November 17, 1996). Attributed to *USA Today*.

15. Richard N. Podell, *When Your Doctor Doesn't Know Best: Medical Mistakes that Even the Best Doctors Make and How to Protect Yourself* (New York: Simon and Schuster, 1995).

16. Paul Sheldon Black and Elaine Fantle Shimberg, *How to Get Out of the Hospital Alive* (New York: Macmillan, 1997).

17. "February Almanac," *Atlantic Monthly* (February 1998): 14.

18. Michael Pretzer, "Protecting patients' privacy isn't coming easy," *Medical Economics* 77, no. 8 (April 24, 2000): 31.

19. Forest Lang, "The Evolving Role of Patient and Physician," *Archives of Family Medicine* 9, no. 1 (January 2000).

20. Ibid.

21. "Explosive Growth of Cyberchondriacs Continues," The Harris Poll #47, (August 5, 1999) <www.harrisinteractive.com>

22. Jon Ferry, "Virtual Doctors on the Horizon in Seattle," *The Lancet* 354, no. 9182 (September 11, 1999): 926.

23. "Harris Interactive Study Reveals a Lack of Information Technology Use in Medicine," Press Release (March 28, 2000). <www.harrisinteractive.com>.

24. "AMA to Provide Online Initiatives for America's Physicians, Patients," *The Journal of the American Medical Association* 282, no. 20 (November 24, 1999): S1.

Physician Contacts by Age, 1996

(number and percent distribution of physician contacts and number per person per year, by age and type of contact, 1996; numbers in thousands)

	total	telephone	office	hospital	other
Total contacts	**1,566,513**	**191,245**	**845,720**	**188,401**	**325,666**
Under age 5	130,232	18,969	73,504	14,519	21,913
Aged 5 to 17	167,708	23,917	94,691	18,474	29,626
Aged 18 to 24	101,620	13,273	53,024	15,871	18,181
Aged 25 to 44	412,501	53,589	235,584	50,173	68,042
Aged 45 to 64	383,812	46,773	207,742	52,278	73,936
Aged 65 to 74	188,048	20,348	101,858	18,173	45,791
Aged 75 or older	182,592	14,376	79,317	18,913	68,177

Percent distribution by type of contact

	total	telephone	office	hospital	other
Total contacts	**100.0%**	**12.2%**	**54.0%**	**12.0%**	**20.8%**
Under age 5	100.0	14.6	56.4	11.1	16.8
Aged 5 to 17	100.0	14.3	56.5	11.0	17.7
Aged 18 to 24	100.0	13.1	52.2	15.6	17.9
Aged 25 to 44	100.0	13.0	57.1	12.2	16.5
Aged 45 to 64	100.0	12.2	54.1	13.6	19.3
Aged 65 to 74	100.0	10.8	54.2	9.7	24.4
Aged 75 or older	100.0	7.9	43.4	10.4	37.3

Percent distribution by age

	total	telephone	office	hospital	other
Total contacts	**100.0%**	**100.0%**	**100.0%**	**100.0%**	**100.0%**
Under age 5	8.3	9.9	8.7	7.7	6.7
Aged 5 to 17	10.7	12.5	11.2	9.8	9.1
Aged 18 to 24	6.5	6.9	6.3	8.4	5.6
Aged 25 to 44	26.3	28.0	27.9	26.6	20.9
Aged 45 to 64	24.5	24.5	24.6	27.7	22.7
Aged 65 to 74	12.0	10.6	12.0	9.6	14.1
Aged 75 or older	11.7	7.5	9.4	10.0	20.9

(continued)

(continued from previous page)

	total	telephone	office	hospital	other
Contacts per person per year					
Total contacts	**5.9**	**0.7**	**3.2**	**0.7**	**1.2**
Under age 5	6.5	0.9	3.7	0.7	1.1
Aged 5 to 17	3.3	0.5	1.8	0.4	0.6
Aged 18 to 24	4.1	0.5	2.2	0.6	0.7
Aged 25 to 44	4.9	0.6	2.8	0.6	0.8
Aged 45 to 64	7.2	0.9	3.9	1.0	1.4
Aged 65 to 74	10.2	1.1	5.5	1.0	2.5
Aged 75 or older	13.7	1.1	5.9	1.4	5.1

Note: Other places of contact include clinics and HMOs not located in hospitals.
Source: National Center for Health Statistics, Current Estimates from the National Health Interview Survey, 1996, *Series 10, No. 200, 1999; calculations by New Strategist*

Health Care Visits by Sex and Age, 1997

(total number, percent distribution, and number per person per year of ambulatory care visits to physician offices, hospital outpatient departments, and emergency rooms, by sex, age, and place of care, 1997; numbers in thousands)

	total	physician offices	hospital outpatient departments	hospital emergency rooms
Number				
Total visits	**959,300**	**787,372**	**76,993**	**94,936**
Female	567,880	471,481	46,112	50,286
Male	391,421	315,891	30,880	44,649
Under age 15	176,294	137,361	18,240	20,693
Aged 15 to 24	85,653	62,488	8,753	14,412
Aged 25 to 44	253,775	203,701	20,677	29,397
Aged 45 to 64	226,064	192,753	17,682	15,629
Aged 65 to 74	112,593	99,714	6,677	6,201
Aged 75 or older	104,922	91,355	4,963	8,604
Percent distribution by place of care				
Total visits	**100.0%**	**82.1%**	**8.0%**	**9.9%**
Female	100.0	83.0	8.1	8.9
Male	100.0	80.7	7.9	11.4
Under age 15	100.0	77.9	10.3	11.7
Aged 15 to 24	100.0	73.0	10.2	16.8
Aged 25 to 44	100.0	80.3	8.1	11.6
Aged 45 to 64	100.0	85.3	7.8	6.9
Aged 65 to 74	100.0	88.6	5.9	5.5
Aged 75 or older	100.0	87.1	4.7	8.2

(continued)

(continued from previous page)

	total	physician's offices	hospital outpatient departments	hospital emergency rooms
Percent distribution by sex and age				
Total visits	**100.0%**	**100.0%**	**100.0%**	**100.0%**
Female	59.2	59.9	59.9	53.0
Male	40.8	40.1	40.1	47.0
Under age 15	18.4	17.4	23.7	21.8
Aged 15 to 24	8.9	7.9	11.4	15.2
Aged 25 to 44	26.5	25.9	26.9	31.0
Aged 45 to 64	23.6	24.5	23.0	16.5
Aged 65 to 74	11.7	12.7	8.7	6.5
Aged 75 or older	10.9	11.6	6.4	9.1
Visits per person per year				
Total visits	**3.6**	**3.0**	**0.3**	**0.4**
Female	4.2	3.5	0.3	0.4
Male	3.0	2.4	0.2	0.3
Under age 15	3.0	2.3	0.3	0.3
Aged 15 to 24	2.3	1.7	0.2	0.4
Aged 25 to 44	3.0	2.4	0.2	0.4
Aged 45 to 64	4.1	3.5	0.3	0.3
Aged 65 to 74	6.2	5.5	0.4	0.3
Aged 75 or older	7.5	6.5	0.4	0.6

Note: For definition of ambulatory care visits, see glossary.
Source: National Center for Health Statistics, Ambulatory Care Visits to Physician Offices, Hospital Outpatient Departments, and Emergency Departments: United States, 1997, *Vital and Health Statistics, Series 13, No. 143, 1999*

Health Care Visits by Type of Provider Seen, 1997

(number and percent distribution of ambulatory care visits by type of provider seen and place of care, 1997; numbers in thousands)

	total	physician's offices	hospital outpatient departments	hospital emergency rooms
Total visits	**959,300**	**787,372**	**76,993**	**94,936**
Physician	913,112	761,907	61,711	89,493
Physician assistant	24,533	19,174	1,629	3,730
Nurse practitioner	14,169	9,212	3,475	1,482
Nurse midwife	1,125	–	553	–
Registered nurse	221,153	107,103	31,303	82,747
Licensed practical nurse	108,277	94,013	8,391	5,873
Medical/nursing assistant	194,591	174,009	13,351	7,232
Emergency medical technician	6,949	–	–	6,949
Other provider	62,102	42,780	12,366	6,955
Total visits	**100.0%**	**100.0%**	**100.0%**	**100.0%**
Physician	95.2	96.8	80.2	94.3
Physician assistant	2.6	2.4	2.1	3.9
Nurse practitioner	1.5	1.2	4.5	1.6
Nurse midwife	0.1	–	0.7	–
Registered nurse	23.1	13.6	40.7	87.2
Licensed practical nurse	11.3	11.9	10.9	6.2
Medical/nursing assistant	20.3	22.1	17.3	7.6
Emergency medical technician	0.7	–	–	7.3
Other provider	6.5	5.4	16.1	7.3

Note: Numbers will not add to total because more than one type of provider could have been seen and "no answer" is not shown; for definition of ambulatory care visits, see glossary; (–) means sample is too small to make a reliable estimate or not applicable.
Source: National Center for Health Statistics, Ambulatory Care Visits to Physician Offices, Hospital Outpatient Departments, and Emergency Departments: United States, 1997, *Vital and Health Statistics, Series 13, No. 143, 1999*

Health Care Visits by Reason, 1997

(number and percent distribution of ambulatory care visits by reason for visit most frequently mentioned by patients, and percent distribution by place of care, 1997; numbers in thousands)

| | total | | place of care | | | |
	number	percent distribution	total	physician's offices	hospital outpatient departments	hospital emergency rooms
Total visits	**959,300**	**100.0%**	**100.0%**	**82.1%**	**8.0%**	**9.9%**
General medical examination	64,804	6.8	100.0	92.3	7.6	–
Progress visit	36,670	3.8	100.0	77.9	21.8	–
Cough	29,603	3.1	100.0	86.9	5.6	7.5
Routine prenatal exam	26,165	2.7	100.0	87.8	11.9	–
Throat symptoms	20,734	2.2	100.0	82.7	7.9	9.4
Postoperative visit	20,443	2.1	100.0	92.3	6.6	1.1
Stomach, abdominal pain	18,785	2.0	100.0	64.3	6.3	29.4
Fever	17,580	1.8	100.0	70.4	5.7	24.0
Well-baby exam	17,148	1.8	100.0	90.5	9.4	–
Earache or ear infection	16,134	1.7	100.0	82.8	6.8	10.4
Back symptoms	15,775	1.6	100.0	81.5	5.3	13.1
Skin rash	14,382	1.5	100.0	85.6	6.3	8.1
Knee symptoms	14,012	1.5	100.0	88.4	5.1	6.4
Chest pain and related symptoms	13,962	1.5	100.0	58.4	3.5	38.1
Vision dysfunctions	13,873	1.4	100.0	96.9	2.0	1.1
Headache, head pain	12,733	1.3	100.0	75.3	4.9	19.8
Depression	12,003	1.3	100.0	87.4	8.2	4.5
Hypertension	11,928	1.2	100.0	91.2	6.8	2.1
Nasal congestion	11,820	1.2	100.0	89.4	5.5	5.2
Head cold, upper respiratory infection	10,262	1.1	100.0	87.4	7.5	5.1
Medications	10,196	1.1	100.0	88.8	8.9	2.3
Blood pressure test	9,152	1.0	100.0	94.1	5.7	–
Low back symptoms	8,797	0.9	100.0	80.4	6.4	13.2
Neck symptoms	8,652	0.9	100.0	80.2	5.2	14.5
Leg symptoms	8,511	0.9	100.0	81.2	6.0	12.7
Shoulder symptoms	8,273	0.9	100.0	83.4	5.9	10.7
Foot and toe symptoms	7,374	0.8	100.0	82.2	5.1	12.7
Anxiety and nervousness	7,168	0.7	100.0	91.4	6.1	2.4
Sinus problems	7,022	0.7	100.0	90.5	6.8	2.6

(continued)

(continued from previous page)

	total		place of care			
	number	percent distribution	total	physician's offices	hospital outpatient departments	hospital emergency rooms
Vertigo, dizziness	7,004	0.7%	100.0%	75.7%	5.9%	18.4%
Hand and finger symptoms	6,770	0.7	100.0	81.0	5.2	13.8
Diabetes	6,673	0.7	100.0	82.4	16.5	–
Shortness of breath	6,217	0.6	100.0	59.3	4.6	36.1
Pain	6,193	0.6	100.0	61.8	5.2	32.9
Other	452,483	47.2	100.0	80.2	8.2	11.6

Note: (–) means sample is too small to make a reliable estimate or not applicable; for definition of ambulatory care visits, see glossary.
Source: National Center for Health Statistics, Ambulatory Care Visits to Physician Offices, Hospital Outpatient Departments, and Emergency Departments: United States, 1997, *Vital and Health Statistics, Series 13, No. 143, 1999*

Health Care Visits by Principal Diagnosis, 1997

(number and percent distribution of ambulatory care visits by principal diagnosis group, and percent distribution by place of care, 1997; numbers in thousands)

	total		place of care			
	number	percent distribution	total	physician's offices	hospital outpatient departments	hospital emergency rooms
Total visits	**959,300**	**100.0%**	**100.0%**	**82.1%**	**8.0%**	**9.9%**
Acute upper respiratory infections	38,067	4.0	100.0	83.9	6.1	10.0
Essential hypertension	33,623	3.5	100.0	88.4	10.1	1.5
Routine infant or child health check	31,654	3.3	100.0	87.1	12.7	–
Normal pregnancy	26,278	2.7	100.0	86.9	12.4	0.7
Otitis media and eustachian tube disorders	24,576	2.6	100.0	81.4	7.8	10.8
Arthropathies and related disorders	23,924	2.5	100.0	87.2	8.6	3.7
General medical exam	22,290	2.3	100.0	93.3	5.7	1.0
Diabetes	21,417	2.2	100.0	83.5	15.1	1.4
Malignant neoplasms	19,990	2.1	100.0	83.0	15.9	0.6
Dorsopathies	19,425	2.0	100.0	81.5	8.1	10.0
Rheumatism, excluding back	18,916	2.0	100.0	86.8	4.8	7.8
Chronic sinusitis	14,933	1.6	100.0	89.4	7.0	3.7
Asthma	12,975	1.4	100.0	75.8	9.4	14.8
Ischemic heart disease	12,432	1.3	100.0	85.9	5.1	8.6
Chronic and unspecified bronchitis	12,159	1.3	100.0	80.0	6.0	14.0
Heart disease, excluding ischemic	11,545	1.2	100.0	79.9	6.2	12.9
Follow-up exam	11,291	1.2	100.0	89.9	8.9	–
Sprains and strains of back	10,057	1.0	100.0	74.0	3.4	22.6
Potential health hazards related to personal and family history	9,946	1.0	100.0	84.0	11.6	4.4
Open wound, excluding head	9,832	1.0	100.0	47.3	4.3	48.5
Acute pharyngitis	9,718	1.0	100.0	77.1	8.9	14.0
Neoplasms of benign, uncertain nature	9,713	1.0	100.0	91.5	7.6	–
Contusion with intact skin surface	9,421	1.0	100.0	49.5	3.0	47.5
Cataract	9,416	1.0	100.0	96.5	3.5	–
Fractures, excluding lower limb	8,555	0.9	100.0	64.6	9.2	26.2
Contact dermatitis and other eczema	8,554	0.9	100.0	87.0	6.4	6.6
Allergic rhinitis	8,342	0.9	100.0	93.1	6.2	–
Urinary tract infection	8,318	0.9	100.0	77.7	7.3	15.0

(continued)

(continued from previous page)

	total		place of care			
	number	percent distribution	total	physician's offices	hospital outpatient departments	hospital emergency rooms
Major depressive disorder	8,184	0.9%	100.0%	88.2%	9.5%	2.4%
Abdominal pain	7,814	0.8	100.0	58.7	5.9	35.3
Obesity	7,795	0.8	100.0	94.5	5.5	–
Psychoses, excluding major depressive disorder	7,707	0.8	100.0	78.4	11.9	9.7
Depressive disorder, not elsewhere classified	7,501	0.8	100.0	85.4	9.1	5.5
Complications of pregnancy, childbirth	7,140	0.7	100.0	70.4	13.8	15.8
Glaucoma	6,974	0.7	100.0	96.4	3.6	–
Chest pain	6,850	0.7	100.0	54.4	4.6	41.1
Disorder of lipoid metabolism	6,824	0.7	100.0	94.1	5.7	–
Gynecological examination	6,623	0.7	100.0	88.8	11.2	–
Artificial opening status and postsurgical states	6,389	0.7	100.0	82.6	16.5	–
Anxiety states	5,747	0.6	100.0	83.0	7.7	9.3
Other	416,388	43.4	100.0	80.9	7.3	11.8

Note: (–) means sample is too small to make a reliable estimate or not applicable; for definition of ambulatory care visits, see glossary.
Source: National Center for Health Statistics, Ambulatory Care Visits to Physician Offices, Hospital Outpatient Departments, and Emergency Departments: United States, 1997, *Vital and Health Statistics, Series 13, No. 143, 1999*

Health Care Visits by Medication Therapy, 1997

(number and percent distribution of ambulatory care visits by medication therapy status and place of care, 1997; numbers in thousands)

	total	physician's offices	hospital outpatient departments	hospital emergency rooms
Total visits	**959,300**	**787,372**	**76,993**	**94,936**
Medication therapy provided or prescribed				
Yes	613,551	498,930	46,786	67,834
No	345,749	288,442	30,206	27,101
Number of medications provided or prescribed				
None	345,749	288,442	30,206	27,101
One	283,344	235,687	19,219	28,438
Two	162,906	131,433	11,471	20,002
Three	77,628	60,992	6,786	9,850
Four	37,020	28,833	3,593	4,594
Five	22,240	17,875	2,087	2,278
Six	30,412	24,110	3,629	2,672
Total visits	**100.0%**	**100.0%**	**100.0%**	**100.0%**
Medication therapy provided or prescribed				
Yes	64.0	63.4	60.8	71.5
No	36.0	36.6	39.2	28.5
Number of medications provided or prescribed				
None	36.0	36.6	39.2	28.5
One	29.5	29.9	25.0	30.0
Two	17.0	16.7	14.9	21.1
Three	8.1	7.7	8.8	10.4
Four	3.9	3.7	4.7	4.8
Five	2.3	2.3	2.7	2.4
Six	3.2	3.1	4.7	2.8

Note: For definition of ambulatory care visits, see the glossary.
Source: National Center for Health Statistics, Ambulatory Care Visits to Physician Offices, Hospital Outpatient Departments, and Emergency Departments: United States, 1997, *Vital and Health Statistics, Series 13, No. 143, 1999*

Medications Prescribed by Therapeutic Classification, 1997

(number and percent distribution of drug mentions during ambulatory care visits by type of drug, and percent distribution by place of care, 1997; numbers in thousands)

| | total | | place of care | | | |
	number	percent distribution	total	hospital physician's offices	hospital outpatient departments	emergency rooms
Total drug mentions	**1,283,795**	**100.0%**	**100.0%**	**80.3%**	**8.5%**	**11.2%**
Cardiovascular-renal drugs	176,382	13.7	100.0	85.7	7.9	6.3
Drugs for relief of pain	173,263	13.5	100.0	66.1	7.9	26.0
Antimicrobial agents	157,724	12.3	100.0	77.9	8.1	14.0
Respiratory tract drugs	126,549	9.9	100.0	79.2	8.7	12.1
Hormones and agents	115,928	9.0	100.0	84.9	9.2	5.9
Central nervous system	107,859	8.4	100.0	84.2	8.7	7.2
Metabolic and nutrient agents	71,596	5.6	100.0	82.3	10.4	7.3
Skin/mucous membrane	66,749	5.2	100.0	88.0	6.6	5.3
Immunologic agents	56,241	4.4	100.0	82.2	12.4	5.4
Gastrointestinal agents	55,915	4.4	100.0	77.9	8.8	13.3
Ophthalmic drugs	39,562	3.1	100.0	91.9	5.0	3.0
Neurologic drugs	32,634	2.5	100.0	78.3	9.0	12.6
Hematologic agents	29,113	2.3	100.0	84.3	7.8	7.9
Anesthetic drugs	13,902	1.1	100.0	60.1	9.9	30.0
Oncolytics	8,765	0.7	100.0	85.1	–	–
Otologic drugs	7,447	0.6	100.0	75.4	9.7	15.0
Radiopharmaceutical/contrast media	5,281	0.4	100.0	88.5	–	–
Antiparasitics	4,933	0.4	100.0	88.3	–	–
Other	33,952	2.6	100.0	83.6	7.3	9.1

Note: (–) means sample is too small to make a reliable estimate; for definition of ambulatory care visits, see glossary.
Source: National Center for Health Statistics, Ambulatory Care Visits to Physician Offices, Hospital Outpatient Departments, and Emergency Departments: United States, 1997, *Vital and Health Statistics, Series 13, No. 143, 1999*

Medications Prescribed by Generic Substance, 1997

(number and percent distribution of drug occurrences during ambulatory care visits by generic substance, and percent distribution by place of care, 1997; numbers in thousands)

| | total | | place of care | | | |
	number	percent distribution	total	physician's offices	hospital outpatient departments	hospital emergency rooms
Total drug occurrences	**1,536,325**	–	**100.0%**	**79.5%**	**9.5%**	**11.0%**
Acetaminophen	63,096	4.9%	100.0	60.2	7.8	32.0
Amoxicillin	39,025	3.0	100.0	80.3	7.7	12.0
Ibuprofen	28,845	2.2	100.0	55.5	9.0	35.5
Albuterol	21,980	1.7	100.0	68.4	12.2	19.4
Aspirin	20,924	1.6	100.0	79.6	11.4	9.0
Hydrochlorothiazide	19,096	1.5	100.0	88.0	10.0	2.0
Hydrocodone	18,686	1.4	100.0	68.6	4.3	27.1
Estrogens	17,970	1.4	100.0	86.6	10.3	3.1
Furosemide	17,499	1.3	100.0	78.9	10.2	10.9
Guaifenesin	15,818	1.2	100.0	85.7	8.4	5.9
Prednisone	13,605	1.0	100.0	77.0	11.3	11.7
Levothyroxine	13,557	1.0	100.0	85.5	10.9	3.6
Naproxen	12,844	1.0	100.0	82.4	7.3	10.3
Influenza virus vaccine	12,546	1.0	100.0	88.5	11.4	–
Loratadine	12,029	0.9	100.0	91.2	7.1	1.6
Insulin	11,899	0.9	100.0	72.3	20.4	7.3
Trimethoprim	11,747	0.9	100.0	72.0	12.2	15.8
Digoxin	11,670	0.9	100.0	87.7	5.4	6.9
Triamcinolone	11,415	0.9	100.0	87.2	8.7	4.2
Estradiol	11,048	0.9	100.0	92.9	6.5	0.6
Sulfamethoxazole	11,043	0.9	100.0	70.8	12.7	16.5
Atenolol	11,018	0.8	100.0	86.5	10.4	3.1
Cephalexin	10,875	0.8	100.0	70.6	6.7	22.7
Codeine	10,740	0.8	100.0	67.0	6.9	26.1
Potassium replacement solutions	10,566	0.8	100.0	82.8	6.8	10.4
Lisinopril	10,315	0.8	100.0	89.2	7.2	3.4
Phenylephrine	10,050	0.8	100.0	88.6	7.2	4.3
Pseudoephedrine	9,923	0.8	100.0	86.8	8.8	4.4
Alprazolam	9,876	0.8	100.0	90.8	4.3	4.9
Medroxyprogesterone	9,861	0.8	100.0	86.8	11.1	2.1
Lidocaine	9,791	0.8	100.0	71.3	7.5	21.2

(continued)

(continued from previous page)

	total		place of care			
	number	percent distribution	total	physician's offices	hospital outpatient departments	hospital emergency rooms
Clarithromycin	9,560	0.7%	100.0%	85.0%	6.3%	8.7%
Warfarin	9,423	0.7	100.0	88.1	7.1	4.8
Fluoxetine hydrocholoride	9,275	0.7	100.0	88.7	8.5	2.8
Naproxen	9,212	0.7	100.0	83.7	9.2	7.1

Note: The number of drug occurrences is larger than the number of drug mentions in the previous table because mentions combine single-ingredient agents with agents as an ingredient in a combination drug; (–) means sample is too small to make a reliable estimate or not applicable; for definition of ambulatory care visits, see glossary. Source: National Center for Health Statistics, Ambulatory Care Visits to Physician Offices, Hospital Outpatient Departments, and Emergency Departments: United States, 1997, *Vital and Health Statistics, Series 13, No. 143, 1999*

Health Care Visits by Primary Source of Payment, 1997

(number and percent distribution of ambulatory care visits by primary expected source of payment, patient's HMO status, and place of care, 1997; numbers in thousands)

	total		physician's offices		hospital outpatient departments		emergency department	
	number	percent distrib.	number	percent distrib.	number	percent distrib.	number	percent distrib.
Primary expected source of payment								
Total visits	**959,300**	**100.0%**	**787,372**	**100.0%**	**76,993**	**100.0%**	**94,936**	**100.0%**
Private insurance	479,699	50.0	417,744	53.1	26,289	34.1	35,666	37.6
Medicare	188,972	19.7	163,263	20.7	11,026	14.3	14,684	15.5
Medicaid	102,496	10.7	64,047	8.1	21,439	27.8	17,010	17.9
Self-pay	83,450	8.7	60,869	7.7	7,245	9.4	15,336	16.2
Worker's Compensation	19,834	2.1	15,595	2.0	945	1.2	3,293	3.5
No charge	11,698	1.2	8,225	1.0	2,432	3.2	1,041	1.1
Other/unknown/blank	73,151	7.6	57,628	7.3	7,617	9.9	7,905	8.3
HMO Status								
Total visits	**959,300**	**100.0**	**787,372**	**100.0**	**76,993**	**100.0**	**94,936**	**100.0**
HMO member	251,750	26.2	220,478	28.0	15,492	20.1	15,779	16.6
Not an HMO member	578,605	60.3	488,291	62.0	43,963	57.1	46,351	48.8
Unknown/blank	128,945	13.4	78,602	10.0	17,537	22.8	32,805	34.6

Note: For definition of ambulatory care visits, see glossary.
Source: National Center for Health Statistics, Ambulatory Care Visits to Physician Offices, Hospital Outpatient Departments, and Emergency Departments: United States, 1997, *Vital and Health Statistics, Series 13, No. 143, 1999*

Physician Office Visits by Sex and Age, 1998

(total number, percent distribution, and number of physician office visits per person per year, by sex and age, 1998; numbers in thousands)

	total	percent distribution	average visits per year
Total visits	**829,280**	**100.0%**	**3.1**
Under age 15	145,842	17.6	2.4
Aged 15 to 24	71,283	8.6	1.9
Aged 25 to 44	211,775	25.5	2.6
Aged 45 to 64	203,296	24.5	3.6
Aged 65 to 74	102,306	12.3	5.7
Aged 75 or older	94,779	11.4	6.6
Visits by females	**500,365**	**60.3**	**3.6**
Under age 15	68,018	8.2	2.3
Aged 15 to 24	48,750	5.9	2.6
Aged 25 to 44	144,827	17.5	3.4
Aged 45 to 64	120,822	14.6	4.1
Aged 65 to 74	58,808	7.1	6.0
Aged 75 or older	59,141	7.1	6.7
Visits by males	**328,916**	**39.7**	**2.5**
Under age 15	77,825	9.4	2.5
Aged 15 to 24	22,532	2.7	1.2
Aged 25 to 44	66,948	8.1	1.6
Aged 45 to 64	82,474	9.9	3.0
Aged 65 to 74	43,498	5.2	5.4
Aged 75 or older	35,638	4.3	6.4

Source: National Center for Health Statistics, National Ambulatory Medical Care Survey: 1998 Summary, *Advance Data No. 315, 2000*

Physician Office Visits by Major Reason for Visit, 1998

(number and percent distribution of physician office visits by age, sex, race, and major reason for visit, 1998; numbers in thousands)

	total	acute problem	chronic problem, routine	chronic problem, flareup	pre- or post-surgery/injury followup	nonillness care
Total visits	**829,280**	**307,542**	**220,744**	**75,977**	**62,650**	**149,382**
Under age 5	145,842	81,775	15,057	6,213	5,339	35,228
Aged 15 to 24	71,283	27,982	10,501	4,655	3,742	23,263
Aged 25 to 44	211,775	77,337	45,551	20,254	16,000	49,503
Aged 45 to 64	203,296	67,245	69,010	22,023	17,005	25,126
Aged 65 to 74	102,306	29,488	40,151	11,098	10,369	9,459
Aged 75 or older	94,779	23,715	40,475	11,735	10,196	6,803
Female	500,365	176,082	126,427	46,317	36,515	106,628
Male	328,916	131,460	94,317	29,660	26,135	42,754
Black	89,832	33,926	23,544	7,497	5,060	18,727
White	702,190	256,618	189,454	65,344	55,634	123,332
Other	37,259	16,998	7,746	3,136	1,956	7,332
Total visits	**100.0%**	**37.1%**	**26.6%**	**9.2%**	**7.6%**	**18.0%**
Under age 5	100.0	56.1	10.3	4.3	3.7	24.2
Aged 15 to 24	100.0	39.3	14.7	6.5	5.2	32.6
Aged 25 to 44	100.0	36.5	21.5	9.6	7.6	23.4
Aged 45 to 64	100.0	33.1	33.9	10.8	8.4	12.4
Aged 65 to 74	100.0	28.8	39.2	10.8	10.1	9.2
Aged 75 or older	100.0	25.0	42.7	12.4	10.8	7.2
Female	100.0	35.2	25.3	9.3	7.3	21.3
Male	100.0	40.0	28.7	9.0	7.9	13.0
Black	100.0	37.8	26.2	8.3	5.6	20.8
White	100.0	36.5	27.0	9.3	7.9	17.6
Other	100.0	45.6	20.8	8.4	5.2	19.7

Note: Numbers will not add to total because blank and unknown are not shown.
Source: National Center for Health Statistics, National Ambulatory Medical Care Survey: 1998 Summary, Advance Data No. 315, 2000

Physician Office Visits by Detailed Reason for Visit, 1998

(number and percent distribution of physician office visits by the 20 principal reasons most frequently mentioned by patients for visit, 1998; numbers in thousands)

	number	percent distribution
Total visits	**829,280**	**100.0%**
General medical exam	59,340	7.2
Cough	29,564	3.6
Routine prenatal exam	29,014	3.5
Progress visit, not otherwise specified	27,768	3.3
Symptoms referable to throat	17,025	2.1
Postoperative visit	16,622	2.0
Vision dysfunctions	15,189	1.8
Fever	13,554	1.6
Well-baby exam	13,470	1.6
Stomach pain, cramps, and spasms	13,134	1.6
Earache or ear infection	12,417	1.5
Skin rash	11,988	1.4
Back symptoms	11,888	1.4
Headache, pain in head	11,403	1.4
Chest pain and related symptoms	11,040	1.3
Knee symptoms	10,792	1.3
Nasal congestion	10,167	1.2
Medication	9,770	1.2
Depression	9,708	1.2
Hypertension	8,929	1.1
All other reasons	486,498	58.7

Source: National Center for Health Statistics, National Ambulatory Medical Care Survey: 1998 Summary, Advance Data No. 315, 2000

Physician Office Visits by Specialty and Referral Status, 1998

(number and percent distribution of physician office visits by specialty, referral status, and prior-visit status, 1998; numbers in thousands)

| | number | percent | referred by another physician or health plan for this visit | | not referred by another physician or health plan for this visit | |
			new patient	old patient	new patient	old patient
Total visits	**829,280**	**100.0%**	**5.8%**	**10.3%**	**6.2%**	**72.8%**
General and family practice	201,946	100.0	1.0	3.0	7.9	83.7
Internal medicine	141,702	100.0	1.2	3.2	5.3	83.7
Pediatrics	95,538	100.0	–	3.6	4.2	87.6
Obstetrics and gynecology	83,827	100.0	2.7	9.6	7.8	76.0
Ophthalmology	49,817	100.0	9.8	11.6	9.4	64.7
Orthopedic surgery	39,910	100.0	16.4	27.9	6.8	42.2
Dermatology	33,409	100.0	13.8	17.5	10.4	54.1
Psychiatry	19,886	100.0	5.5	21.3	–	67.9
General surgery	20,039	100.0	18.9	30.4	2.9	41.6
Otolaryngology	20,401	100.0	17.8	23.1	9.7	44.9
Cardiovascular diseases	18,420	100.0	8.9	14.5	–	72.3
Urology	14,834	100.0	16.1	19.4	4.2	54.7
Neurology	9,057	100.0	26.4	31.9	–	34.7
All other specialties	80,496	100.0	12.5	20.8	3.4	57.2

Note: Percentages will not add to 100 because unknown and blank are not shown. Nonresponses for prior-visit status have been removed from the total; (–) means sample is too small to make a reliable estimate.
Source: National Center for Health Statistics, National Ambulatory Medical Care Survey: 1998 Summary, *Advance Data No. 315, 2000*

Physician Office Visits by Primary Source of Payment, 1998

(number and percent distribution of physician office visits by primary expected source of payment, 1998; numbers in thousands)

	number	percent distribution
Primary expected source of payment		
Total visits	**829,280**	**100.0 %**
Private insurance	457,328	55.1
Medicare	159,442	19.2
Medicaid	71,642	8.6
Self-pay	55,883	6.7
Worker's Compensation	17,255	2.1
No charge	7,904	1.0
Other/unknown/blank	59,827	7.2

Source: National Center for Health Statistics, National Ambulatory Medical Care Survey: 1998 Summary, *Advance Data No. 315, 2000*

Physician Office Visits by Services Provided, 1998

(number and percent distribution of physician office visits by services ordered or provided, 1998; numbers in thousands)

	number	percent
Total visits	**829,280**	**100.0%**
Examinations		
Skin	70,107	8.5
Pelvic	65,115	7.9
Breast	57,199	6.9
Visual	52,203	6.3
Rectal	32,135	3.9
Hearing	29,610	3.6
Glaucoma	13,592	1.6
Tests		
Blood pressure	377,180	45.5
Urinalysis	89,835	10.8
Hematocrit/hemoglobin	46,613	5.6
Pap test	40,601	4.9
Cholesterol	30,176	3.6
EKG	23,035	2.8
Strep test	13,234	1.6
Prostate specific antigen (PSA)	9,992	1.2
Pregnancy test	5,018	0.6
Blood lead level	3,536	0.4
HIV serology	3,038	0.4
Other STD test	6,237	0.8
Other blood test	100,623	12.1
Imaging		
X-ray	49,622	6.0
Ultrasound	21,291	2.6
Mammography	15,335	1.8
CAT scan/MRI	9,889	1.2

(continued)

(continued from previous page)

	number	percent
Counseling/education		
Diet/nutrition	122,858	14.8%
Exercise	85,713	10.3
Injury prevention	25,073	3.0
Tobacco use/exposure	24,003	2.9
Prenatal instruction	23,084	2.8
Stress management	21,313	2.6
Breast self-exam	20,225	2.4
Growth/development	19,421	2.3
Mental health	17,970	2.2
Skin cancer prevention	15,177	1.8
Family planning/contraception	12,958	1.6
HIV/STD transmission	8,980	1.1
Other therapy		
Physiotherapy	21,927	2.6
Psychotherapy	16,112	1.9
Psychopharmacotherapy	15,750	1.9
Other	64,912	7.8

Source: National Center for Health Statistics, National Ambulatory Medical Care Survey: 1998 Summary, *Advance Data No. 315, 2000*

Physicians by Medical Specialty, 1990 and 1998

(number of professionally active doctors of medicine by medical specialty, 1990 and 1998; percent change by specialty, 1990–98)

	1998	1990	percent change 1990–98
Total active doctors of medicine	**667,000**	**547,310**	**21.9%**
NONFEDERAL	**648,009**	**526,835**	**23.0**
Patient care	**606,425**	**487,796**	**24.3**
Office-based practice	468,788	359,932	30.2
General and family practice	64,588	57,571	12.2
Cardiovascular diseases	15,112	10,670	41.6
Dermatology	7,641	5,996	27.4
Gastroenterology	7,948	5,200	52.8
Internal medicine	83,270	57,799	44.1
Pediatrics	38,359	26,494	44.8
Pulmonary diseases	4,927	3,659	34.7
General surgery	27,509	24,498	12.3
Obstetrics and gynecology	31,194	25,475	22.4
Ophthalmology	15,560	13,055	19.2
Orthopedic surgery	18,479	14,187	30.3
Otolaryngology	7,498	6,360	17.9
Plastic surgery	5,303	3,835	38.3
Urological surgery	8,424	7,392	14.0
Anesthesiology	26,218	17,789	47.4
Diagnostic radiology	14,241	9,806	45.2
Emergency medicine	13,253	8,402	57.7
Neurology	8,458	5,587	51.4
Pathology, anatomical/clinical	9,970	7,269	37.2
Psychiatry	24,962	20,048	24.5
Radiology	6,353	6,056	4.9
Other specialty	29,521	22,784	29.6
Hospital-based practice	137,637	127,864	7.6
Residents and interns	92,332	89,913	2.7
Full-time hospital staff	45,305	37,951	19.4
Other professional activity	**41,584**	**39,039**	**6.5**

(continued)

(continued from previous page)

	1998	1990	percent change 1990–98
FEDERAL	**18,991**	**20,475**	**−7.2%**
Patient care	**15,311**	**15,632**	**−2.1**
Hospital-based practice	15,311	14,569	5.1
Other professional activity	**3,680**	**4,843**	**−24.0**

Note: (−) means data not available or category not applicable.
Source: Statistics from the American Medical Association, published in Health, United States, 2000; *calculations by New Strategist*

Employees at Health Service Sites, 1990 to 1999

(total number of employed civilians, and number and percent distribution of those employed at health service sites by type of site, 1990 and 1999; percent change in number and percentage point change in distribution, 1990–99; numbers in thousands)

	1999	1990	percent change 1990–99
Total employed	**133,488**	**117,914**	**13.2%**
Total employed at health service sites	**11,646**	**9,447**	**23.3**
Offices and clinics of physicians	1,624	1,098	47.9
Offices and clinics of dentists	694	580	19.7
Offices and clinics of chiropractors	142	90	57.8
Hospitals	5,117	4,690	9.1
Nursing and personal care facilities	1,786	1,543	15.7
Other health service sites	2,283	1,446	57.9

	1999	1990	percentage point change, 1990–99
Total employed	**100.0%**	**100.0%**	**–**
Percent employed at health service sites	**8.7**	**8.0**	**0.7**
Total employed at health service sites	**100.0**	**100.0**	**–**
Offices and clinics of physicians	13.9	11.6	2.3
Offices and clinics of dentists	6.0	6.1	–0.2
Offices and clinics of chiropractors	1.2	1.0	0.3
Hospitals	43.9	49.6	–5.7
Nursing and personal care facilities	15.3	16.3	–1.0
Other health service sites	19.6	15.3	4.3

Note: (–) means not applicable.
Source: National Center for Health Statistics, Health, United States, 2000; *calculations by New Strategist*

Dental Visits, 1998

(percent of people with a dental visit in the past year by sex, race, Hispanic origin, and age, 1998)

	aged 2 or older	aged 2–17	aged 18–64	aged 65 or older
Total	**66.2%**	**73.5%**	**65.6%**	**56.4%**
Sex				
Male	63.6	72.0	61.7	57.8
Female	68.8	75.1	69.2	55.4
Race				
White	67.8	74.9	67.2	58.2
Black	58.0	69.8	58.3	36.9
American Indian	56.1	72.6	53.7	41.1
Asian	65.5	67.8	63.4	67.4
Hispanic origin				
White, non-Hispanic	69.5	77.1	68.9	58.7
Black, non-Hispanic	58.0	69.8	58.1	37.3
Hispanic	54.1	62.4	52.2	46.8

Source: National Center for Health Statistics, Health, United States, 2000

Trust Doctor's Judgment, 1998

"I trust my doctor's judgments about my medical care. Do you agree or disagree?"

(percent of people aged 18 or older responding by sex, race, age, and education, 1998)

	agree	uncertain	disagree
Total	**81%**	**11%**	**7%**
Men	81	10	7
Women	80	12	7
Black	80	12	8
White	81	11	7
Other	79	15	3
Aged 18 to 29	78	11	9
Aged 30 to 39	75	15	10
Aged 40 to 49	82	11	6
Aged 50 to 59	79	14	7
Aged 60 to 69	84	8	6
Aged 70 or older	91	4	4
Not a high school graduate	81	9	7
High school graduate	79	12	7
Bachelor's degree	82	10	8
Graduate degree	76	14	8

Note: Numbers may not add to 100 because "don't know" and no answer are not shown.
Source: 1998 General Social Survey, National Opinion Research Center, University of Chicago; calculations by New Strategist

Doctors Don't Do All They Should, 1998

"I feel my doctor does not do everything s/he should for my
medical care. Do you agree or disagree?"

(percent of people aged 18 or older responding by sex, race, age, and education, 1998)

	agree	uncertain	disagree
Total	**20%**	**15%**	**63%**
Men	21	16	61
Women	19	14	65
Black	20	17	61
White	19	14	65
Other	33	16	49
Aged 18 to 29	23	18	56
Aged 30 to 39	24	19	57
Aged 40 to 49	18	15	66
Aged 50 to 59	18	12	68
Aged 60 to 69	13	9	76
Aged 70 or older	18	9	71
Not a high school graduate	21	12	60
High school graduate	20	16	63
Bachelor's degree	17	14	69
Graduate degree	22	13	62

Note: Numbers may not add to 100 because "don't know" and no answer are not shown.
Source: 1998 General Social Survey, National Opinion Research Center, University of Chicago; calculations by New Strategist

Worry That Doctors Consider Cost over Care, 1998

"I worry that my doctor will put cost considerations above
the care I need. Do you agree or disagree?"

(percent of people aged 18 or older responding by sex, race, age, and education, 1998)

	agree	uncertain	disagree
Total	**24%**	**15%**	**59%**
Men	25	15	58
Women	23	14	60
Black	24	17	57
White	23	14	62
Other	32	18	42
Aged 18 to 29	28	18	51
Aged 30 to 39	29	17	53
Aged 40 to 49	23	13	62
Aged 50 to 59	25	13	61
Aged 60 to 69	18	10	72
Aged 70 or older	13	12	74
Not a high school graduate	26	18	51
High school graduate	24	15	59
Bachelor's degree	21	11	67
Graduate degree	19	15	65

Note: Numbers may not add to 100 because "don't know" and no answer are not shown.
Source: 1998 General Social Survey, National Opinion Research Center, University of Chicago; calculations by New Strategist

Doctors Put Medical Needs First, 1998

"I trust my doctor to put my medical needs above all other considerations when treating my medical problems. Do you agree or disagree?"

(percent of people aged 18 or older responding by sex, race, age, and education, 1998)

	agree	uncertain	disagree
Total	**72%**	**15%**	**11%**
Men	71	15	11
Women	73	15	10
Black	70	15	13
White	73	15	10
Other	66	15	13
Aged 18 to 29	70	16	11
Aged 30 to 39	65	19	13
Aged 40 to 49	76	14	9
Aged 50 to 59	71	14	12
Aged 60 to 69	79	11	9
Aged 70 or older	80	10	8
Not a high school graduate	69	14	11
High school graduate	73	15	11
Bachelor's degree	72	17	9
Graduate degree	64	20	13

Note: Numbers may not add to 100 because "don't know" and no answer are not shown.
Source: 1998 General Social Survey, National Opinion Research Center, University of Chicago; calculations by New Strategist

Doctors Ignore Patient History, 1998

"The medical problems I've had in the past are ignored when I seek care for a new medical problem. Do you agree or disagree?"

(percent of people aged 18 or older responding by sex, race, age, and education, 1998)

	agree	uncertain	disagree
Total	**18%**	**14%**	**64%**
Men	17	16	63
Women	17	13	65
Black	19	14	63
White	17	14	65
Other	20	17	56
Aged 18 to 29	23	16	56
Aged 30 to 39	17	17	60
Aged 40 to 49	17	15	67
Aged 50 to 59	17	12	69
Aged 60 to 69	17	13	68
Aged 70 or older	11	12	72
Not a high school graduate	30	11	53
High school graduate	17	16	63
Bachelor's degree	11	14	71
Graduate degree	11	18	65

Note: Numbers may not add to 100 because "don't know" and no answer are not shown.
Source: 1998 General Social Survey, National Opinion Research Center, University of Chicago; calculations by New Strategist

Doctors Are Careful, 1998

"Doctors are very careful to check everything when examining their patients. Do you agree or disagree?"

(percent of people aged 18 or older responding by sex, race, age, and education, 1998)

	agree	uncertain	disagree
Total	34%	20%	44%
Men	35	22	42
Women	33	20	46
Black	34	20	43
White	33	20	46
Other	47	21	30
Aged 18 to 29	34	24	38
Aged 30 to 39	33	20	46
Aged 40 to 49	31	19	48
Aged 50 to 59	24	24	52
Aged 60 to 69	42	10	48
Aged 70 or older	45	20	33
Not a high school graduate	43	18	37
High school graduate	32	20	46
Bachelor's degree	33	22	45
Graduate degree	31	21	47

Note: Numbers may not add to 100 because "don't know" and no answer are not shown.
Source: 1998 General Social Survey, National Opinion Research Center, University of Chicago; calculations by New Strategist

Doctors Aren't Thorough Enough, 1998

"Doctors aren't as thorough as they should be.
Do you agree or disagree?"

(percent of people aged 18 or older responding by sex, race, age, and education, 1998)

	agree	uncertain	disagree
Total	**50%**	**14%**	**34%**
Men	48	15	35
Women	52	13	34
Black	46	18	31
White	50	13	35
Other	56	11	28
Aged 18 to 29	51	19	28
Aged 30 to 39	49	14	34
Aged 40 to 49	49	14	36
Aged 50 to 59	54	11	32
Aged 60 to 69	53	9	36
Aged 70 or older	48	11	40
Not a high school graduate	52	12	32
High school graduate	54	13	32
Bachelor's degree	42	20	38
Graduate degree	52	13	33

Note: Numbers may not add to 100 because "don't know" and no answer are not shown.
Source: 1998 General Social Survey, National Opinion Research Center, University of Chicago; calculations by New Strategist

Rarely See Same Doctor Twice, 1998

"I hardly ever see the same doctor when I go for
medical care. Do you agree or disagree?"

(percent of people aged 18 or older responding by sex, race, age, and education, 1998)

	agree	uncertain	disagree
Total	**19%**	**4%**	**75%**
Men	23	6	69
Women	15	3	80
Black	23	4	71
White	17	4	77
Other	26	12	62
Aged 18 to 29	27	5	63
Aged 30 to 39	21	7	69
Aged 40 to 49	22	3	73
Aged 50 to 59	15	4	81
Aged 60 to 69	11	2	85
Aged 70 or older	5	2	91
Not a high school graduate	22	5	71
High school graduate	19	4	75
Bachelor's degree	16	6	77
Graduate degree	9	6	82

Note: Numbers may not add to 100 because "don't know" and no answer are not shown.
Source: 1998 General Social Survey, National Opinion Research Center, University of Chicago; calculations by New Strategist

Doctors Don't Explain Medical Problems, 1998

"Doctors cause people to worry a lot because they don't explain
medical problems to patients. Do you agree or disagree?"

(percent of people aged 18 or older responding by sex, race, age, and education, 1998)

	agree	uncertain	disagree
Total	**41%**	**16%**	**43%**
Men	38	18	42
Women	42	14	43
Black	42	15	42
White	41	16	43
Other	28	22	47
Aged 18 to 29	41	20	37
Aged 30 to 39	38	19	41
Aged 40 to 49	41	14	45
Aged 50 to 59	47	14	39
Aged 60 to 69	40	10	48
Aged 70 or older	37	13	48
Not a high school graduate	44	14	38
High school graduate	41	15	41
Bachelor's degree	32	19	49
Graduate degree	46	20	33

Note: Numbers may not add to 100 because "don't know" and no answer are not shown.
Source: 1998 General Social Survey, National Opinion Research Center, University of Chicago; calculations by New Strategist

Doctors Don't Explain All Options, 1998

"I worry that my doctor is being prevented from telling me the full range of options for my treatment. Do you agree or disagree?"

(percent of people aged 18 or older responding by sex, race, age, and education, 1998)

	agree	uncertain	disagree
Total	**21%**	**17%**	**58%**
Men	24	17	56
Women	20	17	60
Black	18	21	57
White	22	16	59
Other	23	23	45
Aged 18 to 29	23	22	50
Aged 30 to 39	22	22	54
Aged 40 to 49	25	15	59
Aged 50 to 59	24	11	62
Aged 60 to 69	20	12	65
Aged 70 or older	12	14	70
Not a high school graduate	26	19	51
High school graduate	21	18	58
Bachelor's degree	21	14	64
Graduate degree	27	12	58

Note: Numbers may not add to 100 because "don't know" and no answer are not shown.
Source: 1998 General Social Survey, National Opinion Research Center, University of Chicago; calculations by New Strategist

Doctors Try Not to Worry Patients, 1998

"Doctors always do their best to keep the patient from worrying. Do you agree or disagree?"

(percent of people aged 18 or older responding by sex, race, age, and education, 1998)

	agree	uncertain	disagree
Total	**51%**	**20%**	**28%**
Men	55	19	25
Women	48	20	29
Black	63	15	19
White	49	20	30
Other	57	21	20
Aged 18 to 29	49	23	25
Aged 30 to 39	50	20	30
Aged 40 to 49	49	20	31
Aged 50 to 59	45	21	34
Aged 60 to 69	51	17	29
Aged 70 or older	69	14	15
Not a high school graduate	62	14	20
High school graduate	52	19	28
Bachelor's degree	47	21	31
Graduate degree	34	30	35

Note: Numbers may not add to 100 because "don't know" and no answer are not shown.
Source: 1998 General Social Survey, National Opinion Research Center, University of Chicago; calculations by New Strategist

Doctors Treat Patients with Respect, 1998

"Doctors always treat their patients with
respect. Do you agree or disagree?"

(percent of people aged 18 or older responding by sex, race, age, and education, 1998)

	agree	uncertain	disagree
Total	**51%**	**14%**	**34%**
Men	52	17	30
Women	50	12	37
Black	57	15	27
White	49	14	36
Other	60	16	23
Aged 18 to 29	50	15	33
Aged 30 to 39	46	17	36
Aged 40 to 49	45	14	40
Aged 50 to 59	45	13	41
Aged 60 to 69	55	14	30
Aged 70 or older	73	7	19
Not a high school graduate	59	12	25
High school graduate	52	14	33
Bachelor's degree	43	18	38
Graduate degree	41	11	47

Note: Numbers may not add to 100 because "don't know" and no answer are not shown.
Source: 1998 General Social Survey, National Opinion Research Center, University of Chicago; calculations by New Strategist

Doctors Avoid Unnecessary Patient Expenses, 1998

"Doctors always avoid unnecessary patient
expenses. Do you agree or disagree?"

(percent of people aged 18 or older responding by sex, race, age, and education, 1998)

	agree	uncertain	disagree
Total	**22%**	**20%**	**55%**
Men	20	21	55
Women	23	20	55
Black	22	19	55
White	22	20	56
Other	18	28	46
Aged 18 to 29	18	25	54
Aged 30 to 39	17	21	59
Aged 40 to 49	19	18	61
Aged 50 to 59	24	19	52
Aged 60 to 69	27	20	51
Aged 70 or older	38	18	41
Not a high school graduate	35	22	37
High school graduate	22	18	57
Bachelor's degree	16	25	58
Graduate degree	15	23	60

Note: Numbers may not add to 100 because "don't know" and no answer are not shown.
Source: 1998 General Social Survey, National Opinion Research Center, University of Chicago; calculations by New Strategist

Doctors Avoid Unnecessary Surgery, 1998

"Doctors never recommend surgery (an operation) unless there is no other way to solve the problem. Do you agree or disagree?"

(percent of people aged 18 or older responding by sex, race, age, and education, 1998)

	agree	uncertain	disagree
Total	**43%**	**19%**	**34%**
Men	45	21	31
Women	41	18	38
Black	42	22	32
White	42	19	36
Other	51	24	16
Aged 18 to 29	48	21	28
Aged 30 to 39	38	21	37
Aged 40 to 49	41	18	40
Aged 50 to 59	37	20	41
Aged 60 to 69	42	19	36
Aged 70 or older	54	17	24
Not a high school graduate	52	19	24
High school graduate	44	20	34
Bachelor's degree	36	22	40
Graduate degree	32	16	48

Note: Numbers may not add to 100 because "don't know" and no answer are not shown.
Source: 1998 General Social Survey, National Opinion Research Center, University of Chicago; calculations by New Strategist

Doctors Take Unncessary Risks, 1998

"Sometimes doctors take unnecessary risks in treating their patients. Do you agree or disagree?"

(percent of people aged 18 or older responding by sex, race, age, and education, 1998)

	agree	uncertain	disagree
Total	**34%**	**24%**	**39%**
Men	31	25	39
Women	35	24	38
Black	41	27	31
White	33	24	41
Other	33	29	30
Aged 18 to 29	34	28	34
Aged 30 to 39	31	28	39
Aged 40 to 49	37	22	39
Aged 50 to 59	34	23	40
Aged 60 to 69	40	20	39
Aged 70 or older	28	20	43
Not a high school graduate	39	25	30
High school graduate	34	25	38
Bachelor's degree	28	24	45
Graduate degree	35	19	44

Note: Numbers may not add to 100 because "don't know" and no answer are not shown.
Source: 1998 General Social Survey, National Opinion Research Center, University of Chicago; calculations by New Strategist

Trust Doctors to Reveal Mistakes, 1998

"I trust my doctor to tell me if a mistake was made
about my treatment. Do you agree or disagree?"

(percent of people aged 18 or older responding by sex, race, age, and education, 1998)

	agree	uncertain	disagree
Total	**60%**	**16%**	**21%**
Men	60	16	20
Women	60	16	21
Black	55	17	23
White	61	15	21
Other	56	23	15
Aged 18 to 29	60	17	19
Aged 30 to 39	54	19	24
Aged 40 to 49	62	15	21
Aged 50 to 59	57	15	25
Aged 60 to 69	67	15	16
Aged 70 or older	70	13	13
Not a high school graduate	65	12	18
High school graduate	60	15	22
Bachelor's degree	57	22	19
Graduate degree	59	18	20

Note: Numbers may not add to 100 because "don't know" and no answer are not shown.
Source: 1998 General Social Survey, National Opinion Research Center, University of Chicago; calculations by New Strategist

4

Growing Diversity in Health Care

In determining health care needs, race is only one of many dimensions of difference and often not the most important. Age and sex, for example, are more important than race in determining demand for health care. Those characteristics are addressed throughout the book, while this chapter focuses on differences in health care needs by race and ethnicity.

Most differences in the health status of Americans by sex and age are biologically determined. Although the role of biology is less clear for differences by race and ethnicity, medical researchers are beginning to focus on important biological differences among the races that have a major impact on health.

Many of the health problems from which blacks, Hispanics, and other minorities suffer disproportionately are the result of higher poverty rates, lower educational levels, and a more limited access to health care. Cultural factors also greatly influence relationships between minorities and health care providers.

Hispanics are most likely to be without health insurance

(percent of people not covered by health insurance, by race and Hispanic origin, 1997)

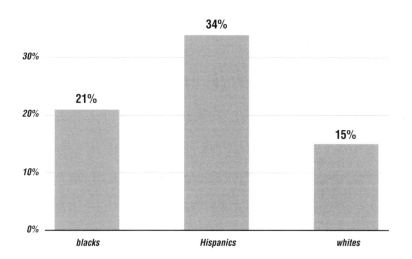

According to many medical researchers, socioeconomic factors are more important than race in determining health status. An article in *Hispanic Journal of Behavioral Sciences*, for example, found that depression was linked to socioeconomic status and gender more than to ethnic identity.[1] Similarly, low birth weight is a socioeconomic rather than a racial phenomenon, according to *The New England Journal of Medicine*.[2] Between 1993 and 1997, the Centers for Disease Control and Prevention tracked the number of "unhealthy days" experienced by adults in every county of the United States. (Unhealthy days are those in which people feel poorly either physically or mentally.) The number was greatest in counties with the lowest socioeconomic status.[3]

Discrimination also affects the health of minorities. Because discrimination is stressful, and because stress causes high blood pressure, discrimination can lead to poor health. At least one study backs up this theory with science. University of Michigan researchers found racism and income disparities to be the primary causes of health differences between blacks and whites. After controlling for important health factors such as income or education, African Americans are still more likely to report poorer health than whites, says David R. Williams, associate research scientist at the University of Michigan Institute for Social Research, in *Jet* magazine.[4]

In their relationships with medical professionals, minority health care consumers must grapple with issues that non-Hispanic whites do not experience. One is the long-standing lack of trust between minorities and the medical community. America as a whole is losing confidence in the health care system, and for blacks the roots of doubt run deep. The United States Office of Minority Health, part of the Public Health Service, speculates that the Tuskegee Syphilis Study has been a contributing factor. Between 1932 and 1972, the United States Public Health Service, in a study of the long-term effects of syphilis, withheld treatment from 399 poor black men from Macon County, Alabama. By the time media attention brought an end to the study in 1972, only 74 participants were still alive, many of them crippled or blinded by the disease. The government settled out of court with survivors for more than $10 million.[5]

The confidence of blacks in the medical community has plummeted over the past few decades—as has the confidence of whites. Only 44 percent of blacks and whites felt a "great deal" of confidence in the people running medicine in 1998, according to the General Social Survey of the University of Chicago's National Opinion Research Center.

The lack of trust in the medical profession affects black health. Black men have the highest mortality rate for all cancers, and black women have the second highest rate, according to the Office of Special Populations Research at the National Cancer Institute of the National Institutes of Health. While mortality rates among whites are declining for many kinds of cancer, including liver, pancreas, and kidney, rates are not declining as rapidly among blacks.[6] Prominent among the reasons for the disparity is the distrust black men feel toward the medical community, according to *Jet* magazine.[7]

The psychological distance between minorities and the medical profession has serious implications for health care consumption. Minorities are less likely to be aware of new treatments for disease, for example. And because they are less informed about their conditions, they have more difficulty evaluating whether new products or services may be right for them. This is more than just a knowledge gap. African Americans and Hispanics are less likely to receive the latest pharmaceutical treatments for AIDS, for example. Among AIDS victims who need drug combination therapy, 56 percent of blacks and 44 percent of Hispanics did not receive it compared with a smaller 32 percent of whites.[8] This lack of treatment has serious implications since African American and Hispanic men with AIDS outnumber non-Hispanic white men with the disease.[9]

The lack of trust of blacks and Hispanics toward the medical community increases their vulnerability to fraudulent medical claims. Hispanics, especially, are a target because of language and cultural barriers, writes Andre A. Skolnick in the *Journal of the American Medical Association*.[10] Because of the tenuous relationship between Hispanics and medical profes-

Minorities are less likely to see physicians

(annual number of physician office visits per person, by race, 1998)

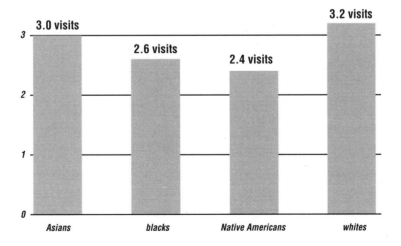

sionals, there is rampant quackery on Hispanic radio and television, he says. Skolnick reports on the efforts to combat this by Dr. Elmer H. Huerta, who broadcasts accurate health information to Hispanics on Spanish-language radio stations across the country. With so many fraudulent health claims being made on Hispanic media, marketers of legitimate products need to take the shady competitors into consideration when planning marketing campaigns. As the legitimate health care industry begins to target Hispanic American consumers in earnest, it will have to distinguish itself from the fakers.

Adding to the problem is the fact that many Hispanic consumers, as well as other minorities, do not have a doctor to ask about the latest medical procedures. According to *American Health Line*, some minority neighborhoods in Los Angeles have only one physician per 24,505 residents—a ratio comparable to those in third world nations. On the other hand, Beverly Hills has one doctor per 254 residents. The California Latino Medical Association is considering a variety of strategies to help solve the problem, including encouraging minority students to go into the health professions and developing a medical school loan forgiveness program.[11]

Health differences

Whites fare better than blacks, Hispanics, and Native Americans on a variety of health indicators ranging from infant mortality to the incidence of AIDS, according to the National Center for Health Statistics. Whites have a higher suicide rate than blacks and Hispanics, however, and they have a higher rate of cardiovascular disease than Hispanics or Native Americans. Asian Americans fare even better than whites with some exceptions such as their incidence of tuberculosis.

At every age, whites are more likely than blacks to say their health is "excellent" or "very good" (69 percent of whites versus 61 percent of blacks). Whites are less likely than blacks to feel only "fair" or "poor" (10 versus 14 percent). Among Hispanics, an even smaller 59 percent feel excellent or very good while an even larger 15 percent feel only fair or poor.

Whites are more likely to have health insurance than blacks or Hispanics. While just 15 percent of whites were uninsured in 1997, the rate was 21 percent among blacks and 34 percent among Hispanics. Because they are less likely to have health insurance, blacks are more likely than whites to depend on hospital outpatient departments and emergency rooms for medical care. Blacks are more likely than whites to visit emergency rooms for minor health problems. While 20 percent of white emergency room visits were classified as emergencies (i.e., the patient should be seen in less than 15 minutes), only 15 percent of black emergency room visits fell into the category.

Blacks contact physicians less frequently than whites, an average of 5.4 physician contacts per person per year for blacks compared with 6.1 for whites. When seeing a doctor, blacks are less likely than whites to go to a doctor's office. Among whites, fully 84 percent of health care visits are to a doctor's office compared with only 67 percent of the health care visits of blacks. Discrimination on the part of doctors could play a role in these numbers. A Johns Hopkins School of Public Health Study found minorities waited longer to be seen during appointments than whites.[12] Sixteen percent of health care visits by blacks are to hospital outpatient departments, more than double the 7 percent among whites. Eighteen percent of black health care visits are to emergency rooms versus 9 percent among whites.

Whites have higher rates of acute conditions than blacks, including colds, flu, and injuries. One factor behind the statistical difference may be the less-frequent contact blacks have with physicians, since the acute conditions reported by the National Center for Health Statistics are only those for which people see a doctor or which restrict their activity for at least half a day. (Comparable data on acute conditions for Hispanics and other minorities are not available.)

Many chronic health problems are more common among blacks than whites. At all ages, for example, blacks are much more likely to have diabetes. High blood pressure is also

Native Americans are most likely to be disabled

(percent of people aged 15 or older with any disabilities, by race and Hispanic origin, 1994–95)

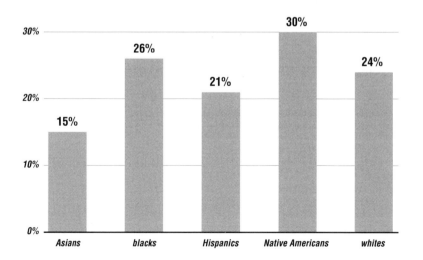

more common among blacks than whites. But whites are more likely to suffer from heart disease. (Comparable data on chronic conditions for Hispanics and other minorities are not available.)

Blacks and Native Americans are more likely to be disabled than whites, and they are more likely to report activity limitations due to chronic conditions. Whites have higher disability rates and are more likely to report limitations than Hispanics or Asians—in part because the white population is, on average, older than the Hispanic or Asian population.

Despite differences in health status by race and Hispanic origin, heart disease and cancer are the leading causes of death for every group. Other major causes of death differ by race and Hispanic origin, however. Accidents are the third leading cause of death among Hispanics, while they rank fourth among blacks and sixth among non-Hispanic whites. HIV infection is the ninth leading cause of death among blacks but does not even appear in the top-ten list for Hispanics or whites.

Among all Americans, Asians have the highest life expectancy. At birth, Asian-American males can expect to live to age 80.9 years, while their female counterparts have a life expectancy of 86.5 years. Blacks have the lowest life expectancy—just 68.4 years for black males and 75.1 years for black females.

A tale of two countries

The differences in health status by race have led some to observe that the state of health care in the U.S. is a tale of two countries, referring to the disparity between white and black health. But in the future, health care will be a tale of too many countries to count. The differences are not just among whites, blacks, Hispanics, and Asians. Within each minority group, disparities in health care needs exist.

The black population is not as segmented as the Hispanic population, but at least two distinct health care consumers are emerging among blacks. The improvement in the socioeconomic status of blacks is creating a sizable black health care market no longer in need of the intense outreach required by a disenfranchised group. The black middle class should continue to grow as blacks gain in education and income.

The need for outreach programs in the black community has not disappeared, however. A large proportion of blacks live in poverty, particularly women and children. They need low-cost health care products and services. Health education opportunities exist in the hospital setting, where blacks are more likely than whites to receive medical care.

Even well-off blacks face serious discrimination problems in access to health care. A study of 720 physicians found that when black patients complain of chest pain, doctors were only 60 percent as likely to order cardiac catheterization—an important detection test for heart disease—as for whites.[13] In another study, differences in cardiac care were found between blacks and whites even after controlling for the type of heart disease and insurance status. Blacks, for example, are 60 percent less likely than whites to have heart bypass surgery.[14]

It's not just heart disease either. Blacks have a lower survival rate than whites for colon cancer, which could be the result of late detection, inadequate treatment, or socioeconomic factors.[15] Another study found that blacks were less likely to be offered analgesics for a bone fracture in an emergency room.[16]

While discrimination is clearly behind many of the discrepancies, research is also revealing important biological differences that affect health status by race. A National Heart Lung and Blood Institute survey found that black patients were at a higher risk for congestive heart failure than similarly treated white patients. The NHLBI thinks the discrepancy may be due to physiological differences.

New attention to researching biological differences between whites and blacks should begin to eliminate the biologically based outcome discrepancies.[17] In 1999, for example, the Agency for Health Care Policy and Research announced a five-year initiative to eliminate

Blacks and Hispanics account for most AIDS cases

(percent distribution of people diagnosed with AIDS by race and Hispanic origin, through June 1999)

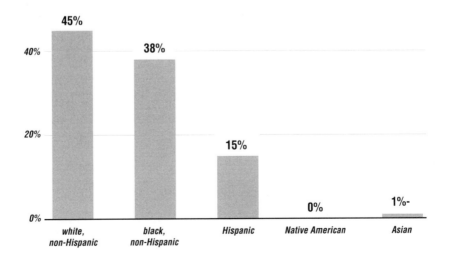

ethnic and racial disparities in health. This effort will likely be spurred by a new wealth of genetic information. Discrimination, on the other hand, will not find its cure in genetic information or a government program.

The need for culturally tailored programs is especially acute in the Hispanic population because so many Hispanics are immigrants, which makes them difficult to reach because of language and cultural barriers. Hispanic immigrants have different attitudes toward health than native-born Hispanics, according to a National Cancer Institute survey. Attracted by the rapidly growing population, many health care marketers are beginning to reach out to Hispanic consumers. Pharmaceutical companies, for example, are rolling out major advertising campaigns for over-the-counter products because many Hispanics self-treat. Drug manufacturer Hoechst sponsored an educational campaign about diabetes for Hispanics, which included four half-hour cable television shows hosted by a Hispanic physician.[18]

To be sure, marketers—and politicians—have to take care to avoid stereotypes. Texas Health Commissioner Dr. William Archer, for example, reportedly commented that the high teen birth rate in Texas could be blamed on Latino approval of teen births. In a witty op-ed piece that ran on the Knight Ridder news service, Russell Contreras writes, "Obviously, Archer has never been to a Latino family reunion. If 11-year-old Maria was breastfeeding junior, that sure would be the talk of the fiesta. Archer's comments are dead wrong. These stereotypes see Latinos as more sexually deviant and quick to get pregnant while other groups strive to get law degrees."[19]

Because many Asian Americans are highly educated, they have greater access to health care than other minority groups. But large numbers of recent Asian immigrants have little education, presenting the same acculturation problems as Hispanic immigrants. In fact, there are significant health differences among Asian American segments. The infant mortality rate among Chinese Americans, for example, is just 3.6 infant deaths per 1,000 live births, while the infant mortality rate for American Samoans is a much higher 12.4. Just 18 percent of Japanese Americans are smokers compared to fully 72 percent of Laotians. And Vietnamese women are seven times as likely as Japanese Americans to develop cervical cancer.[20] Many health differences depend on the length of time immigrants have lived in the United Sates. Asians in the U.S. face higher risks of cancer, for example, than Asians living in other countries—and the longer they have lived in the U.S., the higher the risk.[21]

The widespread poverty and lack of education among Native Americans creates not only health problems but also difficulties in delivering health care to the population. A study from the Kaiser Family Foundation found that 37 percent of Native Americans were uninsured, compared with 16 percent of the total U.S. population. A larger percentage of Native Americans are on Medicaid compared with the average American.[22] The introduction of casino gambling on reservations may help boost Native American income and access to health care, however. The Little River Band of Ottawa Indians, for example, is setting aside casino profits for social services like health care, instead of providing cash payouts to tribal members.[23]

The future of diversity

Most of the trends surrounding the growing diversity of health care consumers are moving in the right direction. The biggest problem is that change is occurring too slowly. But at least the American public and the medical community are aware of the need for more research, better communication skills, and greater cultural sensitivity.

TREND 1: MORE RESEARCH WILL MEAN BETTER CARE

The rapidly growing body of knowledge about minority health should greatly improve medical care for blacks, Hispanics, Asians, and Native Americans. In the past, most health care studies focused only on the health of white men. Their applicability to the health of women or minorities was questionable. After growing public protest over the practice, Congress in 1993 passed the National Institute of Health Revitalization Act, which mandates the inclusion of women and minorities in health research. As a result, many federally funded programs have sprung up specifically to study minority health issues. In January 2000, for example, the National Institute of Neurological Disorders and Stroke awarded grants to five minority institutions, including the University of Puerto Rico and Howard University. The stated goal of these grants is to eliminate health care disparities for minority Americans.[24] In 1999, The National Cancer Institute set aside $30 million for projects that would help create and implement cancer control programs for minorities.[25] Now that the human genome has been mapped, genetic research is sure to yield more race-specific knowledge and lead to better health care. Genetic tests are already on the market for hemochromatosis, a genetic disease most commonly affecting people of Celtic origin.[26] Genetic tests are also available for Tay Sachs disease, which mostly affects eastern European Jews.[27]

Genetic research may be a double-edged sword, however. Expect to see the ethical debate surrounding it intensify because linking specific diseases or health conditions to a particular group has the potential of leading to discrimination. Some states already have genetic anti-discrimination laws in place. According to a 1999 Wake Forest University study, however, insurers in states with antidiscrimination laws on the books were not discriminating against people on the basis of genetic tests even before the legislation.[28] As tests become more sophisticated, however, it's likely that underwriters will ignore the results unless forced to by law.

Trend 2: Growing use of minority mediators

Armed with better information about the health care needs of minorities, the medical community still must confront the difficulty of delivering health care to people who distrust medical professionals or whose beliefs prevent them from obtaining adequate health care.

One way to circumvent distrust, especially in the Hispanic community, is to use informal mediators as go-betweens. Health care providers can tap what is called the Natural Support System. NSS uses the resources, earned authority, and respect of the community to influence people's physical, emotional and spiritual health, according to an article in *Addiction Letter*. In doing this, health care professionals enter a community and identify the community leaders, priests, politicians, spiritualists, and so on. They then collaborate with the leaders to deliver health care information to the community. "The advice from the Center for Substance Abuse Prevention for professionals working with Hispanic clients is to find the NSS, work with it, and make it an ally, or all the preventative outreaches, no matter how well planned, will fall short," the article concludes.[29]

Rochester General Hospital in Rochester, New York, for example, developed a successful health improvement program for mothers and children using NSS. The hospital coordinated efforts with the local YWCA, and implemented a peer health consulting program with local leaders, which routed women to appropriate agencies for help. The government is even getting into the act itself. The Bureau of Primary Health Care is establishing a Faith Partnership Initiative, which will link federally funded community health centers with faith-based organizations in order to increase access to primary and preventative health care.

Trend 3: Cultural sensitivity will increase

As minorities become an ever-larger share of the American population, medical professionals will have to pay more attention to cultural differences in communication. The medical community will likely seek out products and services that boost cultural communication skills.

Native Americans, for example, frequently communicate through stories, said Dr. Linda Burhansstipanov, director of the Native American Cancer Research Program in Denver, Colorado, in *Cancer News*. "You ask how a patient is doing and she starts telling a story about her auntie, and through the course of the story you will find out her symptoms," she says.[30]

Health providers must be culturally sensitive, concluded researchers in an article published in *The Western Journal of Medicine*. A study of attitudes toward breast cancer revealed that Hispanic women, particularly those with lower acculturation levels, were less knowledgeable than Anglo women about the risk factors and symptoms of breast cancer. They were also less likely to participate in early detection programs, such as mammography.[31]

Some deeply held beliefs in the Hispanic community are an obstacle to good health practices. A study funded by the National Cancer Institute, for example, found Hispanic women in Orange County, California, more likely to believe cervical cancer was God's punishment for an immoral lifestyle. Forty-three percent of foreign-born Hispanics agreed with the statement, compared with 23 percent of U.S.–born Hispanics and non-Hispanic whites. This belief could cause Hispanic immigrants to shy away from getting pap smears, which are essential to the early detection of cervical cancer.[32] "Disease has always been a taboo topic among Hispanics. . . . Illness seemed to be a cause of shame," notes Yleana Martinez, writing in *Hispanic*.[33] Anyone working with the Hispanic population must take these attitudes into account.

Unfortunately, as the health care needs of minorities rapidly become more important, the minority share of medical professionals is growing with glacial speed. The non-Hispanic white share of students enrolled in medical school fell from 85 percent in 1980-81 to just 66 percent in 1997-98, but the black share rose only from 6 to 8 percent during those years. The Hispanic share climbed from just 4 to 7 percent. Amonng minorities, only Asians have a significant presence in medical school, accounting for 18 percent of students.

Even more troubling, the black and Hispanic share of first-year medical students has fallen over the past few years. The black share of new entrants fell from a high of 8.1 percent in 1994–95 to 7.1 percent in 1997–98. The Hispanic share fell from 6.6 to 6.1 percent.[34] Several factors explain the decline, including the booming economy which provides opportunities elsewhere, the wish to avoid the managed care paperwork headache, and the elimination of affirmative action policies. With minority representation in the health care professions rising slowly, if at all, it will take much longer to achieve equality in health care.

Notes

1. Israel Cuellar and Robert E. Roberts, "Relations of Depression, Acculturation, and Socioeconomic Status in a Latino Sample," *Hispanic Journal of Behavioral Sciences* 19, no. 2 (May 1997): 230–239.

2. Richard J. David and James W. Collins, Jr., "Differing Birthweights among Infants of U.S. Born Blacks, African Born Blacks and U.S. Born Whites," *The New England Journal of Medicine* 337, no. 17 (October 23, 1997): 1209–1214.

3. "Community Indicators of Health-Related Quality of Life—United States 1993-1997," *The Journal of the American Medical Association* 283, no. 6 (April 26, 2000): 2097.

4. "Racist Slights That Blacks Face Every Day Are Linked to Their Higher Illness Rates: Study," *Jet* (October 20, 1997): 24–26.

5. Office of Minority Health Resource Center, "Why Minorities Are Under-Represented in Clinical Studies," *Closing the Gap* (December 1997/January 1998). <www.omhrc.gov>.

6. The Office of Special Populations Research, National Cancer Institute, "The Cancer Burden" (January 28, 2000). <http://ospr.nci.nih.gov/burden.html>.

7. "Black Men Push for More Funding, Education for Prostate Cancer," *Jet* (February 2, 1998): 24–26.

8. Henry J. Kaiser Family Foundation, *Key Facts: Race, Ethnicity and Medical Care* (1999).

9. "Black, Hispanic Gay Men Surpass Whites in US AIDS cases," *Medical Industry Today* (January 17, 2000).

10. Andrew A. Skolnick, "Hard to Reach Hispanics Get Health News Via Physician's Radio, TV Shows," *Journal of the American Medical Association* 278, no. 4 (July 23, 1997): 269–272.

11. "Minority Health: Paucity of Docs in Ethnic Communities," *American Health Line* (June 9, 1999).

12. "Racial Disparities: Whites Get Better Primary Care," *American Health Line* (October 7, 1999).

13. "Study Suggests Poor Cardiac Care Given Blacks and Women Is Fault of Doctors' Prejudices," *Jet* 95, no. 15 (March 15, 1999): 46.

14. Henry J. Kaiser Family Foundation, *Key Facts: Race Ethnicity and Medical Care*

15. James J. Digman, "Outcomes among African Americans and Caucasians in Colon Cancer Adjuvant Therapy Trials: Findings from the National Surgical Adjuvant Breast and Bowel Project," *The Journal of the American Medical Association* 283, no. 5 (February 2, 2000): 583.

16. Knox H. Todd, "Ethnicity and Analgesic Practice," *The Journal of the American Medical Association* 283, no. 11 (March 15, 2000): 1395.

17. Deborah L. Shelton, "Group Focuses on Closing Gap in Minority, White Health," *American Medical News* 42, no. 44 (November 22, 1999): 25.

18. Mary Wagner, "Rx Solution: Hispanic Households Most Attractive, Attentive Target with Proper In-Language Approach," *Advertising Age* (August 30, 1000): s16.

19. Russell Contreras, "Texas Officials Remarks Stereotype Latinos," Knight Ridder/Tribune News Service (April 13, 2000): 1983.

20. R.A. Zaldivar, "Health Statistics Misleading among Members of Asian, Pacific Islander Groups," Knight Ridder/Tribune News Service (July 21, 1998): 721k2570.

21. R.A. Zaldivar, "Long Term Immigrants from Asian, Latin Countries, Gradually Lose Health Advantages," Knight Ridder/Tribune News Service (July 21 1998): 721k2558.

22. The Henry J. Kaiser Family Foundation, *Sources of Financing and the Level of Health Spending for Native Americans* (October 1999).

23. "Tribe Will Use Casino Profits for Housing, Health Care," *Nation's Cities Weekly* 23, no. 13 (April 3, 2000): 12.

24. "NINDS Funds Five Specialized Neuroscience Programs at Minority Institutions," National Institutes of Health press release (January 18, 2000) <www.nih.gov>

25. National Cancer Institute, "New Project Launched to Study Minority Populations" (March 26, 1999). <http://rex.nci.nih.gov>.

26. Wylie Burke, Elizabeth Thomson, et al., "Hereditary Hemochromatosis Gene Discovery and Its Implications for Population Based Screening," *Journal of the American Medical Association* 280, no. 2 (July 8, 1998): 172A.

27. Frederic Golden, "Good Eggs, Bad Eggs: The Growing Power of Prenatal Genetic Tests Is Raising Thorny New Questions about Ethics, Fairness and Privacy," *Time* 153, no. 1 (January 11, 1999): 56.

28. Joan Stephenson, "Genetic Test Information Fears Unfounded," *The Journal of the American Medical Association* 282, no. 23 (Dec 15, 1999): 2197.

29. "Success is Working with the Community's Natural Support System," *The Addiction Letter* 12, no. 4 (April 1996): 1–3.

30. Jane Zanca, "The Challenge of Multiculturality, Or How Do You Say Cancer Care in America?" *Cancer News* 48, no. 1 (Spring 1994): 8–10.

31. F. Allan Jubbel, Leo R. Chavez, Shirz I. Mishra, and R. Burciaga Valdez, "Differing Beliefs about Breast Cancer among Latinas and Anglo Women," *The Western Journal of Medicine* 164, no. 5. (May 1996): 405–410.

32. "California County Women Say Cancer Is God's Punishment," *Cancer Weekly Plus* (January 6, 1997): 14.

33. Yleana Martinez, "Sexual Silence: To Battle Aids, Hispanics Must Overcome Cultural Barriers," *Hispanic* (January-February 1997): 100–104.

34. Karen Scott Collins, Allyson Hall, and Charlotte Neuhaus, *U.S. Minority Health: A Chartbook*, The Commonwealth Fund (May 1999).

Confidence in Medicine by Race, 1974 and 1998

"As far as people running medicine are concerned, would you say
you have a great deal of confidence, only some confidence,
or hardly any confidence at all in them?"

(percent of people aged 18 or older responding "a great deal of confidence," by race, 1974 and 1998)

	1998	1974	percentage point change
Total	44%	60%	−16
Black	44	58	−14
White	44	61	−17

Source: General Social Surveys, National Opinion Research Center, University of Chicago; calculations by New Strategist

Health Indicators by Race and Hispanic Origin, 1996

(selected indicators of health by race and Hispanic origin, and index of indicator by race and Hispanic origin to total population, 1996)

Indicator	total population	Asian	black	Hispanic	Native American	white
Infant mortality rate (deaths before age 1 per 1,000 live births)	7.3	5.2	14.7	6.1	10.0	6.1
Total deaths per 100,000 population	491.6	277.4	738.3	365.9	456.7	466.8
Motor vehicle crash deaths per 100,000 population	16.2	9.4	16.7	16.1	34.0	16.3
Work-related injury deaths per 100,000 people aged 16 or older	3.1	2.3	2.6	3.3	2.3	3.0
Suicides per 100,000 population	10.8	6.0	6.6	6.7	13.0	11.6
Homicides per 100,000 population	8.5	4.6	30.6	12.4	10.1	4.9
Lung cancer deaths per 100,000 population	37.9	16.9	46.1	14.3	23.8	37.6
Female breast cancer deaths per 100,000 population	20.2	8.9	26.5	12.8	12.7	19.8
Cardiovascular disease deaths per 100,000 population	170.7	101.4	251.0	114.5	128.1	163.6
Heart disease deaths per 100,000 population	134.5	71.7	191.5	88.6	100.8	129.8
Stroke deaths per 100,000 population	26.4	23.9	44.2	19.5	21.1	24.5
Reported incidence of AIDS per 100,000 population	27.8	7.6	110.9	48.4	13.4	13.4
Reported incidence of tuberculosis per 100,000 population	8.0	41.6	22.3	16.0	14.5	2.8
Reported incidence of syphilis per 100,000 population	4.3	0.6	30.2	1.9	2.1	0.6
Prevalence of low birth weight, as percent of total live births	7.4	7.1	13.0	6.3	6.5	6.3
Births to girls aged 10 to 17, as percent of total live births	5.1	2.1	10.3	7.3	8.7	4.2
Percent of mothers without care, first trimester of pregnancy	18.1	18.8	28.6	27.8	32.3	16.0
Percent under age 18 living in poverty	20.5	–	39.9	40.3	–	16.3
Percent living in counties exceeding U.S. air quality standards	18.7	35.6	19.2	43.7	16.8	18.1

(continued)

(continued from previous page)

Index	total population	Asian	black	Hispanic	Native American	white
Infant mortality rate (deaths before age 1 per 1,000 live births)	100	71	201	84	137	84
Total deaths per 100,000 population	100	56	150	74	93	95
Motor vehicle crash deaths per 100,000 population	100	58	103	99	210	101
Work-related injury deaths per 100,000 people aged 16 or older	100	74	84	106	74	97
Suicides per 100,000 population	100	56	61	62	120	107
Homicides per 100,000 population	100	54	360	146	119	58
Lung cancer deaths per 100,000 population	100	45	122	38	63	99
Female breast cancer deaths per 100,000 population	100	44	131	63	63	98
Cardiovascular disease deaths per 100,000 population	100	59	147	67	75	96
Heart disease deaths per 100,000 population	100	53	142	66	75	97
Stroke deaths per 100,000 population	100	91	167	74	80	93
Reported incidence of AIDS per 100,000 population	100	27	399	174	48	48
Reported incidence of tuberculosis per 100,000 population	100	520	279	200	181	35
Reported incidence of syphilis per 100,000 population	100	14	702	44	49	14
Prevalence of low birth weight, as percent of total live births	100	96	176	85	88	85
Births to girls aged 10 to 17, as percent of total live births	100	41	202	143	171	82
Percent of mothers without care, first trimester of pregnancy	100	104	158	154	178	88
Percent under age 18 living in poverty	100	–	195	197	–	80
Percent living in counties exceeding U.S. air quality standards	100	190	103	234	90	97

Note: (–) means data are not available. The index for each indicator is calculated by dividing the figure by race or Hispanic origin by the total population figure and multiplying by 100. For example, the index of 71 for Asians in the first row indicates that the Asian death rate is 29 percent below the rate for the total population. The index of 201 for blacks means the black death rate is more than twice the rate for the total population.
Source: National Center for Health Statistics, Health Status Indicators by Race and Hispanic Origin, Healthy People 2000 Review, 1998–99; calculations by New Strategist

Health Status by Race, Hispanic Origin, and Age, 1998

(percent distribution of people by self- and parent-assessed health status, by race, Hispanic origin, and age, 1996)

	excellent	very good	good	fair/poor
Total blacks	**34.5%**	**26.1%**	**25.4%**	**14.0%**
Under age 18	48.1	26.2	21.5	4.2
Aged 18 to 64	29.3	27.0	27.7	16.1
Aged 65 or older	14.3	19.9	25.4	40.4
Total Hispanics	**32.1**	**26.4**	**26.6**	**14.9**
Under age 18	42.8	26.7	22.7	7.8
Aged 18 to 64	26.8	26.8	28.9	17.4
Aged 65 or older	15.8	19.4	27.9	36.9
Total whites	**37.5**	**31.0**	**21.1**	**10.3**
Under age 18	55.3	28.7	13.1	2.9
Aged 18 to 64	34.6	33.0	22.5	9.9
Aged 65 or older	19.1	26.3	29.3	25.3

Source: Agency for Health Care Policy and Research, Health Status and Limitations: A Comparison of Hispanics, Blacks, and Whites, 1996, *MEPS Research Findings No. 10, AHCPR Pub. No. 00-0001, 1999*

Health Insurance Coverage of Blacks by Age, 1997

(number and percent distribution of blacks by age and health insurance coverage status, 1997; numbers in thousands)

| | | covered by private or government health insurance | | | | | | | |
| | | | private health insurance | | government health insurance | | | | |
	total	total	total	group health	total	Medicaid	Medicare	military	not covered
Total blacks	**34,598**	**27,166**	**18,544**	**17,077**	**12,423**	**7,750**	**3,573**	**1,100**	**7,432**
Under 18	11,507	9,333	5,486	5,201	4,682	4,224	156	302	2,174
18 to 24	3,715	2,421	1,773	1,499	867	721	46	100	1,294
25 to 34	5,300	3,825	3,025	2,894	1,034	782	56	196	1,475
35 to 44	5,499	4,250	3,457	3,289	1,129	722	218	189	1,249
45 to 54	3,663	2,930	2,489	2,378	708	388	196	124	733
55 to 64	2,224	1,755	1,269	1,142	801	339	338	124	469
65 or older	2,691	2,653	1,046	675	3,203	574	2,563	66	38

Percent distribution by health insurance coverage status

Total blacks	**100.0%**	**78.5%**	**53.6%**	**49.4%**	**35.9%**	**22.4%**	**10.3%**	**3.2%**	**21.5%**
Under 18	100.0	81.1	47.7	45.2	40.7	36.7	1.4	2.6	18.9
18 to 24	100.0	65.2	47.7	40.3	23.3	19.4	1.2	2.7	34.8
25 to 34	100.0	72.2	57.1	54.6	19.5	14.8	1.1	3.7	27.8
35 to 44	100.0	77.3	62.9	59.8	20.5	13.1	4.0	3.4	22.7
45 to 54	100.0	80.0	67.9	64.9	19.3	10.6	5.4	3.4	20.0
55 to 64	100.0	78.9	57.1	51.3	36.0	15.2	15.2	5.6	21.1
65 or older	100.0	98.6	38.9	25.1	119.0	21.3	95.2	2.5	1.4

Percent distribution by age

Total blacks	**100.0%**	**100.0%**	**100.0%**	**100.0%**	**100.0%**	**100.0%**	**100.0%**	**100.0%**	**100.0%**
Under 18	33.3	34.4	29.6	30.5	37.7	54.5	4.4	27.5	29.3
18 to 24	10.7	8.9	9.6	8.8	7.0	9.3	1.3	9.1	17.4
25 to 34	15.3	14.1	16.3	16.9	8.3	10.1	1.6	17.8	19.8
35 to 44	15.9	15.6	18.6	19.3	9.1	9.3	6.1	17.2	16.8
45 to 54	10.6	10.8	13.4	13.9	5.7	5.0	5.5	11.3	9.9
55 to 64	6.4	6.5	6.8	6.7	6.4	4.4	9.5	11.3	6.3
65 or older	7.8	9.8	5.6	4.0	25.8	7.4	71.7	6.0	0.5

Note: Numbers will not add to total because some people have more than one type of health insurance.
Source: Bureau of the Census, unpublished tables from the 1998 Current Population Survey; calculations by New Strategist

Health Insurance Coverage of Hispanics by Age, 1997

(number and percent distribution of Hispanics by age and health insurance coverage status; 1997; numbers in thousands)

		covered by private or government health insurance							not covered
			private health insurance			government health insurance			
	total	total	total	group health	total	Medicaid	Medicare	military	
Total Hispanics	**30,773**	**20,239**	**13,751**	**12,790**	**8,470**	**5,970**	**1,974**	**526**	**10,534**
Under 18	10,939	7,805	4,542	4,314	3,772	3,529	77	166	3,134
18 to 24	3,791	1,879	1,356	1,234	639	548	20	71	1,912
25 to 34	5,488	3,129	2,596	2,476	647	538	34	75	2,359
35 to 44	4,606	2,938	2,469	2,330	570	438	74	58	1,668
45 to 54	2,700	1,818	1,520	1,412	420	266	101	53	882
55 to 64	1,633	1,122	821	745	429	207	182	40	511
65 or older	1,617	1,548	447	278	1,995	445	1,487	63	69

Percent distribution by health insurance coverage status

Total Hispanics	**100.0%**	**65.8%**	**44.7%**	**41.6%**	**27.5%**	**19.4%**	**6.4%**	**1.7%**	**34.2%**
Under 18	100.0	71.4	41.5	39.4	34.5	32.3	0.7	1.5	28.6
18 to 24	100.0	49.6	35.8	32.6	16.9	14.5	0.5	1.9	50.4
25 to 34	100.0	57.0	47.3	45.1	11.8	9.8	0.6	1.4	43.0
35 to 44	100.0	63.8	53.6	50.6	12.4	9.5	1.6	1.3	36.2
45 to 54	100.0	67.3	56.3	52.3	15.6	9.9	3.7	2.0	32.7
55 to 64	100.0	68.7	50.3	45.6	26.3	12.7	11.1	2.4	31.3
65 or older	100.0	95.7	27.6	17.2	123.4	27.5	92.0	3.9	4.3

Percent distribution by age

Total Hispanics	**100.0%**	**100.0%**	**100.0%**	**100.0%**	**100.0%**	**100.0%**	**100.0%**	**100.0%**	**100.0%**
Under 18	35.5	38.6	33.0	33.7	44.5	59.1	3.9	31.6	29.8
18 to 24	12.3	9.3	9.9	9.6	7.5	9.2	1.0	13.5	18.2
25 to 34	17.8	15.5	18.9	19.4	7.6	9.0	1.7	14.3	22.4
35 to 44	15.0	14.5	18.0	18.2	6.7	7.3	3.7	11.0	15.8
45 to 54	8.8	9.0	11.1	11.0	5.0	4.5	5.1	10.1	8.4
55 to 64	5.3	5.5	6.0	5.8	5.1	3.5	9.2	7.6	4.9
65 or older	5.3	7.6	3.3	2.2	23.6	7.5	75.3	12.0	0.7

Note: Numbers may not add to total because some people have more than one type of health insurance.
Source: Bureau of the Census, unpublished tables from the 1998 Current Population Survey; calculations by New Strategist

Health Insurance Coverage of Whites by Age, 1997

(number and percent distribution of whites by age and health insurance coverage status; 1997; numbers in thousands)

	total	covered by private or government health insurance							not covered
		private health insurance			government health insurance				
		total	total	group health	total	Medicaid	Medicare	military	
Total whites	**221,650**	**188,409**	**161,682**	**140,601**	**57,754**	**19,652**	**31,108**	**6,994**	**33,241**
Under 18	56,312	48,374	39,973	37,298	11,560	9,648	199	1,713	7,938
18 to 24	20,259	14,381	12,783	10,629	2,352	1,715	97	540	5,878
25 to 34	31,779	24,762	22,611	21,269	3,028	1,955	298	775	7,017
35 to 44	36,736	30,793	28,660	26,799	3,376	1,849	639	888	5,943
45 to 54	28,871	25,162	23,460	21,729	3,266	1,280	888	1,098	3,709
55 to 64	19,140	16,619	14,892	12,815	3,422	1,080	1,405	937	2,521
65 or older	28,553	28,318	19,302	10,063	30,753	2,125	27,583	1,045	235

Percent distribution by health insurance coverage status

Total whites	**100.0%**	**85.0%**	**72.9%**	**63.4%**	**26.1%**	**8.9%**	**14.0%**	**3.2%**	**15.0%**
Under 18	100.0	85.9	71.0	66.2	20.5	17.1	0.4	3.0	14.1
18 to 24	100.0	71.0	63.1	52.5	11.6	8.5	0.5	2.7	29.0
25 to 34	100.0	77.9	71.2	66.9	9.5	6.2	0.9	2.4	22.1
35 to 44	100.0	83.8	78.0	73.0	9.2	5.0	1.7	2.4	16.2
45 to 54	100.0	87.2	81.3	75.3	11.3	4.4	3.1	3.8	12.8
55 to 64	100.0	86.8	77.8	67.0	17.9	5.6	7.3	4.9	13.2
65 or older	100.0	99.2	67.6	35.2	107.7	7.4	96.6	3.7	0.8

Percent distribution by age

Total whites	**100.0%**	**100.0%**	**100.0%**	**100.0%**	**100.0%**	**100.0%**	**100.0%**	**100.0%**	**100.0%**
Under 18	25.4	25.7	24.7	26.5	20.0	49.1	0.6	24.5	23.9
18 to 24	9.1	7.6	7.9	7.6	4.1	8.7	0.3	7.7	17.7
25 to 34	14.3	13.1	14.0	15.1	5.2	9.9	1.0	11.1	21.1
35 to 44	16.6	16.3	17.7	19.1	5.8	9.4	2.1	12.7	17.9
45 to 54	13.0	13.4	14.5	15.5	5.7	6.5	2.9	15.7	11.2
55 to 64	8.6	8.8	9.2	9.1	5.9	5.5	4.5	13.4	7.6
65 or older	12.9	15.0	11.9	7.2	53.2	10.8	88.7	14.9	0.7

Note: Numbers may not add to total because some people have more than one type of health insurance.
Source: Bureau of the Census, unpublished tables from the 1998 Current Population Survey; calculations by New Strategist

Health Care Visits by Race, 1997

(total number, percent distribution, and average annual number of ambulatory care visits per 100 persons by race and place of care, 1997; numbers in thousands)

	total	physician offices	hospital outpatient departments	hospital emergency departments
Total visits	**959,300**	**787,372**	**76,993**	**94,936**
White	809,388	681,085	56,138	72,165
Black	117,108	78,106	18,432	20,570
Other	32,804	28,181	2,423	2,200
Percent distribution by place of care				
Total visits	**100.0%**	**82.1%**	**8.0%**	**9.9%**
White	100.0	84.1	6.9	8.9
Black	100.0	66.7	15.7	17.6
Other	100.0	85.9	7.4	6.7
Percent distribution by race				
Total visits	**100.0%**	**100.0%**	**100.0%**	**100.0%**
White	84.4	86.5	72.9	76.0
Black	12.2	9.9	23.9	21.7
Other	3.4	3.6	3.1	2.3
Visits per person				
Total visits	**359.6**	**295.2**	**28.9**	**35.6**
White	367.9	309.6	25.5	32.8
Black	342.2	228.2	53.9	60.1
Other	262.1	225.1	19.4	17.6

Note: For definition of ambulatory care visits, see glossary.
Source: National Center for Health Statistics, Ambulatory Care Visits to Physician Offices, Hospital Outpatient Departments, and Emergency Departments: United States, 1997, *Vital and Health Statistics, Series 13, No. 143, 1999*

Physician Contacts by Blacks, 1996

(total number of physician contacts by blacks and number per person per year, by age and type of contact, 1996; numbers in thousands)

	total	telephone	office	hospital	other
Total contacts	**180,477**	**13,935**	**85,557**	**33,525**	**45,854**
Under age 18	39,363	4,508	17,109	7,508	9,813
Aged 18 to 44	66,027	4,870	34,923	11,761	13,740
Aged 45 to 64	39,761	2,624	20,656	8,149	7,968
Aged 65 or older	35,326	1,933	12,868	6,107	14,334
Contacts per person	**5.4**	**0.4**	**2.6**	**1.0**	**1.4**
Under age 18	3.5	0.4	1.5	0.7	0.9
Aged 18 to 44	4.8	0.4	2.5	0.9	1.0
Aged 45 to 64	7.3	0.5	3.8	1.5	1.5
Aged 65 or older	13.5	0.7	4.9	2.3	5.5

Source: National Center for Health Statistics, Current Estimates from the National Health Interview Survey, 1996, Series 10, No. 200, 1999

Physician Contacts by Whites, 1996

(total number of physician contacts by whites and number per person per year, by age and type of contact, 1996; numbers in thousands)

	total	telephone	office	hospital	other
Total contacts	**1,338,807**	**173,745**	**738,086**	**148,601**	**264,810**
Under age 18	247,287	36,897	146,778	23,957	37,752
Aged 18 to 44	432,260	61,397	244,532	52,462	68,356
Aged 45 to 64	331,044	42,936	181,840	41,952	61,767
Aged 65 or older	328,216	32,514	164,934	30,230	96,934
Contacts per person	**6.1**	**0.8**	**3.4**	**0.7**	**1.2**
Under age 18	4.4	0.6	2.6	0.4	0.7
Aged 18 to 44	4.9	0.7	2.7	0.6	0.8
Aged 45 to 64	7.2	0.9	4.0	0.9	1.4
Aged 65 or older	11.5	1.1	5.8	1.1	3.4

Source: National Center for Health Statistics, Current Estimates from the National Health Interview Survey, 1996, *Series 10, No. 200, 1999*

Physician Office Visits by Race, 1998

(number and percent distribution of physician office visits, and number of visits per person per year by race and age, 1998; number of visits in thousands)

	number of visits	percent distribution	visits per person per year
Blacks			
Total visits	**89,832**	**100.0%**	**2.6**
Under age 15	22,327	24.9	2.3
Aged 15 to 24	8,417	9.4	1.5
Aged 25 to 44	24,238	27.0	2.3
Aged 45 to 64	20,742	23.1	3.5
Aged 65 to 74	8,271	9.2	5.1
Aged 75 or older	5,837	6.5	5.4
Whites			
Total visits	**702,190**	**100.0**	**3.2**
Under age 15	113,358	16.1	2.4
Aged 15 to 24	59,927	8.5	2.0
Aged 25 to 44	177,947	25.3	2.6
Aged 45 to 64	173,822	24.8	3.6
Aged 65 to 74	90,379	12.9	5.7
Aged 75 or older	86,757	12.4	6.7
Asians	**31,495**	**100.0**	**3.0**
Native Americans	**5,764**	**100.0**	**2.4**

Source: National Center for Health Statistics, National Ambulatory Medical Care Survey: 1998 Summary, *Advance Data No. 315, 2000; calculations by New Strategist*

Acute Health Conditions by Race, 1996

(number of acute conditions and rate per 100 people, by type of acute condition and race, 1996; numbers in thousands)

	number		rate	
	black	*white*	*black*	*white*
Total acute conditions	**47,500**	**371,304**	**143.1**	**168.7**
Infective and parasitic diseases	**6,300**	**46,298**	**19.0**	**21.0**
Common childhood diseases	579	2,428	1.7	1.1
Intestinal virus	1,811	13,801	5.5	6.3
Viral infections	2,373	12,201	7.2	5.5
Other	1,536	17,868	4.6	8.1
Respiratory conditions	**22,097**	**179,091**	**66.6**	**81.4**
Common cold	8,644	51,261	26.0	23.3
Other acute upper respiratory infections	2,770	26,169	8.3	11.9
Influenza	9,313	82,048	28.1	37.3
Acute bronchitis	631	11,485	1.9	5.2
Pneumonia	249	4,376	0.8	2.0
Other respiratory conditions	489	3,751	1.5	1.7
Digestive system conditions	**2,279**	**14,971**	**6.9**	**6.8**
Dental conditions	712	2,023	2.1	0.9
Indigestion, nausea, and vomiting	1,053	6,748	3.2	3.1
Other digestive conditions	514	6,199	1.5	2.8
Injuries	**6,898**	**48,607**	**20.8**	**22.1**
Fractures and dislocations	612	7,853	1.8	3.6
Sprains and strains	2,111	10,428	6.4	4.7
Open wounds and lacerations	1,069	7,674	3.2	3.5
Contusions and superficial injuries	1,433	8,229	4.3	3.7
Other current injuries	1,673	14,422	5.0	6.6

(continued)

	number		rate	
	black	white	black	white
Selected other acute conditions	**6,558**	**55,090**	**19.8**	**25.0**
Eye conditions	442	2,875	1.3	1.3
Acute ear infections	1,649	19,823	5.0	9.0
Other ear conditions	293	3,541	0.9	1.6
Acute urinary conditions	923	7,267	2.8	3.3
Disorders of menstruation	–	839	–	0.4
Other disorders of female genital tract	123	1,474	0.4	0.7
Delivery and other conditions of pregnancy	399	2,744	1.2	1.2
Skin conditions	723	4,263	2.2	1.9
Acute musculoskeletal conditions	989	7,082	3.0	3.2
Headache, excluding migraine	498	1,094	1.5	0.5
Fever, unspecified	519	4,089	1.6	1.9
All other acute conditions	**3,369**	**27,247**	**10.2**	**12.4**

Note: The acute conditions shown here are those that caused people to restrict their activity for at least half a day or to contact a physician about the illness or injury. (–) means not applicable or sample is too small to make a reliable estimate.
Source: National Center for Health Statistics, Current Estimates from the National Health Interview Survey, 1996, *Series 10, No. 200, 1999*

Chronic Health Conditions among Blacks by Age, 1996

(number of chronic conditions and rate per 1,000 blacks, by type of chronic condition and age, 1996; numbers in thousands)

	number				rate			
	< 45	45–64	65–74	75+	< 45	45–64	65–74	75+
Selected skin and musculoskeletal conditions								
Arthritis	942	1,390	870	532	37.5	256.5	511.8	583.3
Gout, including gouty arthritis	17	193	75	17	0.7	35.6	44.1	18.6
Intervertebral disc disorders	51	395	85	15	2.0	72.9	50.0	16.4
Bone spur or tendinitis, unspecified	104	22	23	–	4.1	4.1	13.5	–
Disorders of bone or cartilage	39	41	–	21	1.6	7.6	–	23.0
Trouble with bunions	94	54	23	13	3.7	10.0	13.5	14.3
Bursitis, unclassified	102	96	124	49	4.1	17.7	72.9	53.7
Sebaceous skin cyst	64	17	–	–	2.5	3.1	–	–
Trouble with acne	474	–	–	–	18.8	–	–	–
Psoriasis	58	16	–	–	2.3	3.0	–	–
Dermatitis	874	76	18	14	34.7	14.0	10.6	15.4
Trouble with dry skin, unclassified	489	72	15	43	19.4	13.3	8.8	47.1
Trouble with ingrown nails	270	170	95	77	10.7	31.4	55.9	84.4
Trouble with corns and calluses	299	338	101	14	11.9	62.4	59.4	15.4
Impairments								
Visual impairment	505	342	129	85	20.1	63.1	75.9	93.2
Color blindness	53	16	20	–	2.1	3.0	11.8	–

(continued)

(continued from previous page)

	number				rate			
	<45	45–64	65–74	75+	<45	45–64	65–74	75+
Cataracts	69	113	246	166	2.7	20.9	144.7	182.0
Glaucoma	82	82	151	94	3.3	15.1	88.8	103.1
Hearing impairment	478	417	233	173	19.0	77.0	137.1	189.7
Tinnitus	187	169	79	65	7.4	31.2	46.5	71.3
Speech impairment	512	112	–	–	20.4	20.7	–	–
Absence of extremities	18	21	33	27	0.7	3.9	19.4	29.6
Paralysis of extremities, complete or partial	287	173	7	40	11.4	31.9	4.1	43.9
Deformity or orthopedic impairment	1,749	1,114	251	100	69.5	205.6	147.6	109.6
Back	978	527	127	33	38.9	97.3	74.7	36.2
Upper extremities	248	158	25	32	9.9	29.2	14.7	35.1
Lower extremities	850	611	140	41	33.8	112.8	82.4	45.0
Selected digestive conditions								
Ulcer	131	402	69	21	5.2	74.2	40.6	23.0
Hernia of abdominal cavity	58	93	25	–	2.3	17.2	14.7	–
Gastritis or duodenitis	263	137	95	19	10.5	25.3	55.9	20.8
Frequent indigestion	203	204	146	64	8.1	37.6	85.9	70.2
Enteritis or colitis	23	26	10	–	0.9	4.8	5.9	–
Spastic colon	36	9	23	–	1.4	1.7	13.5	–
Diverticula of intestines	–	–	–	67	–	–	–	73.5
Frequent constipation	214	128	42	36	8.5	23.6	24.7	39.5

(continued)

(continued from previous page)

	number				rate			
	< 45	45–64	65–74	75+	< 45	45–64	65–74	75+
Selected conditions of the genitourinary, nervous, endocrine, metabolic, and blood-forming systems								
Goiter or other disorders of the thyroid	222	93	54	41	8.8	17.2	31.8	45.0
Diabetes	211	810	263	257	8.4	149.5	154.7	281.8
Anemias	546	104	49	35	21.7	19.2	28.8	38.4
Epilepsy	153	45	–	–	6.1	8.3	–	–
Migraine headache	968	331	40	74	38.5	61.1	23.5	81.1
Neuralgia or neuritis, unspecified	–	–	35	–	–	–	20.6	–
Kidney trouble	107	51	22	–	4.3	9.4	12.9	–
Bladder trouble	155	70	15	18	6.2	12.9	8.8	19.7
Diseases of prostate	–	56	31	76	–	10.3	18.2	83.3
Diseases of female genital organs	571	80	–	–	22.7	14.8	–	–
Selected circulatory conditions								
Rheumatic fever with or without heart disease	119	8	–	–	4.7	1.5	–	–
Heart disease	881	701	185	208	35.0	129.4	108.8	228.1
Ischemic heart disease	66	187	50	119	2.6	34.5	29.4	130.5
Heart rhythm disorders	633	283	37	24	25.2	52.2	21.8	26.3
Tachycardia or rapid heart	54	90	20	16	2.1	16.6	11.8	17.5
Heart murmurs	544	88	–	–	21.6	16.2	–	–
Other and unspecified heart rhythm disorders	35	105	17	7	1.4	19.4	10.0	7.7

(continued)

(continued from previous page)

	number				rate			
	< 45	45–64	65–74	75+	< 45	45–64	65–74	75+
Other selected diseases of heart, excluding hypertension	182	230	99	65	7.2	42.4	58.2	71.3
High blood pressure (hypertension)	1,194	2,036	849	423	47.5	375.7	499.4	463.8
Cerebrovascular disease	48	135	62	123	1.9	24.9	36.5	134.9
Hardening of the arteries	–	34	–	55	–	6.3	–	60.3
Varicose veins of lower extremities	295	242	88	32	11.7	44.7	51.8	35.1
Hemorrhoids	337	183	110	–	13.4	33.8	64.7	–
Selected respiratory conditions								
Chronic bronchitis	1,290	280	93	9	51.3	51.7	54.7	9.9
Asthma	1,926	275	61	49	76.6	50.7	35.9	53.7
Hay fever or allergic rhinitis without asthma	1,665	350	63	59	66.2	64.6	37.1	64.7
Chronic sinusitis	3,056	978	256	63	121.5	180.5	150.6	69.1
Deviated nasal septum	–	20	–	–	–	3.7	–	–
Chronic disease of tonsils or adenoids	207	14	–	–	8.2	2.6	–	–
Emphysema	–	79	14	12	–	14.6	8.2	13.2

Note: Chronic conditions are those that last longer than three months or belong to a group of conditions considered chronic regardless of when they began.
(–) means not applicable or sample is too small to make a reliable estimate.
Source: National Center for Health Statistics, Current Estimates from the National Health Interview Survey, 1996, Series 10, No. 200, 1999

Chronic Health Conditions among Whites by Age, 1996

(number of chronic conditions and rate per 1,000 whites, by type of chronic condition and age, 1996; numbers in thousands)

	number				rate			
	< 45	45–64	65–74	75+	< 45	45–64	65–74	75+
Selected skin and musculoskeletal conditions								
Arthritis	4,482	11,187	7,296	6,344	30.7	244.6	447.4	517.8
Gout, including gouty arthritis	277	959	509	377	1.9	21.0	31.2	30.8
Intervertebral disc disorders	2,278	2,896	617	305	15.6	63.3	37.8	24.9
Bone spur or tendinitis, unspecified	1,077	1,161	246	251	7.4	25.4	15.1	20.5
Disorders of bone or cartilage	296	491	287	522	2.0	10.7	17.6	42.6
Trouble with bunions	707	783	367	294	4.9	17.1	22.5	24.0
Bursitis, unclassified	1,320	2,207	618	366	9.1	48.3	37.9	29.9
Sebaceous skin cyst	584	441	62	–	4.0	9.6	3.8	–
Trouble with acne	4,092	241	–	–	28.1	5.3	–	–
Psoriasis	1,252	1,086	300	176	8.6	23.7	18.4	14.4
Dermatitis	4,238	1,948	451	295	29.1	42.6	27.7	24.1
Trouble with dry skin, unclassified	2,799	1,302	676	818	19.2	28.5	41.5	66.8
Trouble with ingrown nails	2,845	1,233	530	494	19.5	27.0	32.5	40.3
Trouble with corns and calluses	1,107	965	398	429	7.6	21.1	24.4	35.0
Impairments								
Visual impairment	2,481	2,185	1,152	1,308	17.0	47.8	70.6	106.7
Color blindness	1,261	817	359	219	8.7	17.9	22.0	17.9

(continued)

(continued from previous page)

	number				rate			
	< 45	45–64	65–74	75+	< 45	45–64	65–74	75+
Cataracts	264	1,083	2,506	2,486	1.8	23.7	153.7	202.9
Glaucoma	132	464	708	882	0.9	10.1	43.4	72.0
Hearing impairment	4,827	6,356	4,413	4,736	33.1	139.0	270.6	386.5
Tinnitus	1,727	2,898	1,670	921	11.8	63.4	102.4	75.2
Speech impairment	1,382	216	184	188	9.5	4.7	11.3	15.3
Absence of extremities	346	284	362	196	2.4	6.2	22.2	16.0
Paralysis of extremities, complete or partial	536	542	221	304	3.7	11.9	13.6	24.8
Deformity or orthopedic impairment	12,905	8,047	2,941	1,684	88.5	176.0	180.4	137.4
Back	8,093	4,791	1,346	677	55.5	104.8	82.5	55.3
Upper extremities	1,379	1,336	692	232	9.5	29.2	42.4	18.9
Lower extremities	4,953	3,584	1,262	831	34.0	78.4	77.4	67.8
Selected digestive conditions								
Ulcer	1,207	929	542	256	8.3	20.3	33.2	20.9
Hernia of abdominal cavity	1,189	1,551	680	834	8.2	33.9	41.7	68.1
Gastritis or duodenitis	1,386	1,036	531	232	9.5	22.7	32.6	18.9
Frequent indigestion	2,819	2,014	563	289	19.3	44.0	34.5	23.6
Enteritis or colitis	777	503	143	140	5.3	11.0	8.8	11.4
Spastic colon	861	721	288	145	5.9	15.8	17.7	11.8
Diverticula of intestines	263	935	663	601	1.8	20.4	40.7	49.0
Frequent constipation	1,079	585	397	598	7.4	12.8	24.3	48.8

(continued)

(continued from previous page)

	number				rate			
	< 45	45-64	65-74	75+	< 45	45-64	65-74	75+
Selected conditions of the genitourinary, nervous, endocrine, metabolic, and blood and blood-forming systems								
Goiter or other disorders of the thyroid	1,205	1,501	871	563	8.3	32.8	53.4	45.9
Diabetes	1,091	2,044	1,459	1,041	7.5	44.7	89.5	85.0
Anemias	1,519	435	204	443	10.4	9.5	12.5	36.2
Epilepsy	623	263	99	99	4.3	5.8	6.1	8.1
Migraine headache	6,389	2,670	464	305	43.8	58.4	28.5	24.9
Neuralgia or neuritis, unspecified	45	129	12	131	0.3	2.8	0.7	10.7
Kidney trouble	1,333	627	230	182	9.1	13.7	14.1	14.9
Bladder trouble	1,285	762	352	468	8.8	16.7	21.6	38.2
Diseases of prostate	213	696	868	806	1.5	15.2	53.2	65.8
Diseases of female genital organs	2,115	935	304	161	14.5	20.4	18.6	13.1
Selected circulatory conditions								
Rheumatic fever with or without heart disease	709	546	144	234	4.9	11.9	8.8	19.1
Heart disease	5,021	5,369	4,030	3,916	34.4	117.4	247.1	319.6
Ischemic heart disease	387	2,504	2,294	1,945	2.7	54.8	140.7	158.7
Heart rhythm disorders	3,693	1,880	1,128	953	25.3	41.1	69.2	77.8
Tachycardia or rapid heart	633	552	551	393	4.3	12.1	33.8	32.1
Heart murmurs	2,646	850	339	231	18.2	18.6	20.8	18.9
Other and unspecified heart rhythm disorders	414	478	238	329	2.8	10.5	14.6	26.9

(continued)

(continued from previous page)

	number				rate			
	< 45	45–64	65–74	75+	< 45	45–64	65–74	75+
Other selected diseases of heart, excluding hypertension	942	985	608	1,017	6.5	21.5	37.3	83.0
High blood pressure (hypertension)	4,016	9,165	5,494	4,447	27.6	200.4	336.9	362.9
Cerebrovascular disease	203	530	654	1,205	1.4	11.6	40.1	98.3
Hardening of the arteries	–	320	522	625	–	7.0	32.0	51.0
Varicose veins of lower extremities	2,073	2,184	1,220	1,023	14.2	47.8	74.8	83.5
Hemorrhoids	3,398	2,628	1,165	607	23.3	57.5	71.4	49.5
Selected respiratory conditions								
Chronic bronchitis	7,348	2,810	950	862	50.4	61.4	58.3	70.4
Asthma	8,301	2,168	702	592	56.9	47.4	43.0	48.3
Hay fever or allergic rhinitis without asthma	13,404	5,077	1,020	927	92.0	111.0	62.5	75.7
Chronic sinusitis	16,440	7,999	2,081	1,297	112.8	174.9	127.6	105.9
Deviated nasal septum	990	776	59	139	6.8	17.0	3.6	11.3
Chronic disease of tonsils or adenoids	2,015	109	26	–	13.8	2.4	1.6	–
Emphysema	58	623	580	423	0.4	13.6	35.6	34.5

Note: Chronic conditions are those that last longer than three months or belong to a group of conditions considered chronic regardless of when they began.
(–) means not applicable or sample is too small to make a reliable estimate.
Source: National Center for Health Statistics, Current Estimates from the National Health Interview Survey, 1996, Series 10, No. 200, 1999

People with Disabilities by Type of Disability, Race, and Hispanic Origin, 1994–95

(total number of people aged 15 or older, and percent with a disability, by type of disability, race, and Hispanic origin, 1994–95; numbers in thousands)

	total	Asian	black	Hispanic	Native American	white
Total people	**202,367**	**6,184**	**23,805**	**18,815**	**1,350**	**154,813**
With any disability	**24.0%**	**14.6%**	**26.4%**	**20.6%**	**29.7%**	**24.3%**
Severe	12.5	7.2	17.3	10.9	14.1	12.2
Not severe	11.5	7.4	9.1	9.7	15.6	12.1
With a mental disability	4.8	–	6.4	3.7	–	4.8
Uses wheelchair	0.9	0.5	1.2	0.6	0.1	0.9
Used cane/crutch/walker for six or more months	2.6	1.2	3.3	1.6	2.4	2.6
Difficulty with or unable to perform one or more functional activities	**16.4**	**9.0**	**18.0**	**13.7**	**18.6**	**16.8**
Seeing words and letters	5.8	–	5.5	3.1	–	4.2
Hearing normal conversation	6.2	–	3.2	2.6	–	5.5
Having speech understood	1.0	–	1.4	0.7	–	1.0
Lifting, carrying 10 pounds	7.9	–	9.7	6.8	–	8.0
Climbing stairs without resting	8.9	–	11.7	7.6	–	9.0
Walking three city blocks	9.1	–	11.1	6.9	–	9.4
Difficulty with or unable to perform one or more ADLs	**4.0**	**2.1**	**5.3**	**2.8**	**4.6**	**4.1**
Getting around inside the home	1.7	–	2.6	1.1	–	1.7
Getting in and out of bed or chair	2.7	–	3.4	1.8	–	2.8
Bathing	2.2	–	3.0	1.4	–	2.2
Dressing	1.6	–	2.2	1.3	–	1.6
Eating	0.5	–	0.8	0.4	–	0.5
Getting to/using toilet	0.9	–	1.5	0.6	–	1.0
Difficulty with or unable to perform one or more IADLs	**6.1**	**3.5**	**7.7**	**4.7**	**6.4**	**6.1**
Going outside alone	4.0	–	5.0	2.7	–	4.1
Keeping track of money and bills	1.9	–	2.9	1.2	–	1.9
Preparing meals	2.1	–	2.9	1.2	–	2.1
Doing light housework	3.4	–	4.6	2.8	–	3.3
Taking prescribed medicines	1.5	–	2.2	1.0	–	1.5
Using the telephone	1.3	–	1.4	0.7	–	1.5
Needs personal assistance with an ADL or an IADL	**4.7**	**2.4**	**5.9**	**3.5**	**4.5**	**4.7**

Note: An ADL is an activity of daily living; an IADL is an instrumental activity of daily living. (–) means data not available.
Source: Bureau of the Census, Internet web site <http://www.census.gov/hhes/www/disable/cps/cps199.html>

Limitations Caused by Chronic Conditions by Race and Hispanic Origin, 1997

(percent of people with any activity limitations caused by chronic conditions by race and Hispanic origin, 1997

	with activity limitation
Total people	**13.3%**
Race	
White	13.1
Black	17.1
American Indian or Alaska Native	23.1
Asian	7.5
Hispanic origin	
White, non-Hispanic	13.2
Black, non-Hispanic	17.0
Hispanic	12.8
Mexican	12.5

Source: National Center for Health Statistics, Health, United States, 2000; *calculations by New Strategist*

Prenatal Care by Race and Hispanic Origin, 1998

(percent of women giving birth who obtained prenatal care during the first trimester, by race and Hispanic origin, and index of prenatal care by race and Hispanic origin, 1998)

	percent	index
Total births	**82.8%**	**100**
White	84.8	102
Non-Hispanic white	87.9	106
Black	73.3	89
Non-Hispanic black	73.3	89
Hispanic	74.3	90

Note: The index is calculated by dividing the percentage for each race or Hispanic origin group by the percentage for the total population and multiplying by 100.
Source: National Center for Health Statistics, Births: Final Data for 1998, National Vital Statistics Report, Vol. 48, No. 3, 2000; calculations by New Strategist

Smoking during Pregnancy by Race and Hispanic Origin, 1998

(percent of women giving birth who smoked during pregnancy, and index of smoking, by race and Hispanic origin, 1998)

	percent	index
Total mothers	**12.9%**	**100**
White	14.0	109
Non-Hispanic white	16.2	126
Black	9.5	74
Non-Hispanic black	9.6	74
Hispanic	4.0	31
Mexican	2.8	22
Puerto Rican	10.7	83
Cuban	3.7	29
Central and South American	1.5	12
Other Hispanic	8.0	62

Note: The index is calculated by dividing the percentage for each race or Hispanic origin group by the percentage for the total population and multiplying by 100.
Source: National Center for Health Statistics, Births: Final Data for 1998, *National Vital Statistics Report, Vol. 48, No. 3, 2000; calculations by New Strategist*

Low-Weight Births by Race and Hispanic Origin, 1998

(low-weight births as a percent of total births, and index of low-weight births, by race and Hispanic origin, 1998)

	percent	*index*
Total births	**7.8%**	**100**
White	6.7	86
Non-Hispanic white	6.6	85
Black	13.1	168
Non-Hispanic black	13.3	171
Hispanic	6.9	88
Mexican	6.3	81
Puerto Rican	9.7	124
Cuban	6.4	82
Central and South American	6.5	83
Other Hispanic	7.8	100

Note: Low weight means less than 2,500 grams. The index is calculated by dividing the percentage for each race or Hispanic origin group by the percentage for the total population and multiplying by 100.
Source: National Center for Health Statistics, Births: Final Data for 1998, *National Vital Statistics Report, Vol. 48, No. 3, 2000; calculations by New Strategist*

Overweight and Obese People by Sex, Race, and Hispanic Origin, 1997

(percent of people aged 18 or older who are overweight or obese by sex, race, and Hispanic origin, 1997)

	overweight	obese
Total people	**54.1%**	**19.0%**
White, non-Hispanic	52.6	18.0
Black, non-Hispanic	64.4	28.6
Asian, non-Hispanic	29.8	6.0
Hispanic	61.0	20.5
Total men	**62.2**	**18.9**
White, non-Hispanic	62.4	18.6
Black, non-Hispanic	64.1	22.7
Asian, non-Hispanic	35.2	5.8
Hispanic	64.7	19.5
Total women	**46.4**	**19.2**
White, non-Hispanic	43.0	17.3
Black, non-Hispanic	64.5	33.2
Asian, non-Hispanic	25.2	5.9
Hispanic	56.8	21.2

Note: Overweight is defined as a body mass index of 25 or more. Obesity is defined as a body mass index of 30 or more. BMI is calculated by dividing weight in kilograms by the square of height in meters.
Source: National Center for Health Statistics, data from the 1997 National Health Interview Survey, NCHS Health E-Stats, July 1, 2000, Internet site <http://www.cdc.gov/nchs>

Hypertension by Race and Hispanic Origin, 1988–94

(percent of people aged 20 to 74 who have hypertension, and index of hypertension by sex, race, and Hispanic origin, 1988–94)

	percent	index
Total men	**24.7%**	**100**
White	24.3	98
Black	31.5	128
White, non-Hispanic	25.0	101
Black, non-Hispanic	31.6	128
Mexican	18.0	73
Total women	**21.5**	**100**
White	20.4	95
Black	30.6	142
White, non-Hispanic	20.9	97
Black, non-Hispanic	31.2	145
Mexican	15.8	73

Note: A person with hypertension is someone who either has elevated blood pressure (140/90 or above) or who takes antihypertensive medication. The index is calculated by dividing the percentage for each race or Hispanic orgin group by the percentage for total men or women and multiplying by 100.
Source: National Center for Health Statistics, Health, United States, 2000; *calculations by New Strategist*

High Serum Cholesterol by Race and Hispanic Origin, 1988–94

(percent of people aged 20 to 74 who have high cholesterol, and index of high cholesterol by sex, race, and Hispanic origin, 1988–94)

	percent	*index*
Total men	**17.6%**	**100**
White	18.1	103
Black	14.4	82
White, non-Hispanic	17.9	102
Black, non-Hispanic	14.5	82
Mexican	15.5	88
Total women	**19.9**	**100**
White	20.5	103
Black	16.8	84
White, non-Hispanic	20.9	105
Black, non-Hispanic	17.2	86
Mexican	14.0	70

Note: High serum cholesterol is defined as 240 mg/dl or more. The index is calculated by dividing the percentage for each race or Hispanic origin group by the percentage for total men or women and multiplying by 100.
Source: National Center for Health Statistics, Health, United States, 2000; *calculations by New Strategist*

Cigarette Smoking by Sex, Age, and Race, 1998

(percent of people who smoke cigarettes by sex, age, and race, and percentage point difference between whites and blacks, 1998)

	white	black	percentage point difference
Total men	**26.3%**	**29.0%**	**–2.7**
Aged 18 to 24	34.1	19.7	14.4
Aged 25 to 34	29.2	25.2	4.0
Aged 35 to 44	29.6	36.2	–6.6
Aged 45 to 64	27.0	37.3	–10.3
Aged 65 or older	10.0	16.3	–6.3
Total women	**22.6**	**21.0**	**1.6**
Aged 18 to 24	28.0	8.3	19.7
Aged 25 to 34	26.9	21.5	5.4
Aged 35 to 44	26.7	30.0	–3.3
Aged 45 to 64	22.5	25.3	–2.8
Aged 65 or older	11.2	11.5	–0.3

Source: National Center for Health Statistics, Health, United States, 2000*; calculations by New Strategist*

AIDS Cases by Race, Hispanic Origin, and Sex, through June 1999

(cumulative number and percent distribution of AIDS cases among people aged 13 or older by sex, and among children under age 13, by race and Hispanic origin; through June 1999)

	total	male	female	children
Total cases	**687,863**	**570,211**	**109,459**	**8,193**
White, non-Hispanic	311,292	284,410	25,383	1499
Black, non-Hispanic	262,057	191,919	65,131	5007
Hispanic	106,454	86,988	17,868	1598
American Indian	2,034	1,670	335	29
Asian or Pacific Islander	5,104	4,475	583	46
Percent distribution by race				
Total cases	**100.0%**	**100.0%**	**100.0%**	**100.0%**
White, non-Hispanic	45.3	49.9	23.2	18.3
Black, non-Hispanic	38.1	33.7	59.5	61.1
Hispanic	15.5	15.3	16.3	19.5
American Indian	0.3	0.3	0.3	0.4
Asian or Pacific Islander	0.7	0.8	0.5	0.6
Percent distribution by sex				
Total cases	**100.0%**	**82.9%**	**15.9%**	**1.2%**
White, non-Hispanic	100.0	91.4	8.2	0.5
Black, non-Hispanic	100.0	73.2	24.9	1.9
Hispanic	100.0	81.7	16.8	1.5
American Indian	100.0	82.1	16.5	1.4
Asian or Pacific Islander	100.0	87.7	11.4	0.9

Source: National Center for Health Statistics, Health, United States, 2000; *calculations by New Strategist*

Leading Causes of Death for Asians, 1998

(total number of Asian deaths, and number and percent accounted for by the 10 leading causes of death among Asians, 1998)

		number	*percent*
All causes		**31,987**	**100.0%**
1.	Diseases of heart	8,633	27.0
2.	Malignant neoplasms	8,366	26.2
3.	Cerebrovascular diseases	2,859	8.9
4.	Accidents and adverse effects	1,564	4.9
5.	Pneumonia and influenza	1,497	4.7
6.	Diabetes mellitus	1,022	3.2
7.	Chronic obstructive pulmonary diseases	949	3.0
8.	Suicide	640	2.0
9.	Homicide and legal intervention	383	1.2
10.	Nephritis, nephrotic syndrome, nephrosis	335	1.0
All other causes		5,739	17.9

Source: National Center for Health Statistics, Health, United States, 2000; *calculations by New Strategist*

Leading Causes of Death for Blacks, 1998

(total number of black deaths, and number and percent accounted for by the 10 leading causes of death among blacks, 1998)

	number	percent
All causes	**278,440**	**100.0%**
1. Diseases of heart	78,294	28.1
2. Malignant neoplasms	61,193	22.0
3. Cerebrovascular diseases	18,237	6.5
4. Accidents and adverse effects	12,801	4.6
5. Diabetes mellitus	11,378	4.1
6. Homicide and legal intervention	8,420	3.0
7. Pneumonia and influenza	8,326	3.0
8. Chronic obstructive pulmonary diseases	7,205	2.6
9. Human immunodeficiency virus infection	7,180	2.6
10. Certain conditions originating in perinatal period	4,841	1.7
All other causes	60,565	21.8

Source: National Center for Health Statistics, Deaths: Final Data for 1998, *National Vital Statistics Report, Vol. 48, No. 11, 2000; calculations by New Strategist*

Leading Causes of Death for Hispanics, 1998

(total number of Hispanic deaths, and number and percent accounted for by the 10 leading causes of death among Hispanics, 1998)

		number	*percent*
All causes		**98,406**	**100.0%**
1.	Diseases of heart	24,596	25.0
2.	Malignant neoplasms	19,528	19.8
3.	Accidents and adverse effects	8,248	8.4
4.	Cerebrovascular diseases	5,587	5.7
5.	Diabetes mellitus	4,741	4.8
6.	Pneumonia and influenza	3,277	3.3
7.	Homicide and legal intervention	2,978	3.0
8.	Chronic liver disease and cirrhosis	2,845	2.9
9.	Chronic obstructive pulmonary diseases	2,528	2.6
10.	Certain conditions originating in the perinatal period	1,987	2.0
	All other causes	22,091	22.4

Source: National Center for Health Statistics, Deaths: Final Data for 1998, *National Vital Statistics Report, Vol. 48, No. 11, 2000; calculations by New Strategist*

Leading Causes of Death for Native Americans, 1998

(total number of Native American deaths, and number and percent accounted for by the 10 leading causes of death among Native Americans, 1998)

		number	percent
All causes		**10,845**	**100.0%**
1.	Diseases of heart	2,383	22.0
2.	Malignant neoplasms	1,834	16.9
3.	Accidents and adverse effects	1,292	11.9
4.	Diabetes mellitus	645	5.9
5.	Cerebrovascular diseases	497	4.6
6.	Chronic liver disease and cirrhosis	467	4.3
7.	Pneumonia and influenza	389	3.6
8.	Chronic obstructive pulmonary diseases	369	3.4
9.	Suicide	310	2.9
10.	Homicide and legal intervention	228	2.1
All other causes		2,431	22.4

Source: National Center for Health Statistics, Health, United States, 2000*; calculations by New Strategist*

Leading Causes of Death for Whites, 1998

(total number of white deaths, and number and percent accounted for by the 10 leading causes of death among whites, 1998)

		number	percent
All causes		**2,015,984**	**100.0%**
1.	Diseases of heart	635,549	31.5
2.	Malignant neoplasms	470,139	23.3
3.	Cerebrovascular diseases	136,855	6.8
4.	Chronic obstructive pulmonary diseases	104,061	5.2
5.	Accidents and adverse effects	82,178	4.1
6.	Pneumonia and influenza	81,659	4.1
7.	Diabetes mellitus	51,706	2.6
8.	Suicide	27,648	1.4
9.	Chronic liver disease and cirrhosis	21,771	1.1
10.	Nephritis, nephrotic syndrome, nephrosis	21,369	1.1
All other causes		383,049	19.0

Source: National Center for Health Statistics, Deaths: Final Data for 1998, *National Vital Statistics Report, Vol. 48, No. 11, 2000; calculations by New Strategist*

Leading Causes of Death for Non-Hispanics, 1998

(total number of non-Hispanic deaths, and number and percent accounted for by the 10 leading causes of death among non-Hispanics, 1998)

	number	percent
All causes	**2,230,127**	**100.0%**
1. Diseases of heart	697,516	31.3
2. Malignant neoplasms	520,483	23.3
3. Cerebrovascular diseases	152,418	6.8
4. Chronic obstructive pulmonary diseases	109,703	4.9
5. Accidents and adverse effects	89,069	4.0
6. Pneumonia and influenza	88,280	4.0
7. Diabetes mellitus	59,808	2.7
8. Suicide	28,721	1.3
9. Nephritis, nephrotic syndrome, nephrosis	25,139	1.1
10. Septicemia	22,754	1.0
All other causes	436,236	19.6

Source: National Center for Health Statistics, Deaths: Final Data for 1998, *National Vital Statistics Report, Vol. 48, No. 11, 2000; calculations by New Strategist*

Leading Causes of Death for Non-Hispanic Blacks, 1998

(total number of non-Hispanic black deaths, and number and percent accounted for by the 10 leading causes of death among non-Hispanic blacks, 1998)

	number	percent
All causes	**275,264**	**100.0%**
1. Diseases of heart	77,434	28.1
2. Malignant neoplasms	60,642	22.0
3. Cerebrovascular diseases	18,067	6.6
4. Accidents and adverse effects	12,617	4.6
5. Diabetes mellitus	11,278	4.1
6. Homicide and legal intervention	8,282	3.0
7. Pneumonia and influenza	8,246	3.0
8. Chronic obstructive pulmonary diseases	7,131	2.6
9. Human immunodeficiency virus infection	7,055	2.6
10. Certain conditions originating in perinatal period	4,674	1.7
All other causes	59,838	21.7

Source: National Center for Health Statistics, Deaths: Final Data for 1998, *National Vital Statistics Report, Vol. 48, No. 11, 2000; calculations by New Strategist*

Leading Causes of Death for Non-Hispanic Whites, 1998

(total number of non-Hispanic white deaths, and number and percent accounted for by the 10 leading causes of death among non-Hispanic whites, 1998)

	number	percent
All causes	**1,912,802**	**100.0%**
1. Diseases of heart	609,256	31.9
2. Malignant neoplasms	449,785	23.5
3. Cerebrovascular diseases	131,039	6.9
4. Chronic obstructive pulmonary diseases	101,274	5.3
5. Pneumonia and influenza	78,174	4.1
6. Accidents and adverse effects	73,669	3.9
7. Diabetes mellitus	46,884	2.5
8. Suicide	25,846	1.4
9. Alzheimer's disease	20,834	1.1
10. Nephritis, nephrotic syndrome, nephrosis	20,372	1.1
All other causes	355,669	18.6

Source: National Center for Health Statistics, Deaths: Final Data for 1998, *National Vital Statistics Report, Vol. 48, No. 11, 2000; calculations by New Strategist*

Life Expectancy at Birth by Race and Hispanic Origin, 1999

(average number of years of life remaining at birth by race, Hispanic origin, and sex, 1999)

	male	female
Asian	80.9	86.5
Black	68.4	75.1
Hispanic	77.2	83.7
Native American	72.9	82.0
White, non-Hispanic	74.7	80.1

Source: Bureau of the Census, Projections of the Resident Population by Age, Sex, Race, and Hispanic Origin: 1999 to 2100, *Internet web site <http://www.census.gov/population/www/projections/natproj.html>; calculations by New Strategist*

Students Enrolled in Schools for Health Occupations by Race and Hispanic Origin, 1997–98

(number and percent distribution of students enrolled in schools for selected health occupations, by race and Hispanic origin, 1997–98)

	number	percent
ALLOPATHIC MEDICINE		
Total enrolled	**66,900**	**100.0%**
White, non-Hispanic	44,310	66.2
Black, non-Hispanic	5,303	7.9
Hispanic	4,423	6.6
Native American	561	0.8
Asian	12,303	18.4
DENTISTRY		
Total enrolled	**16,926**	**100.0**
White, non-Hispanic	11,246	66.4
Black, non-Hispanic	883	5.2
Hispanic	825	4.9
Native American	96	0.6
Asian	3,876	22.9
OPTOMETRY		
Total enrolled	**5,075**	**100.0**
White, non-Hispanic	3,705	73.0
Black, non-Hispanic	120	2.4
Hispanic	200	3.9
Native American	23	0.5
Asian	1,027	20.2
OSTEOPATHIC MEDICINE		
Total enrolled	**9,434**	**100.0**
White, non-Hispanic	7,404	78.5
Black, non-Hispanic	386	4.1
Hispanic	378	4.0
Native American	82	0.9
Asian	1,184	12.6

(continued)

(continued from previous page)

	number	percent
PHARMACY		
Total enrolled	**32,529**	**100.0%**
White, non-Hispanic	22,166	68.1
Black, non-Hispanic	2,632	8.1
Hispanic	1,130	3.5
Native American	150	0.5
Asian	6,451	19.8
PODIATRY		
Total enrolled	**2,471**	**100.0**
White, non-Hispanic	1,820	73.7
Black, non-Hispanic	148	6.0
Hispanic	92	3.7
Native American	9	0.4
Asian	402	16.3
REGISTERED NURSES		
Total enrolled	**238,244**	**100.0**
White, non-Hispanic	193,061	81.0
Black, non-Hispanic	23,611	9.9
Hispanic	9,227	3.9
Native American	1,816	0.8
Asian	10,529	4.4

Source: National Center for Health Statistics, Health, United States, 2000*; calculations by New Strategist*

5

Making Sense of Health Information

Information is the lifeblood of the new health care consumer. Increasingly educated Americans hunger for information about their physical well-being, and the Internet brings that information home, to the office, or wherever consumers want it. In fact, it's the Internet's democratization of information that has tipped the balance of power in medical relationships, handing the reins to consumers. According to *The New York Times*, patients are beginning to switch doctors when their doctor is unwilling to review information they've gathered on the Internet. Physicians are feeling frustrated because they do not have time to sift through web site information patients bring into the office.[1] Clearly, information is not only the lifeblood of the new health care consumer—it's the force transforming modern medicine.

Health information is big business both on and off the Internet. Health ranks second only to crime as the news topic people are most likely to follow "very closely," according to

Top news interests of Americans

(percent of people aged 18 or older who follow each type of news "very closely," 2000)

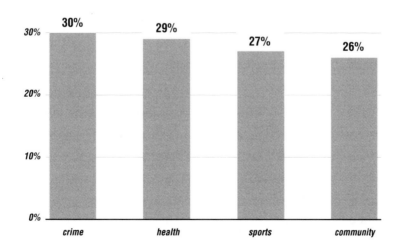

the Pew Research Center for the People & the Press.[2] Among those who go online for the news, health ranks second only to weather news as the topic people research most.

Americans today are increasingly likely to get their news online rather than from television or newspapers, according to the Pew survey. Between 1998 and 2000, the percentage of people who regularly watch the nightly network news fell from 38 to 30 percent, while the percentage of those who regularly get their news online rose from 13 to 23 percent. Even more startling, the percentage of college graduates who regularly get their news online is now greater (40 percent) than the percentage of those who regularly watch the nightly network news (28 percent).

Seventy-four percent of people who go online use the Internet to look up health information, according to a Harris poll. Forty-three percent of those online look for health information "often" or "sometimes." The majority who research health topics online are looking for information about specific diseases, and most of the time they want the information for themselves or a family member. The diseases consumers are most interested in include depression, allergies or sinus problems, cancer, bipolar disorder, arthritis/ rheumatism, high blood pressure, and migraines.[3]

The number of consumers with access to the Internet continues to soar. According to Nielsen//NetRatings, the number of Americans with Internet access at home grew 23 percent in 1999, to 119 million.[4] Soon, access to health information via the Internet will no longer be confined to home or office—it will become portable. The number of wireless devices with Internet access is projected to increase an astonishing 728 percent between 1999 and 2003, when 61.5 million mobile devices will be accessing the Internet, according to IDC, a company that analyzes the information technology industry.[5] In the future, if a man walking down the street notices a rash on his arm, he may attempt to diagnose it instantly using his wireless web gadget.

Although millions of consumers are getting health information online, traditional media are still an important source of health advice. Television, for example, is still the number one source of nutrition information, according to the American Dietetic Association, but its influence is declining. Forty-eight percent of adults said they got nutrition information from television in 1999, down from 57 percent in 1997.[6] Forty-seven percent said they got nutrition information from magazines in 1999, up from 44 percent in 1997. Newspapers were cited by 18 percent, followed by books (12 percent), doctors (11 percent) the Internet (6 percent), and radio (5 percent).

The ADA also asked consumers to identify their most valued sources of nutrition information. Doctors came out on top (cited by 92 percent), followed by registered dietitians, and nutritionists. Magazines were mentioned by 87 percent, TV news by 79 percent, and the Internet by 61 percent.[7]

Other studies show the media ranking much lower as a trusted source of health care information, however. A 1998 study by Time, Inc., found two-thirds of consumers turning to doctors and pharmacists for health care advice compared with a much smaller 28 percent who relied on newspapers and magazines and 26 percent who depended on television news.[8] Similarly, when buying over-the-counter drugs, the sources of information trusted "a lot" by the largest share of consumers were doctors (67 percent) and pharmacists (66 percent). On the credibility scale, product labels followed (43 percent), then friends and family (38 percent). Books were trusted a lot by 27 percent, advertising by just 12 percent, and magazines by only 11 percent.[9]

Despite the public's wariness of the health advice they see on TV or read in newspapers or magazines, the media have been successful in alerting Americans to health problems. One topic frequently covered by the media are health problems caused by poor eating habits. Thanks to this coverage, more than 8 in 10 men and women know of the harmful effects of eating too much fat. Seventy-nine percent of women know that a lack of calcium can lead to osteoporosis, and the same percentage of men associate eating too much cholesterol with heart disease, according to government surveys.

To avoid these health problems, millions of Americans rely on the information supplied by food labels. Women are especially likely to use nutritional information on labels when purchasing products, with over half often or always examining the fat content of a product. Forty-four percent of women often or always look at the calorie count. While men are less likely than women to examine food labels when buying products, a large proportion check the fat, cholesterol, and sodium content of the food they buy.

The public knows what to look for on food labels thanks to media coverage of health risks. Coverage has begun to emphasize the health benefits of food rather than the risks that predominated coverage during the mid to late-1990s. To assess the quality and quantity of diet and nutrition coverage, the International Food Information Council measures news coverage of food issues. Between 1995 and 1999, its surveys revealed a marked shift toward coverage of the health benefits of food rather than the diseases linked to food consumption.[10] The leading food news topic in 1999 was disease prevention, while it was food-borne illness in 1997 and fat intake in 1995. IFIC attributes the shift to the increased coverage of functional foods and biotechnology. This shift doesn't mean negative stories about food and health have disappeared, however. Food-borne illness was the second leading topic of discussion in food news of 1999, while fat intake ranked fourth.

The same studies also show that much of the media's nutritional information is presented out of context. Stories about healthy foods, for example, rarely specify how much or how often the foods should be eaten. Context in nutrition stories is actually on the decline, says the IFIC. It estimates that 18 percent of health coverage in 1999 provided appropriate context, down from 34 percent in 1997. But reporters are seeking out more independent scientific experts to bolster their stories, which may lead to gradual improvement in the coverage of nutritional information. Food stories were more user-friendly in 1999 than in 1995, linking nutrient information to the foods that supply them, turning abstract concepts into shopping lists. Between 1995 and 1997, the number of stories initiated by activist groups declined because of the changing nature of food issues. That number was even lower in 1999, but the fact that the Center for Science in the Public Interest (a major source of activist alerts) did not release any studies that year could be behind the decline.[11]

The media also play an important and growing role in boosting awareness of health issues to meet public health goals. An example of the media's effectiveness in this area is the publicizing of the ultraviolet index. During the summers of 1994 and 1995, hundreds of television stations and newspapers across the nation received ultraviolet index information from the Centers for Disease Control and disseminated it to their viewers and readers. The message reached 13 million adults each day, according to follow-up survey estimates. After the media campaign, 64 percent of Hispanics and non-Hispanic whites (the populations most at risk of melanoma) had heard of the ultraviolet index, with 54 percent hearing or read about it at least five times. Television accounted for the largest share of respondents having been exposed to the index (40 percent), followed by newspapers. Although there was no difference in the level of awareness between men and women, women were more likely to change their behavior after learning about the indicator. Among men, younger ones were more likely to change their behavior than older ones. The media campaign did not work well on people aged 60 or older, who were least aware of the ultraviolet index despite the campaign.[12]

Although more research is needed, the follow-up survey results suggest the media can be effective in reaching younger generations of Americans. Mobilizing young and middle-aged adults around health issues may not require official health messages. But for older people, formal messages may be necessary. This finding is supported by survey results published in the journal *Cancer*, which showed that women aged 50 or older were more likely to get mammograms when the test was suggested by health care professionals rather than promoted through the media. As well-educated and media-savvy baby boomers age, however, it will become much easier to reach older Americans through skillful media use.[13]

As boomers age, so do boomer celebrities. Because these celebrities are not immune to the risks of aging, they will become powerful spokespersons for health issues. One example is the "Today Show's" Katie Couric, whose husband died of colon cancer at age 42. Using her clout, Couric launched a public information campaign about the disease, making the cover of *Time* magazine. She also founded The National Colorectal Cancer Research Alliance, which released a study about the public's lack of awareness about the disease. The study found that 86 percent of adults were aware of colorectal cancer, the second leading cause of death in the United States. But only 6 percent of those aged 50 or older thought that it was very likely they would develop the disease—although 93 percent of all cases occur to those aged 50 or older.[14] The study was conducted in January 2000, and a follow-up will be needed to determine whether Couric's efforts have had a lasting impact.

Health care advertising

Although consumers claim they are not influenced by health care advertising, in fact the influence of marketing is greater than they think. Each day, Americans are exposed to dozens of advertising messages about over-the-counter medications, prescription drugs, nutritional products, doctors, hospitals, and other medical services and facilities. These messages guide consumers to advertised products in drugstores and supermarkets and even influence their choice of doctors and hospitals.

Americans spend billions of dollars each year on over-the-counter and prescription medications, and much of their spending is directed by advertising. The majority of adults aged 18 or older consume pain relief medication, antacids, and allergy and cold medicines each year, according to the Prevention/APhA survey. In addition, 46 percent of Americans currently use prescription drugs.[15]

The pharmaceutical industry spent more than $1 billion in 1998 on direct-to-consumer advertising of prescription medications in an attempt to get patients to ask their doctors for particular drugs, reports *Advertising Age*.[16] According to a 1999 *Prevention* survey, 31 percent of consumers who saw ads for prescription drugs asked their doctors about the medication.[17] A 1999 study of physicians found 47 percent feeling "a little" pressure to prescribe drugs requested by patients, while 6 percent felt "a lot" of pressure. Only 9 percent said they felt no pressure.[18]

With patients requesting prescription medications by brand name, the balance of power has shifted again. Consumers are wresting control away from physicians. Many doctors and pharmacists are not happy about this turn of events. Michael Dillon, director of pharmacy services for Community Health Plan/Kaiser Permanente Northeast Division, complains in *Drug Benefit Trends* that prescription advertising has contributed to what he calls disease creation. "In my facility," he says, "there's been a rather sudden increase in anti-fungal prescriptions written for patients with toenail fungus.... Has there been an epidemic of toenail fungus? I don't think so. But there has been a plethora of TV and print ads featuring people with cruddy toenails."[19] A 1998 survey of physicians' attitudes toward consumer advertising of prescription drugs by Time, Inc., found 79 percent of doctors concerned that relaxed advertising guidelines would have patients asking for unnecessary or incorrect drugs. A 40 percent minority thought it would help them provide the best treatment for patients.[20] Other health professionals worry that direct-to-consumer (or DTC) ads will lead consumers to believe they do not have to change their lifestyle to cure what ails them, according to Michael Wilkes, M.D., on WebMD's web site (www.webmd.com). These ads "may cultivate the belief among the public that there's a pill for every ill and contribute to the medicalization of trivial ailments, leading to an even more 'overmedicated society,'" he says.[21]

But DTC advertising is only as effective as any kind of advertising—which means it's not going to hit the mark all the time. According to a study by Morpace Pharma Group, a market research firm in Farmington Hills, Michigan, only 4 percent of adults have requested a drug because of a DTC ad.[22] Although many consumers are aware of drug brands thanks to DTC ads, a study of 18 prescription brands by CME Health—the health marketing division of Campbell Mithun Esty, a marketing communications firm in Minneapolis—consumers were twice as likely to strongly dislike rather than strongly like the ads.[23] More than half of consumers surveyed by *Drug Topics* magazine found DTC ads useful, while 29 percent said they were not useful and 20 percent were unsure. Only 29 percent wanted to see more DTC ads, while half did not want more.[24]

The future of health information

Overwhelmed with information, but at least partly protected by a good dose of skepticism, today's health care consumers are much more aware of health risks, disease symptoms, and medical treatments. The flow of information will only increase, continuing to change the relationship between doctors and patients, the health care industry and its consumers.

Trend 1: Medicine by modem

The Internet will become the primary source of health information. A substantial share of Americans already go online for news. One-third of Americans go online for news at least once a week, up from 20 percent in 1998. Fifteen percent say they receive daily news reports from the Internet, up from 6 percent two years ago, according to the Pew Research Center for the People & the Press.[25] Baby Boomers, Gen Xers, and Millennials are the ones most likely to go online for news—46 percent of people under age 30 do so at least once a week, as do 37 percent of those aged 30 to 49. This compares with just 20 percent of people aged 50 or older. As the computer-savvy younger generations age and encounter more health problems, they will turn increasingly to the Internet to investigate health problems and seek advice.

Thousands of web sites are devoted to health, with more coming online every day. Medical journals have their own web sites, while other sites are devoted to specific diseases. Online support groups are common. Some sites offer directories of doctors and hospitals, while others provide information about specific drugs. One of the best sites for information about health is Medline (www.nlm.nih.gov), which offers abstracts from articles published in thousands of medical journals.

Because information on the Internet is not regulated, the greatest challenge for consumers is determining the credibility of what pops up on their screens. "It's about 90

Many people search for health information online

(percent distribution of people aged 18 or older with Internet access by frequency with which they look for health information online, 1999)

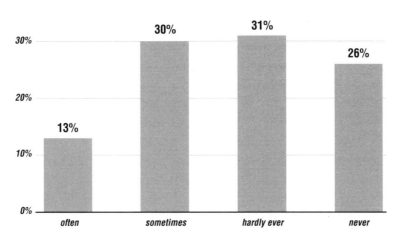

percent 'Jerry Springer' and 10 percent 'Masterpiece Theater," explains Jennifer Wayne-Doppke, author of the Annual Healthcare Guide to the Internet, in *The Wall Street Journal*. "Finding the 'Masterpiece Theater' part is really hard because there's no *TV Guide* for the Internet," she says.[26] Consumer magazines as diverse as *Men's Health* and *PC/Computing* all sound a cautionary note about the quality of health care information on the Internet. Many companies are trying to fill the credibility gap. The American Medical Association and six other medical industry groups have joined together to form a for-profit web portal called Medem (www.medem.com), which provides links to licensed physicians and accurate online information as well as allows patients and doctors to e-mail one another.[27] Other health portals, like WebMD and DrKoop.com are duking it out for becoming the number-one online brand for consumer health information.

But many consumers do not have time to sort it all out themselves, even with the help of a good portal. This is why some employers have contracted with health information specialists—physicians and researchers whose sole purpose is to sort through the abundance of health data and provide customized, credible information to consumers.[28] For these researchers—and the companies that employ them—liability is a concern that will have to be addressed by legislation before such services can become widespread.

TREND 2: MEDIA-SAVVY MEDICAL PROFESSIONALS

Medical professionals will become more savvy about using the media to their advantage. "The medical profession has a lot to learn about how to pass on news of [medical] advances in useful form. It will not do it by reciting mantras about 'evidence based medicine' or complaining about public misunderstanding of risk. There is not much risk of the public listening, for one thing," writes Tim Radford in the British journal *The Lancet*.[29]

According to a survey of 620 public health administrators published in the *Journal of the American Medical Association*, one-third of the administrators thought the media and medical community had an adversarial relationship as a result of inaccurate reporting. And despite all indicators pointing to television as the number one source of medical news, health administrators dealt with the print media 63 percent of the time and television just 19 percent.[30]

As the health care system shakes out, medical professionals will be forced to develop a closer relationship with the media. To attract customers, they will have to become much more sophisticated marketers. Targeted marketing is one avenue that will be traveled with increasing frequency as the health care industry reaches out to customers. The pharmaceutical industry is already skilled at targeting individual consumers using an arsenal of devices ranging from videos and newsletters to 800 numbers, self-monitoring calendars, and mail reminders. Many are building relationships online as well. The makers of Xenical, the weight loss drug, successfully launched XeniCare, a web site that supports patients using the drug. The company has discovered that patients who use the web site stay with the program longer—and thus refill their prescriptions more often. Brochures are no longer enough for today's savvy Internet consumer.

Increasingly, medical professionals will use technology, such as the telephone and e-mail, to reach out to individual patients. Research shows that patients are more likely to follow a prescribed self-care regimen, such as taking medication, when a doctor calls to check up on them. But research also shows that this communication does not necessarily have to come from a human being. Computerized calls work just as well, says Dr. Robert Freidman, chief of the Medical InfoSystems Unit at Boston University Medical Center. Adherence to a medical regimen improved 18 percent for patients who received a weekly computerized reminder, he announced at an American Psychological Association conference in 1996.[31] For such communication to become common, managed care companies will have to see it as a cost containment strategy. Doctors will resist handling issues over the phone or by e-mail if they are not compensated for their time.

Another effective way to deliver health information, particularly to young people, is through "edutainment." Important messages about health have a greater impact when sugar-coated with fun, like the story lines of popular programs such as "ER" and "General Hospital." The Henry Kaiser Family Foundation and Johns Hopkins University have teamed up to produce "Following ER," a 90-second television news segment that provides follow-up information for people concerned about medical problems spotlighted by the popular NBC drama.

More information is available on the Johns Hopkins web site (http://er.jhsph.edu), which explains the mission quite well. "Through 'Following ER,' for the first time, entertainment television will be the driving force behind a multimedia initiative designed to link scientific information and community resources to educate and motivate viewers to take action on a series of personal and public health topics," explains the site. It continues: "For each episode, the writers at ER talk with staff at the School and the Foundation about the plot line. Working together they decide upon the health theme for the week. For instance, an ER episode that dealt with teen pregnancy was followed by a segment featuring a teenage boy who talked about making good choices about sex and contraception. In addition to the television news segment, viewers will be able to receive more detailed information on a specific health topic immediately following each episode and throughout the week via a toll-free interactive voice response system audiotext service. And viewers who have access to the Internet, either at home, school, or work, will be able to receive more information at their own convenience with this user friendly Internet Web site."[32]

TREND 3: MORE COMPARATIVE DATA

One of the most important trends in health information is the growing availability of comparative information about doctors, hospitals, and other suppliers in the health care industry. Just as *Consumer Reports* publishes information helpful for choosing a car, soon doctors and hospitals will be required to disclose their track records.

The comparative databases available to the public today are mostly proprietary in nature. Reference books and, increasingly, web sites offer guidance to the best physicians in a particular specialty—for a price.

Health plans also gather their own data in the form of "report cards." One example is HEDIS, or Health Plan Employer Data and Information Set. HEDIS is a standardized set of 60 performance measures regarding quality, access, patient satisfaction, membership, and other areas of importance to health plans. HEDIS is not meant for consumers, however. "Our interest lies in the performance of our health plans and not in the community's health," explains a Prudential Health Plan manager.[33] This is why the quality measures aren't as meaningful to consumers as they could be.

Health care by legislation will ensure that report cards will become available to the public more often and in clearer language. As the era of consumer-driven health care moves forward, comparative data will no longer be limited to health care professionals and insurers. But it will take marketing to get consumers to pay attention, says Mark Legnini, President of the Health Care Decisions Group, which received federal government funding to study quality measures. "There's the idea that a doctor is a doctor is a doctor. We know that's not true. It's been proved time and time again that there's an enormous gap between the quality of care that the average person receives and the quality of care that some other people receive. There's a pretty large gap between what most people get and the gold standard that's available at the Mayo Clinic. People are not aware of the degree of variation, that the average care is not up to the highest standard. Consumers need that information," he says.[34]

Notes

1. Gina Kolata, "Web Research Transforms Visit to the Doctor," *The New York Times Online* (March 6, 2000). <www.nytimes.com>.

2. The Pew Research Center for The People & The Press, "Investors Now Go Online for Quotes, Advice—Internet Sapping Broadcast News Audience" (June 11, 2000). <http://www.people-press.org>.

3. "Explosive Growth of Cyberchondriacs Continues," The Harris Poll #47 (August 5, 1999). <www.harrisinteractive.com>.

4. Nielsen//NetRatings, "Nielsen//NetRatings Reports on Internet Year 1999 in Review" (January 20, 2000). < www.nielsentnetratings.com>.

5. IDC, "The Internet Goes Wireless" (February 8, 2000). <www.idc.com>.

6. American Dietetic Association, "Americans' Food and Nutrition Attitudes and Behaviors—American Dietetic Association's Nutrition and You: Trends 2000" (January 3, 2000). <www.eatright.org>.

7. Ibid.

8. Stuart Elliot, "A Seminar Examines the Plethora of Prescription Drug Pitches Since Regulations Were Loosened," *The New York Times* (June 15, 1998): c11.

9. Prevention Magazine and the American Pharmaceutical Association, *Navigating the Medication Marketplace* (1997).

10. International Food Information Council Foundation and the Center for Media and Public Affairs, *Food for Thought III, A Quantitative and Qualitative Content Analysis of Diet, Nutrition and Food Safety Reporting* (February 2000).

11. Ibid.

12. The Centers for Disease Control and Prevention, "Media Dissemination of and Public Response to the Ultra Violet Index," *Mortality and Morbidity Weekly Report* 46, no. 17 (May 2, 1997): 370-374.

13. Victoria Champion, "Relationship of Age to Mammography Compliance," *Cancer* 74, no. 1 (July 1, 1994): 329-337.

14. "Prevention Magazine Teams with National Colorectal Cancer Research Alliance on Colorectal Cancer Awareness Survey," *PR Newswire* (May 22, 2000).

15. *Prevention Magazine.*

16. "DTC Drug Ads Should Hit $1 Bil for 1998," *Advertising Age* (January 4, 1999): 1.

17. David Goetzl, "Second Magazine Study Touts Value of DTC Drug Ads," *Advertising Age* (June 28, 1999): 22.

18. "US Doctors under Pressure from DTC Ads," *Chemist and Druggist* (November 27, 1999): 11.

19. Robert McCarthy, "Rx Ads Hit Consumer Bull's Eye," *Drug Benefit Trends* 10, no. 1 (January 1998): 23.

20. Elliot.

21. Sean Martin, "Drug Ads for Consumers Hurt Quality of Care, Article Says. Pharmaceutical Firms Say the Spots Empower Patients," WebMD (April 18, 2000). <www.webmd.com>.

22. "Are DTC Ads Losing Their Punch?" *Drug Topics* 144, no. 6. (March 20, 2000): 8.

23. "National Study Finds Most Pharmaceutical Advertising Ineffective with Consumers," *PR Newswire* (December 2, 1998).

24. Michael F. Conlan, "Consumers Speak Out—Our Exclusive Survey Reveals How Consumers Rate Herbals, Internet Pharmacies, DTC Ads and Rheir Own Rx and More," *Drug Topics* 44, no. 6 (March 20, 2000): 71.

25. The Pew Research Center.

26. Rebecca Quick, "CybeRx: Getting Medical Advice and Moral Support on the Web," *The Wall Street Journal Interactive Edition* (April 30, 1998). <www.wsj.com>.

27. Joseph Goedert, "Medical Societies Enter Web Portal Wars," *Health Data Management* (December 1999): pITEM00088008.

28. Milt Freudenheim, "Advice is the Newest Prescription for Health Costs," *The New York Times Online* (April 9, 2000). <www.nytimes.com>.

29. Tim Radford, "Public Understanding and Biomedical Advance," *The Lancet* 349, no. 9070 (July 5, 1997): 55–57.

30. George A. Gellert, Kathleen V. Higgins, Rosann M. Lowery, et al., "A National Survey of Public Health Officer's Interactions with Media," *Journal of the American Medical Association* 271, no. 16 (April 27, 1994): 1285-1291.

31. Jean McCann, "Friendly Computer Voice Gets People to Take Their Medicine," *Drug Topics* 140, no. 18 (September 16, 1996): 50–52.

32. "Following ER," Johns Hopkins School of Public Health web site (June 28, 2000). <http://er.jhsph.edu>.

33. Allyson M. Pollock and Dorothy P. Rice, "Monitoring Health Care in the United States—A Challenging Task," *Public Health Reports* 112, no. 2 (March–April 1997): 108–114.

34. Interview with Mark Legnini (May 31, 2000).

News Interests, 2000

(percent of people aged 18 or older who follow news stories "very closely," by topic, 2000)

	percent
Crime	30%
Health	29
Sports	27
Community	26
Religion	21
Local government	20
Science and technology	18
Washington news	17
Entertainment news	14
International affairs	14
Business and finance	14
Consumer news	12
Culture and arts	10

Source: "Investors Now Go Online for Quotes, Advice—Internet Sapping Broadcast News Audience," The Pew Research Center for the People & the Press, June 11, 2000; Internet site <http://www.people-press.org>

Online News Topics, 2000

(percent of people aged 18 or older who go online for news, by topic they seek online, 2000)

	percent
Weather news	66%
Science/health news	63
Technology news	59
Business news	53
World news	45
Entertainment news	44
Sports news	42
Political news	39
Local news	37

Source: "Investors Now Go Online for Quotes, Advice—Internet Sapping Broadcast News Audience," The Pew Research Center for the People & the Press, June 11, 2000; Internet site <http://www.people-press.org>

Broadcast News versus Online News, 1998 and 2000

(percent of people aged 18 or older who regularly watch nightly network news or go online for news at least 3 days a week, by sex and education, 1998 and 2000; percentage point change, 1998–2000)

	nightly network news			online news		
	1998	*2000*	*percentage point change 1998–2000*	*1998*	*2000*	*percentage point change 1998–2000*
Total	**38%**	**30%**	**–8**	**13%**	**23%**	**10**
Men	34	29	–5	17	28	11
Women	40	31	–9	9	18	9
College graduate	40	28	–12	24	40	16
Some college	39	30	–9	16	29	13
High school graduate	39	32	–7	7	13	6
Not a high school graduate	29	30	1	6	8	2

Source: "Investors Now Go Online for Quotes, Advice—Internet Sapping Broadcast News Audience," The Pew Research Center for the People & the Press, June 11, 2000; Internet site <http://www.people-press.org>

Getting Health Information Online, 1999

(number and percent of people aged 18 or older with Internet access who have used the Internet to get health information in the previous 12 months, 1999)

Number of people using the Internet to get health information: 70 million

Percent of Internet users who look for information about health online:

Total seeking health information	74%
Often	13
Sometimes	30
Hardly ever	31
Never	26

Those using the Internet to get health information seek information about specific medical conditions:

Often	19
Sometimes	43
Hardly ever	23
Never	15

Those using the Internet to get health information are generally looking for information for:

Myself	55
Family member	57
Friend	15

Particular disease researched the last time they were on the Internet seeking health information:

Depression	19
Allergies or sinus	16
Cancer	15
Bipolar disorder	14
Arthritis/rheumatism	10
High blood pressure/hypertension	10
Migraine	9
Anxiety disorder	9
Heart disease	8
Sleep disorders	8
Asthma	6
Thyroid disorder	6
Diabetes (Type 2)	6
Alzheimer's	6
Chronic back problems	5

Source: "Explosive Growth of 'Cyberchondriacs' Continues," The Harris Poll, No. 47, August 5, 1999

Top Health Sites on the Internet, 1999

(number of unique visitors in October 1999 for the 15 most visited health information web sites; numbers in thousands)

rank	site	visitors
1	AOL Health Channel	3,567
2	ONHEALTH.COM	2,949
3	DRKOOP.COM	2,367
4	WEBMD.COM	1,608
5	NIH.GOV	1,453
6	PLANETRX.COM	1,349
7	MOTHERNATURE.COM	1,213
8	DRUGSTORE.COM	1,186
9	HEALTHSHOP.COM	1,100
10	THRIVEONLINE.COM	1,099
11	MAYOHEALTH.ORG	717
12	INTELIHEALTH.COM	699
13	MEDSCAPE.COM	517
14	HEALTHCENTRAL.COM	363
15	AMA-ASSN.ORG	324

Source: Media Metrix, *October 1999*

Source of Nutrition Information, 1999

(percent of people aged 18 or older citing media/professional as primary source of nutrition information and as most valued source of nutrition information, 1999)

Primary source of nutrition information

Television	48%
Magazines	47
Newspapers	18
Reference/general books	12
Family and friends	11
Doctors	11
Internet	6
Radio	5

Most valued source of nutrition information

Doctors	92
Registered dieticians	90
Nutritionists	90
Magazines	87
Nurses	85
Newspapers	82
TV news	79
Family and friends	69
Radio news	65
Non-news TV	61
Internet	61

Source: American Dietetic Association, Americans' Food and Nutrition Attitudes and Behaviors—American Dietetic Association's Nutrition and You: Trends 2000, *January 3, 2000; Internet site <http://www.eatright.org/pr/2000/010300a.html>*

Media Reporting on Food Safety and Nutrition, 1995 to 1999

(leading food safety and nutrition topics in the media, 1995 to 1999)

1999	1997	1995
1. Disease prevention	1. Foodborne illness	1. Fat intake
2. Foodborne illness	2. Fat intake	2. Disease prevention
3. Biotechnology	3. Disease prevention	3. Foodborne illness
4. Fat intake	4. Disease causation	4. Vitamin/mineral intake
5. Functional foods	5. Food trends	5. Disease causation
6. Disease causation	6. Vitamin/mineral intake	6. Caloric intake
7. Vitamin/mineral intake	7. Caloric intake	7. Antioxidants
8. Fiber intake	8. Food labels	8. Cholesterol intake
9. Antioxidants	9. Antioxidants	9. Sugar intake
10. Caloric intake	10. Weight loss	10. Fiber intake

Source: International Food Information Council Foundation and the Center for Media and Public Affairs, Food for Thought III, A Quantitative and Qualitative Content Analysis of Diet, Nutrition and Food Safety Reporting, *February 2000*

6

The Emerging Self-Care Industry

A trip to the hospital, or to the doctor, is an expensive proposition. In this era of managed care, it is no surprise, then, that efforts are being made to remove medical care from a medical setting. This cost-cutting trend, combined with the changing attitudes of Americans, is behind the shift from hospitals to homes, from waiting rooms to living rooms, as the preferred setting for medical care.

This shift is transforming both the hospital and nursing home industries. Institutions are emptying out as patients increasingly care for themselves at home. The deinstitutionalization of medical care is greatly favored by the nation's new health care consumers, within reason. The furor over shortened hospital stays for childbirth and same-day surgery for mastectomies shows the trend can only go so far before it meets consumer resistance.

Although it is getting more attention today, self-care is nothing new. Most medical problems are minor and recurring in nature, allowing the ailing to treat themselves rather than go to a doctor. The most common health problems experienced by adults are muscle aches and pains, headaches, and colds.[1] Usually, the only treatment these problems require is the application of an over-the-counter medication. According to a 1997 survey by Kline & Company for the Nonprescription Drug Manufacturers Association, 81 percent of consumers use over-the-counter medications for headaches. Three in four self-treat for colds, and more than half do so for allergies and yeast infections.[2]

Self-care is growing in popularity because of the rise in chronic conditions caused by the aging of the population. Younger Americans are the ones most likely to suffer from acute conditions, such as colds and injuries. Older Americans are the ones most likely to experience chronic conditions. Consequently, as the population ages, attitudes among health care providers and consumers are shifting from a "cure" to a "care" mentality. The long-term care required by chronic conditions means patients must become involved in treating themselves.

Another factor behind the increase in self-care is the growing list of health care products available to consumers. Each year the government is allowing more formerly prescription-only drugs to be sold over-the-counter, such as those that treat vaginal yeast infections and baldness. These new options are one reason why retail sales of OTC drugs have been so strong: $18.9 billion in 1999, up from $10.3 billion in 1990.[3]

This trend is just the beginning. Today, drugs can be sold without a prescription when they are intended to treat mild conditions, like headaches or upset stomach. The Food and Drug Administration may expand the category of drugs that can be bought over-the-counter to include drugs that patients take for chronic conditions—like hypertension or high cholesterol. Also under consideration for the move outside the pharmacists' domain are oral contraceptives and antibiotics. In a *New York Times* interview, Dr. Robert DeLap, who is heading the FDA's review, noted that "the health care environment has changed tremendously in recent years—people are much more interested in self-care and being able to manage minor conditions themselves."[4]

This move would dramatically change the economics of the pharmaceutical industry since over-the-counter drugs are cheaper than prescription drugs. It is also not without controversy. But whether or not the FDA dramatically changes its over-the-counter regulations, there's no doubt DeLap is correct—and that consumers will continue to look for ways to eliminate the people in white coats when it comes to minor ailments.

"With new opportunities in self-medication come. . .a growing need for knowledge," notes a pamphlet distributed by the Food and Drug Administration and the Nonprescription Drug Manufacturers Association.[5] Led by the baby-boom generation, Americans are becoming more educated about health and medical care, creating greater consumer participation not only in health care decisions but also in medical treatment itself. A growing variety of diagnostic tests are available to consumers, ranging from pregnancy kits to glucose monitoring equipment. Tests such as these allow consumers to diagnose and monitor conditions without seeing a doctor. Consumers can buy otoscopes to check children's ears for infection. They can buy genetic test kits to determine paternity, and they can buy kits to check for urinary tract infections. Coming soon are kits for hepatitis C, strep throat, and osteoporosis, according to *American Medical News*. In fact, noninvasive home tests for ovarian, colon, and testicular cancer may not be far in the future.[6] And in this age of wellness, there may be no reason to wait for results. A company called LifeShirt.com, in Ojai, California, sells shirts equipped with six types of sensors woven into the fabric, measuring such things as blood pressure and heart beat. The shirt connects to a handheld computer, which beams the information to a web site where it can be reviewed by physicians. "Being able to create a medical movie of a patient, any time of day or night, rather than relying on a few snapshots taken under clinical conditions, promises a far more accurate diagnosis," *The Economist* reports.[7]

With people able to diagnose themselves at home or on the road, health care providers will need to reinvent their relationship with health care consumers.

Alternative Medicine

Although many consumers depend on conventional medicine to treat their ailments—such as aspirin, digestive aids, and other over-the-counter options—millions of Americans turn to alternative medicine.

Alternative medicine is no longer on the fringes of the health care industry. Studies show the size of the alternative market rivals that of traditional medicine. Today, alternative treatments for problems ranging from the common cold to fatal diseases can be found not only in specialty shops but also in Main Street groceries and drugstores.

Alternative medicine encompasses many different practices, from bee sting therapy to yoga. The best description of alternative medicine, and one commonly used by medical professionals, is any treatment or therapy not commonly taught in medical school. Increas-

Americans spend big on alternative health care

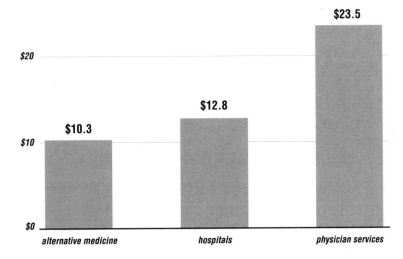

(out-of-pocket spending on alternative health care, hospitalizations, and physician services, 1990; in billions of dollars)

ingly, many medical professionals regard alternative therapy as complementary to conventional medicine. In fact, it is sometimes referred to as complementary alternative medicine.

Alternative medical treatments have been in use throughout human history, but what accounts for the current popularity of homeopathy, aroma therapy, feng shui, acupuncture, and other alternative treatments? Multiculturalism, for one. As the American population becomes more diverse, immigrants bring with them traditional medicines and folk treatments. Another reason for the growing popularity of alternative therapy is a backlash against the increasingly high-tech delivery of conventional medicine, where vision can be corrected with lasers, organs transplanted routinely, and fertility coolly manipulated. Alternative medicine puts a human face on medical care, offering a high-touch rather than a high-tech experience.

Another reason for the popularity of alternative medicine is the rising educational level of the population. The biggest fans of alternative medicine are the most educated Americans, the ones most likely to eschew authority and to investigate and treat health problems themselves.

Another factor driving growth in alternative treatments is the fallibility of modern medicine itself. Every day, it seems, headlines announce yet another problem with modern medicine. Antibiotics are overprescribed and create disease resistant bacteria. Mammograms can give false positive results. Heroic medical efforts can lead to machine-dependent lives.

The well-educated are most likely to use alternative health care

(percent of people aged 18 or older having used alternative health care in the past 12 months, 1998)

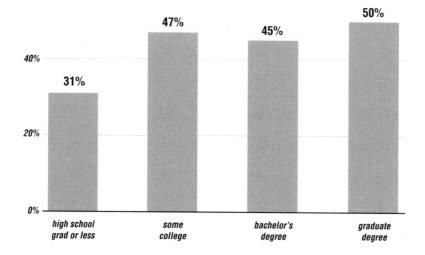

The lessons learned from headlines such as these is that conventional medicine can harm as well as help. Today's new health care consumers are not willing to accept illness, disability, or death. They want answers, solutions, and cures. Alternative medicine allows these educated activists to feel that they control their physical well-being.

How many Americans turn to alternative treatments? Despite the ubiquitous presence of nontraditional medicine in the consumer marketplace—from drugstore shelves to best-seller lists—few studies have attempted to determine the characteristics of the users of alternative medicine.

The first representative survey of Americans' use of alternative health care was done in 1991 by a group of doctors led by David M. Eisenberg, published in *The New England Journal of Medicine* in 1993.[8] After listing 16 alternative therapies—including chiropractic, herbal medicines, homeopathy, and spiritual healing—Eisenberg et al. asked survey respondents whether they had used any of the treatments in the past 12 months. They also asked whether respondents had seen a provider of alternative medicine, and if so how much they paid for treatment. The results were astounding. The study found 34 percent of people aged 18 or older had used at least one unconventional therapy in 1990. During the year, Americans visited alternative care providers an estimated 425 million times, a figure that exceeded the number of visits to all primary care physicians in the U.S. The public paid these providers $11.7 billion—70 percent of it out-of-pocket. According to the researchers, this figure is nearly equivalent to the amount Americans spend out-of-pocket on hospitalizations, and is about half of what they spend out-of-pocket on physician visits. Patients paid an average of $27.60 per visit to alternative therapists in 1990, with charges ranging from under $20 for some treatments to more than $100 for others. These are impressive numbers and probably underestimated, the researchers note, because the study underrepresented the sick—who are more likely to use alternative treatments. And the estimates did not include the billions of dollars Americans spend on over-the-counter alternative remedies, books, and supplies.

The biggest surprise of the 1991 study was that "the use of unconventional therapy was not confined to any narrow segment of U.S. society," according to the researchers. Those most likely to turn to alternative therapies were people aged 25 to 49 (38 percent), those with household incomes of $35,000 or more (39 percent), college graduates (44 percent), and people living in the West (44 percent). "Unconventional medicine has an enormous presence in the U.S. health care system," the researchers concluded.

A 1997 study found that 42 percent of people aged 18 or older with health insurance had used alternative therapies, according to Landmark Healthcare, an alternative health insurer.[9] Herbal therapy was the type of alternative medicine most commonly used, cited by 17 percent, followed by chiropractic (16 percent), massage (14 percent), and vitamin therapy (13 percent).

In 1998, John A. Astin updated the Eisenberg et al. study, publishing his findings in the *Journal of the American Medical Association*.[10] While not strictly comparable with the earlier research, the 1998 study found 40 percent of people aged 18 or older having used alternative medicine in the past 12 months—somewhat higher than the 34 percent of 1990. Those most likely to use alternative medicine were the most educated adults, including 50 percent of people with graduate degrees. Education was the most important determinant of the use of alternative medicine, according to Astin. Another important predictor was attitude. People having a holistic philosophy of health (defined as those who agree with the statement, "The health of my body, mind, and spirit are related, and whoever cares for my health should take that into account") were much more likely to use alternative medicine than others—46 versus 33 percent.

Interestingly, Astin's study showed that users of alternative medicine did not do so because they were dissatisfied with conventional medicine. In fact, nearly three-quarters of those who use alternative medicine simultaneously use conventional care, according to the Landmark study. Only 15 percent use alternative treatments as a replacement for traditional care.

Chronic conditions are the main reason people turn to unconventional therapy— chronic pain being the number one problem for which people seek alternative therapy, according to the 1998 study. The second-most-commonly reported problem is anxiety, followed by chronic fatigue syndrome, sprains and muscle strains, addictive problems, arthritis, headaches, depression, digestive problems, and diabetes. To treat these problems, people turn to exercise, chiropractic, massage, herbs, self-help groups, homeopathy, diet change, and a variety of other therapies.

The importance of chronic conditions in driving people to alternative medicine explains why older Americans seek alternative treatments. Although people aged 65 or older are less likely to use alternative medicine than younger consumers, when they do go to an alternative provider they are more likely to make frequent visits—an average of ten visits for older Americans versus three for younger consumers, according to a study by D. F. Foster, M.D., reported in *The Back Letter*.[11] The most common alternative therapies used by people aged 65 or older were chiropractic (11 percent), herbal remedies (8 percent), relaxation techniques (5 percent), high-dose or megavitamins (4 percent), and religious or spiritual healing (4 percent). Arthritis, back pain, heart disease, allergy, and diabetes were the most common reasons why older Americans sought alternative therapies. Interestingly, Foster's study also showed that older consumers who had a primary care provider were about five times more likely to use alternative medicines than those without a provider.

The question surrounding many alternative medicines is not whether to use it, but how to integrate its use with traditional treatment. Doctors today are grappling with ways to combine alternative and traditional medical treatments to improve patient outcomes. Many consumers don't tell their doctor when they use alternative remedies, according to *Medical Economics*.[12] In a study of women with breast cancer conducted by the University of California at San Francisco, 70 percent of women in the study had used alternative therapies. Many of those using alternative therapies did not discuss this fact with their physicians because they thought it wasn't relevant to their treatment, or they thought their doctor didn't care or would disapprove. A University of Pennsylvania Cancer Center study found that about 40 percent of patients taking unconventional medications for cancer did not tell their physicians about it unless they were specifically asked.[13]

Hospital care

The rise of self-care, including home health care, has transformed the hospital industry. Between 1980 and 1998, the average length of a hospital stay has declined by more than two days. This shift has had a big financial impact on the bottom line of the hospital industry. Hospital admissions fell 13 percent between 1980 and 1998. Consequently, the hospital industry is shrinking. There were 14 percent fewer hospitals in 1998 than in 1980. The number of hospital beds is down 26 percent. Nevertheless, the hospital occupancy rate also fell— declining from 78 percent in 1980 to 65 percent in 1998.

Hospitals discharged 32 million customers in 1998. The average length of stay was 5.1 days. Men have longer average stays than women—5.5 versus 4.7 days. Women's stays are shorter because many are in the hospital only to give birth. Deliveries accounted for 4 million hospital discharges in 1998, with an average length of stay of just 2.5 days.

Hospitals are in a dilemma. To be attractive to managed care, they must cut costs. But to attract patients, they need to provide high-quality service. Differences in the quality of care among hospitals are critically important to patients. When Yale University researchers studied the records of more than 150,000 heart attack patients, they discovered that patients at hospitals ranked high in the field of cardiology were 17 percent more likely to survive than those at less advanced hospitals.[14]

The balance between efficiency and quality is difficult to achieve. Teaching hospitals, which provide medical education and conduct research, for example, are often more expensive than nonteaching hospitals. This places them at a competitive disadvantage in the era of managed care. But the quality of care may be better at teaching hospitals than at nonteaching hospitals. After examining 30 hospitals and nearly 90,000 discharged patients in northeastern Ohio, researchers found teaching hospitals had a lower death rate and shorter length of stay than nonteaching hospitals.[15]

Public hospitals face a similar dilemma. Because public hospitals overwhelmingly serve the poor, they must compete fiercely in order to retain their paying customers, who help subsidize indigent care. The consequences of this competition are serious. In a Hastings Center Report, author Peter MacPherson examined the consequences in Las Vegas, where five of the seven community hospitals are for-profit companies. MacPherson describes Las Vegas's public University Medical Center as the "poor person's hospital." To attract paying patients, writes MacPherson, "The hospital has spent lavishly improving its labor and delivery suite. Childbirth is an important source of revenue to almost all hospitals. . . UMC needed to protect this business line."[16] Ironically, however, the hospital's focus on attracting paying patients to subsidize indigent care has shifted assets away from caring for the indigent themselves.

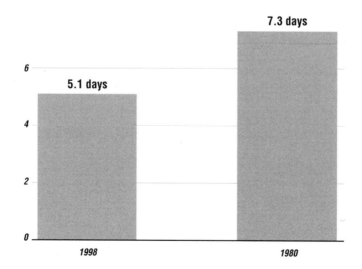

Hospital stays are shorter

(average length of stay in nonfederal, short-stay hospitals, 1980 and 1998)

For poor patients, then, hospital options are increasingly limited. One way in which hospitals are pulling in more paying patients is by offering a greater variety of outpatient services. These include convenient care centers where walk-in patients can be seen at any time of day without an appointment. They also include same-day surgery centers as an alternative to overnight hospital stays.

A growing area of competition within the hospital industry are ambulatory surgery centers set up by doctors. These centers siphon money and patients away from hospitals and their outpatient departments. Because ambulatory centers can be highly specialized, their expenses are lower. Consequently, they can charge as much as 20 to 25 percent less than a hospital.[17] This competition is a serious problem for hospitals, which increasingly depend on outpatient revenue. Between 1980 and 1998, the number of outpatient hospital visits more than doubled, rising from 263 million to 545 million. Today, fully 62 percent of surgeries are performed on outpatients, up from only 16 percent in 1980.

For patients who can pay, hospitals are willing to jump through hoops. Increasingly, the hospital experience includes new facilities and the latest in technology. In Buffalo's Mercy Hospital, for example, computer terminals allow patients to get information about illnesses and possible treatments.[18] Columbia Hospital for Women in Washington, D.C., hired a Four Seasons Hotel vice president to train staff and suggest ways to improve the

Hospital occupancy rate is down

(percent of hospital beds occupied, 1980 and 1998)

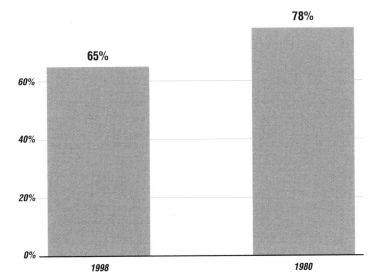

atmosphere.[19] This is a nod to the power of the new health care consumer. Hospitals like Columbia are hoping patients will select a managed care plan based on a positive hospital experience, and that managed care plans will take notice.

Hospitals believe consumers are the ultimate market drivers, according to a study by KPMG, but they are frustrated by the fact that insurers come between hospitals and consumers.[20] Some hospitals are revamping their information technology capabilities to smooth the process of third-party payments. Scripps Health, for example, which has six hospitals in San Diego, is upgrading its information technology to the tune of $75 million to link medical and administrative information through a broadband-enabled web hook-up.[21]

Home health care

Shorter hospital stays mean more patients must recover at home, giving rise to the home health care industry. Home health care is growing so rapidly that it accounts for two of the fastest growing occupational categories in the United States, according to projections by the Bureau of Labor Statistics. Between 1998 and 2008, it projects the number of personal and home care aides to increase 58 percent, making it the seventh-fastest-growing occupation in the nation. During the coming decade, health services figure to be the second-fastest-growing industry in the U.S.

Most surgeries are now performed on outpatients

(percent of total surgeries performed on outpatients, 1980 and 1998)

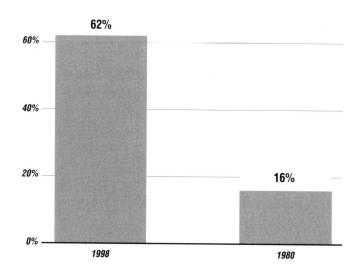

The home health care industry included 13,500 agencies in 1996, up from just 8,000 in 1992, according to the National Center for Health Statistics—a 69 percent increase. The 54 percent majority of home health care agencies are privately owned, while 34 percent are nonprofit organizations and 11 percent are owned by governments or some other type of organization. Almost half (48 percent) are part of a group or chain of agencies, and 27 percent are owned by hospitals.

Behind the rapid growth in home health care are several important trends, according to the National Center for Health Statistics: (1) advances in medical technology that allow people to be cared for at home at a much lower cost than in an institution; (2) Medicare's inclusion of home health care services in its benefits; (3) the increase in the elderly population; and (4) the preference of consumers for home health care.

Millions of Americans are customers of the home health care industry. In 1996, at any one time, 2.4 million patients were under the care of a home health care agency. During the entire year, home health care agencies discharged 7.8 million customers. Most home health care patients are elderly—72 percent are aged 65 or older and half are aged 75 or older. Because most older Americans are women, so too are two out of three home health care patients. Thirty-five percent of home health care patients are widowed and another 19 percent have never married. These statistics explain why millions of people need the help of a home health care agency. Many have no one at home to help them recover from illness.

Most home health care patients are elderly

(percent distribution of home health care patients, by age, 1996)

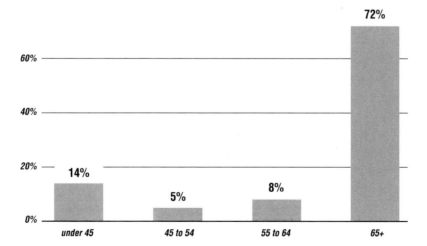

Hospital patients are often discharged to home health care agencies to complete their rehabilitation. This is one reason why hospitals have been able to shorten lengths of stay. Diseases of the circulatory system are the most common diagnosis for home health care patients, with 22 percent recovering from cardiovascular surgery. Another 27 percent of home health care patients are recovering from broken bones, hip replacements, and so on. Diabetes is also a common diagnosis.

Home health care's popularity has forced hospitals and nursing homes to become more competitive to attract patients. Hospitals are redesigning their floors to include family rooms, softer lighting, and home furnishings. Nursing homes are remaking themselves to look more like private residences, with doors that lock and kitchenettes. The impact of home health care can also be seen in statistics on nursing home residents. Until the late 1980s, the nursing home business enjoyed rapid growth. The number of nursing home residents climbed 37 percent between 1973–74 and 1985. But between 1985 and 1997, the number of residents rose only 11 percent. During those years, the number of nursing home residents per 1,000 people aged 65 or older dropped from 46.2 to 43.4.

"Everyone is more comfortable in their own home," explains Tami Gazzero, director of nursing at Genesis Home Health Agency in Watertown, New York, about the popularity of home health care services. "There's time to do one-on-one that you don't have in the hospital," she says.[22] Home care allows nurses and aides the chance to see patients in context, she says, which may alert health care providers to problems such as abuse. Home health care workers can also act as patient advocates in dealing with physicians, she says.

Nursing home care is less likely for older Americans

(number of nursing home residents per 1,000 people in age group, 1973–74 and 1997)

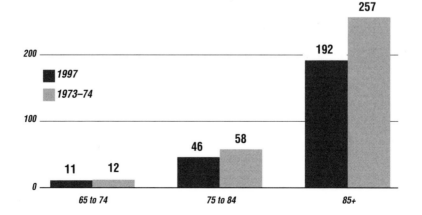

The deinstitutionalization of medical care is likely to continue because health care consumers prefer to be cared for at home. But the rapid growth in home health care cannot be sustained, especially with the federal government stepping in to regulate services. The 1998 balanced budget agreement included $16 billion in cuts to Medicare's home health care budget over the next five years. And indeed, Medicare spending on home health care dropped from $17.5 billion in 1997 to $9.7 billion in 1999, according to the Congressional Budget Office. Some Medicare patients have had to spend more time in the hospital because they have not been able to afford home care, and some elderly patients have not gotten the care they need.[23] As baby boomers age, pressure will grow on Congress to loosen restrictions on home care.

The growing home health care industry is already confronting the same problems hospitals face today—the need to attract insurers through lower costs while attracting patients with high-quality service. However this paradox is resolved, home health care is here to stay, certain to become an increasingly important component of medical care—especially in later life.

The future of self-care

The economic and demographic trends all point in one direction: Increasingly, the ailing will be cared for at home. Hospitals and nursing homes will become facilities of last resort, reserved for the sickest. This has profound implications for all Americans, requiring us to become more involved in caring not only for ourselves, but also for our loved ones.

Trend 1: Technology to the rescue

The technological revolution is certain to come to the aid of the home health care industry. New technologies will allow patients to care for themselves or aid families in caring for their loved ones. An *Annals of Internal Medicine* survey found that most patients with pneumonia preferred to be treated at home, but hesitated to do so because of concerns over how their family would cope with the burden.[24] As technologies become available to ease the duties of caregivers, more patients will opt for home care.

One technology certain to revolutionize home care is telemedicine—or health care at a distance. Telemedicine is already well received by the medical community. The *American Journal of Obstetrics and Gynecology* reported in 1997 that fetal ultrasounds transmitted via modem were just as good, if not better, than videotaped recordings.[25,26] Not only can telemedicine bring doctors closer to patients located far from medical facilities, it can also be cost-effective—especially as the price of technology falls.

Telemedicine will make even more financial sense once greater numbers of homes go online. In the future, consumers could perform medically accredited self-diagnostics at home, then shop their symptoms via the Internet for suggested treatments. This practice would reduce the number of unnecessary office visits and eliminate the lag time in procuring second or third opinions. It could also reduce the time doctors spend taking vital signs, which could be e-mailed ahead or brought in on a disk, much like bringing in a urine sample today.

As telemedicine becomes mainstream, it will change the face of medicine entirely. Doctors and nurses will spend less time collecting data and more time analyzing it. This will place even greater importance on the evolving relationship between health care providers and consumers.

Telemedicine is not home free. Many obstacles to its growth remain, including licensing difficulties, concerns among some doctors about the erosion of their patient base, the expense of equipment, and liability issues. Payment is also a problem, since presently most insurers only cover face-to-face consultations.

TREND 2: MORE SUPPORT FOR CAREGIVERS

The National Association of Home Care estimates that from 9 million to 11 million Americans need home health care services, a number that far surpasses the 2.5 million current patients. This disparity means that most Americans in need of care receive it informally from friends and family members. A Bureau of the Census study found 9.3 million Americans providing regular, unpaid care to a family member or friend in 1996. Those caring for people in their home provided an average of 42 hours of care per week, while those caring for people living elsewhere provided 16 hours of care per week. Two-thirds of informal caregivers are women.

As boomers age, this kind of informal care may not be readily available. Many boomers do not have children, while others have only one or two, limiting the number of potential caregivers. In addition, the boomer propensity to divorce means many will be alone in old age. Products and services to assist informal caregivers, such as adult day care, as well as options for those who live alone will grow in popularity.

TREND 3: ALTERNATIVE MEDICINE WILL BECOME MAINSTREAM

When well-educated baby boomers encounter more health problems as they age, demand for alternative medical care will grow. As alternative treatments gain acceptance, many of them will lose their radical image. The first sign of the mainstreaming of alternative medicine came in 1992, when the Department of Health and Human Services created the Office of Alternative Medicine. Today, doctors and hospitals are offering acupuncture, therapeutic touch, and biofeedback. Alternative therapies are gaining ground in other ways as well. The vanguard of conventional medicine, The National Institutes of Health, has issued the opinion that acupuncture is effective in treating nausea and pain. New York State now requires insurers to cover chiropractic care. The *Journal of the American Medical Association* gave megavitamin therapy a favorable review for reducing the risk of heart disease.[27]

But how can alternative medicine survive on Main Street? Certainly not in its current form. When a trend moves from the fringes to the center of society, it is transformed in much the same way as a business when it grows from an entrepreneurial organization to an established bureaucracy. The organic food industry is an example of what happens when a marginal operation moves into the mainstream. Organic foods were barely a blip in the agricultural industry until sales in the category began to grow more than 20 percent per year. By the early 1990s, the organic food industry had become large enough to merit attention, particularly because the term "organic" did not have a legal definition. Thus began a huge political debate over the definition of organic. Did it include irradiated food? Did it include biologically enhanced foods? When the government invited public discussion, it received an estimated 150,000 comments. The final rules haven't been released yet.

If organic foods had remained a fringe product, they would not have attracted the attention of food industry giants like Gerber. As big corporations enter the fray, executives replace ideologues as industry leaders. The CEOs of profit-making businesses act differently than freethinkers on a spiritual quest. With money to be made, regulations are sure to follow. The organic food industry had no choice but to become organized—and to lose some of what made it special in the first place.

Alternative medicine is guaranteed to experience similar growing pains, especially because many of its features appeal to profit-making businesses. Unlike conventional medicine, which is closely monitored and directed by insurance companies, alternative medicine is directed by individual consumers and practitioners. Because insurance doesn't yet pay for most alternative therapies, there are no insurance limitations on the number of visits allowed or brands of medications to be used. And because so much alternative treatment is provided on a fee-for-service basis, it bypasses costly paperwork and third-party billing processes—boosting profits.

Today, alternative medicine is largely unregulated. It will not remain so for long. As alternative medicine becomes more popular and gains credibility in the medical community, the Food and Drug Administration will be obligated to put alternative medications through the same rigorous evaluation process that conventional treatments must pass. This will lead to greater lag time between innovation and consumer use, as is the case for conventional treatments. Practitioners will need certification, which raises their fees. Insurance paperwork, research and testing expenses, and certification requirements will drive up the cost of alternative medicine, making it more difficult for consumers to pay for it out-of-pocket. Alternative medicine will have become mainstream.

TREND 4: THE BACKLASH AGAINST ALTERNATIVE MEDICINE

Many in the medical community are not happy with the growing number of alternative enthusiasts, or with its growing acceptance in the medical establishment. Some are trying to debunk alternative therapies. One debunking study, conducted by nine-year-old Emily Rosa and published in the *Journal of the American Medical Association*, disputed the effectiveness of therapeutic touch therapy.[28] This practice involves manipulating an energy field said to hover above the body. In her study, Rosa found therapeutic touch practitioners able to detect energy fields only 44 percent of the time, which is less than pure guesswork. Rosa was encouraged to publish her study—originally intended as a school project—by Stephen Barret, psychiatrist and professional skeptic. While the dissenters are fighting the far stronger tide of growing acceptance of alternative medicine, they make at least one point on which all agree: There's plenty of snake oil out there. As alternative medicine becomes mainstreamed, research will reveal what works and what doesn't, causing a much-needed shake-out in the industry.

The consumers of alternative medicine will not be happy about the mainstreaming process either. Already, major companies are running into problems marketing alternative medical products, such as Campbell Soup's Intelligent Quisine. Although Intelligent Quisine had a variety of problems, the fatal blow may have been that the product did not give consumers enough control. A diet is a diet, regardless of whether it is conventional or alternative medicine. Also, the program cost $80 a week, making drug therapy not only easier but cheaper. Companies marketing alternative health care must make sure their products offer the benefits that draw consumers to alternative medicine in the first place, such as individual control and lower costs.

Alternative medicine will never be for the masses. It will remain the province of the well-educated and well-off because staying abreast of alternative therapies requires time and research skills. In addition, because so many alternative medical treatments are self-directed, users must be highly self-motivated. Consequently, most alternative therapies would be extremely difficult to implement as public health initiatives.

Alternative medicine will face greater competition from conventional medicine in the years ahead as well. Drugs such as Propecia for baldness and Viagra for impotence are a direct challenge to alternative medicine because they help users take control of lifestyle issues typically left to alternative treatments. As pharmaceuticals become more sophisticated, they may erode the alternative market. And if conventional medicine achieves a real breakthrough—such as a cure for cancer—consumers are likely to abandon alternative therapy and embrace conventional treatment.

Notes

1. Nonprescription Drug Manufacturers Association, *Self-Medication in the '90's: Practices and Perceptions* (November 1992): 23–32.

2. Kline and Company Inc., *Economic Benefits of Self-Medication—A Final Report to the Nonprescription Drug Manufacturers Association* (May 15, 1997): 13.

3. Consumer Healthcare Products Association, *OTC Retail Sales 1964–1999* (July 11, 2000). <www.nmdainfo.org>.

4. Sheryl Gay Stolberg, "FDA Considers Switching Some Prescription Drugs to Over-the-Counter Status," *New York Times* Online (June 28, 2000). <www.nytimes.com>.

5. United States Food and Drug Administration and Nonprescription Drug Manufacturers Association, "Nonprescription Medicines: What's Right for You?" Publication 621-C. (Pueblo, Colorado, Consumer Information Center).

6. Deborah L. Shelton, "Home Tests Test Doctor's Role," *American Medical News* 42, no. 13 (April 5, 1999): 26.

7. "Medical Monitoring: Web Shirts," *The Economist* 353, no. 8148 (December 4, 1999): 78.

8. David M. Eisenberg, Ronald C. Kessler, Cindy Foster, et al., "Unconventional Medicine in the United States—Prevalence, Cost and Patterns of Use," *The New England Journal of Medicine* 328, no. 4 (January 28, 1993): 246–52.

9. Landmark Healthcare Inc., *The Landmark Report on Public Perceptions of Alternative Care* (January 1998): 12, 18.

10. John A. Astin, "Why Patients Use Alternative Medicine," *Journal of the American Medical Association* 279, no. 19 (May 20, 1998): 1548–1554.

11. "Alternative Medicine Use Common among the Elderly," *The Back Letter* 14, no. 14 (May 1999): 50.

12. Joan R. Rose, "Who Else Is Treating Your Patients," *Medical Economics* 77, no. 7 (April 10, 2000): 33.

13. Rebecca Voelker, "Do Ask, Do Tell," *Journal of the American Medical Association* 283, no. 24 (June 28, 2000): 3189.

14. Avery Camarow Chrof, Richard Folkers, et al., "The Best Hospitals are the Best," *US News and World Report* 126, no. 5 (February 8, 1999): 67.

15. Gary E. Rosenthal, Dwain L. Harper, Linda M. Quinn, and Gregory S. Cooper, "Severity-adjusted Mortality and Length of Stay in Teaching and Nonteaching Hospitals: Results of a Regional Study," *Journal of the American Medical Association* 278, no. 6 (August 13, 1997): 485–491.

16. Peter MacPherson, "Is This Where We Want to Go?" *The Hastings Center Report* 27, no. 6 (November-December 1997): 17–23.

17. Judith Messina, "Hospital Fights Surgery Sights," *Crain's New York Business* 16 (April 30, 2000): 3.

18. "Computer Terminal Aids Hospital Patients," *Business First of Buffalo* (February 14, 2000): 3

19. Suz Redfearn, "Hospitals Look to Hotels for Business Tips," *Baltimore Business Journal* 16, no 47 (April 9, 1999): 20.

20. "Balance of Power Needed in Industry," *Health Management Technology* 19, no. 1 (December 1998): 8.

21. Alan Joch, "Getting a Network Transplant," *eWeek* (June 26, 2000): 74.

22. Interview with Tami Gazzero, November 1997.

23. J.P. Bender, "Medicare Home Health Care Plunges," *South Florida Business Journal* 20 (May 26, 2000): 1.

24. A. Russell Localio, Bruce H. Hamory, Tonya J. Sharp, Susan L. Weaver, Thomas R. TenHave, and J. Richard Landis, "Comparing Hospital Mortality in Adult Patients with Pneumonia: A Case Study of Statistical Methods in a Managed Care Program," *Annals of Internal Medicine* 122, no. 2 (January 15, 1995): 125–133.

25. Fergal D. Malone, Jose A. Nores, and Achilles Athanassiou, et al. "Validation of Fetal Telemedicine as a New Obstetric Technique," *American Journal of Obstetrics and Gynecology* 177, no. 3 (September 1997): 626–629.

26. Joseph B. Landwher, Ivan E. Zador, and Honor M. Wolfe et al., "Telemedicine and Fetal Ultrasonography: Assessment of Technical Performance and Clinical Feasibility," *American Journal of Obstetrics and Gynecology* 177, no. 3 (September 1997): 846-849.

27. Eric B. Rimm, Walter C. Willet, Frank B. Hu, and Laura Sampson, et al., "Folate and Vitamin B6 from Diet and Supplements in Relation to Risk of Coronary Heart Disease among Woman," *Journal of the American Medical Association* 279, no. 5 (February 4, 1998): c15.

28. Linda Rosa, Emily Rosa, Larry Sainer, and Stephen Barret, "A Close Look at Therapeutic Touch," *Journal of the American Medical Association* 279, no. 13 (April 1, 1998) 1005–1011.

Top 25 Health Problems in an Average Two-Week Period: Adults

(percent of people aged 18 or older reporting health problems during the past two weeks, by type of problem, 1992; ranked by percent reporting problem)

	percent reporting
Muscle aches/pains	34%
Headache	33
Common cold	31
Lip problems	31
Overweight problems	30
Upset stomach	29
Minor cuts/scratches	26
Sinus problems	25
Acne/pimples	23
Eye problems	23
Sleep problems	23
Fatigue	22
Teeth problems	21
Back problems	20
Arthritis/rheumatism	19
Painful dry skin	18
Bruises	14
Anxiety	14
Premenstrual problems	12
Constipation	11
Overindulgence of food	11
Bunions/corns/calluses	11
Diarrhea	10
Sore throat not associated with a cold	10
Hay fever	10

Source: Consumer Healthcare Products Association, Self-Medication in the '90s: Practices and Perceptions, *1992*

Top 25 Health Problems in an Average Two-Week Period: Children

(percent of people under age 18 self-reporting or parent-reporting health problems during the past two weeks, by type of problem; ranked by percent reporting problem, 1992)

	percent reporting
Common cold	26%
Minor cuts/scratches	21
Lip problems	19
Bruises	16
Diarrhea	12
Upset stomach	10
Teeth problems	10
Sore throat not associated with a cold	8
Headache	7
Sinus problems	7
Acne/pimples	6
Eye problems	6
Painful dry skin	5
Constipation	5
Hay fever	5
Muscle aches/pains	4
Overweight problems	4
Sleep problems	4
Overindulgence of food	2
Fatigue	1
Back problems	1
Anxiety	1
Arthritis/rheumatism	–
Premenstrual problems	–
Bunions/corns/calluses	–

Note: (–) means not applicable or sample too small to make a reliable estimate.
Source: Consumer Healthcare Products Association, Self-Medication in the '90s: Practices and Perceptions, *1992*

Top 25 Health Problems in an Average Two-Week Period: Men and Women

(percent of people aged 18 or older reporting health problems during the past two weeks, by type of problem and sex, 1992; ranked by percent of total population reporting problem)

	men	women
Muscle aches/pains	35%	34%
Headache	32	34
Common cold	34	28
Lip problems	26	35
Overweight problems	22	36
Upset stomach	27	30
Minor cuts/scratches	35	17
Sinus problems	22	28
Acne/pimples	20	25
Eye problems	24	22
Sleep problems	22	24
Fatigue	17	25
Teeth problems	24	18
Back problems	18	22
Arthritis/rheumatism	16	22
Painful dry skin	17	19
Bruises	14	15
Anxiety	10	18
Premenstrual problems	–	22
Constipation	7	15
Overindulgence of food	12	9
Bunions/corns/calluses	6	15
Diarrhea	9	10
Sore throat not associated with a cold	8	12
Hay fever	8	11

Note: (–) means not applicable.
Source: Consumer Healthcare Products Association, Self-Medication in the '90s: Practices and Perceptions, 1992

Top 25 Health Problems in an Average Two-Week Period: Age Groups

(percent of people aged 18 or older reporting health problems during the past two weeks, by type of problem and age, 1992; ranked by percent of total population reporting problem)

	aged 18–34	*aged 35–54*	*aged 55–64*	*aged 65+*
Muscle aches/pains	33%	37%	37%	32%
Headache	41	37	20	17
Common cold	40	28	24	19
Lip problems	41	30	24	17
Overweight problems	23	35	40	26
Upset stomach	30	31	30	22
Minor cuts/scratches	38	24	16	6
Sinus problems	26	31	21	15
Acne/pimples	40	18	6	3
Eye problems	22	22	26	21
Sleep problems	22	19	30	29
Fatigue	23	28	13	11
Teeth problems	21	25	17	13
Back problems	21	22	18	14
Arthritis/rheumatism	5	22	34	38
Painful dry skin	19	20	15	14
Bruises	20	13	10	8
Anxiety	13	18	14	10
Premenstrual problems	16	14	–	–
Constipation	10	10	13	17
Overindulgence of food	10	14	10	6
Bunions/corns/calluses	5	12	16	20
Diarrhea	12	11	7	5
Sore throat not associated with a cold	13	9	9	3
Hay fever	10	13	7	6

Note: (–) means sample is too small to make a reliable estimate.
Source: Consumer Healthcare Products Association, Self-Medication in the '90s: Practices and Perceptions, *1992*

Minor Health Problems Treated by Over-the-Counter Medications, 1997

(percent of people with minor health problems who self-treat with over-the-counter medications, by type of problem, 1997; ranked by percent who self-treat)

	percent treating with over-the-counter medication
Jock itch	100.0%
Athlete's foot	85.5
Heartburn/indigestion	82.2
Headache	81.3
Common cold	73.9
Acne	59.2
Allergy	56.3
Rash/itchy skin	55.3
Vaginal yeast infection	52.6
Arthritis	49.2
Backache	42.7
Sinusitis	31.9

Source: Kline & Company, Inc., Economic Benefits of Self-Medication—A Final Report to the Nonprescription Drug Manufacturers Association, *May 15, 1997*

Alternative Health Care Use, 1990

(percent of people aged 18 or older who used alternative health care in the past 12 months, percent seeing professional providers, and average number of visits per user, by type of care, 1990)

	percent using	percent seeing provider	average number of visits per user in past 12 months
Total using one or more therapies*	**34%**	**36%**	**19**
Relaxation techniques	13	9	19
Chiropractic	10	70	13
Massage	7	41	15
Imagery	4	15	14
Spiritual healing	4	9	14
Commercial weight-loss programs	4	24	23
Lifestyle diets	4	13	8
Herbal medicine	3	10	8
Megavitamin therapy	2	12	13
Self-help groups	2	38	21
Energy healing	1	32	8
Biofeedback	1	21	6
Hypnosis	1	52	3
Homeopathy	1	32	6
Acupuncture	< 1	91	38
Folk remedies	< 1	0	0
Exercise**	26	–	–
Prayer**	25	–	–

* Excluding exercise or prayer.
** Users of exercise or prayer were not asked about providers or visits.
Source: The New England Journal of Medicine, *"Unconventional Medicine in the United States—Prevalence, Costs, and Patterns of Use," David M. Eisenberg et al., January 28, 1993. Copyright © 1993 Massachusetts Medical Society.*

Spending on Alternative Health Care, 1990

(selected characteristics of expenditures on alternative health care, 1990)

Average spending

Average charge per visit to provider	$27.60
Average out-of-pocket payment per visit	19.39

Total spending (in billions)

Alternative medical care, total*	$13.7
Services of providers	11.7
Megavitamin supplements	0.8
Commercial diet supplements	1.2

Percent of spending

Unreimbursed by third-party payer	55%
Partially reimbursed by third-party payer	31
Totally reimbursed by third-party payer	14
Percent of total charges paid out-of-pocket	70

Comparative spending (in billions)

Out-of-pocket spending on alternative medicine	$10.3
Out-of-pocket spending on hospitalizations	12.8
Out-of-pocket spending on physicians' services	23.5

* Total spending includes only services of providers, over-the-counter vitamins, and diet supplements. It does not include spending on herbs, medical equipment, devices, books, or other material.
Source: The New England Journal of Medicine, "Unconventional Medicine in the United States—Prevalence, Costs, and Patterns of Use," David M. Eisenberg et al., January 28, 1993. Copyright © 1993 Massachusetts Medical Society.

Alternative Health Care Use, 1997

(percent of people aged 18 or older with health insurance who used alternative care in the previous 12 months, and percent of participants who use professional providers, by type of care, 1997)

	percent using	percent seeing provider
Any therapy	**42%**	–
Herbal therapy	17	15%
Chiropractic	16	99
Massage therapy	14	84
Vitamin therapy	13	21
Homeopathy	5	27
Yoga	5	40
Acupressure	5	31
Biofeedback	2	65
Acupuncture	2	94
Hypnotherapy	1	80
Naturopathy	1	38

Note: (–) means data not available.
Source: Landmark Healthcare, Inc., The Landmark Report on Public Perceptions of Alternative Care, *1998*

Likelihood of Using Alternative Health Care, 1997

(percent of people aged 18 or older with health insurance who are aware of alternative care by likelihood of ever using care, 1997; ranked by percent saying "very likely")

	very likely	somewhat likely	not likely
Massage therapy	38%	42%	20%
Vitamin therapy	35	45	20
Chiropractic	33	40	26
Herbal therapy	33	42	25
Homeopathy	20	41	40
Naturopathy	20	38	41
Acupressure	18	49	33
Biofeedback	15	41	44
Yoga	12	26	61
Acupuncture	10	32	58
Hypnotherapy	9	27	63

Source: Landmark Healthcare, Inc., The Landmark Report on Public Perceptions of Alternative Care, *1998*

Characteristics of the Users of Alternative Health Care, 1998

(percent of people aged 18 or older who used alternative health care during the past 12 months by selected characteristics, 1998)

	percent
Total	**40%**
Age	
Aged 18 to 24	35
Aged 25 to 34	41
Aged 35 to 49	42
Aged 50 to 64	44
Aged 65 or older	35
Race and Hispanic origin	
White	41
Black	29
Hispanic	40
Asian	44
Native American	71
Other	44
Sex	
Male	39
Female	41
Education	
High school graduate or less	31
Some college	47
Bachelor's degree	45
Graduate degree	50
Household income	
Under $12,500	33
$12,500 to $24,999	42
$25,000 to $39,999	36
$40,000 to $59,999	44
$60,000 or more	44

Source: Journal of the American Medical Association, *"Why Patients Use Alternative Medicine—Results of a National Study," John A. Astin, May 29, 1998*

Health Problems Treated with Alternative Therapies, 1998

(ten health problems most likely to be treated by alternative therapies, by most common type of therapies used, 1998)

1. **Chronic pain**
    Exercise
    Chiropractic
    Massage

2. **Anxiety**
    Relaxation
    Exercise
    Herbs
    Art/music therapy
    Massage

3. **Chronic fatigue syndrome**
    Massage
    Exercise
    Self-help group
    Megavitamins

4. **Sprains/muscle strains**
    Chiropractic
    Exercise
    Massage
    Relaxation
    Herbs

5. **Addictive problems**
    Psychotherapy
    Self-help group

6. **Arthritis or rheumatism**
    Exercise
    Chiropractic
    Homeopathy
    Herbs

7. **Severe headaches**
    Chiropractic
    Massage
    Exercise
    Relaxation

8. **Depression**
    Relaxation
    Exercise
    Herbs

9. **Digestive problems**
    Lifestyle diet
    Relaxation
    Herbs
    Chiropractic

10. **Diabetes**
    Lifestyle diet
    Exercise

Source: Journal of the American Medical Association, *"Why Patients Use Alternative Medicine—Results of a National Study," John A. Astin, May 29, 1998*

Hospital Discharges and Length of Stay, 1980 and 1998

(number of hospital discharges, discharge rate per 10,000 population, and average length of stay in days, for inpatients from nonfederal short-stay hospitals by age, 1980 and 1998; percent change in number and rate and percentage point change in length of stay, 1980–98; excludes newborn infants)

	1998	1980	percent change 1980–98
Total discharges (in 000s)	**31,827**	**37,832**	**–15.9%**
Under age 15	2,299	3,672	–37.4
Aged 15 to 44	10,376	15,635	–33.6
Aged 45 to 64	6,696	8,660	–22.7
Aged 65 or older	12,456	9,864	26.3
Discharge rate (per 10,000 population)	**1,165**	**1,677**	**–30.5**
Under age 15	383	716	–46.5
Aged 15 to 44	851	1,501	–43.3
Aged 45 to 64	1,173	1,948	–39.8
Aged 65 or older	3,653	3,837	–4.8

	1998	1980	change 1980–98
Average length of stay (days)	**5.1**	**7.3**	**–2.2**
Under age 15	4.6	4.4	0.2
Aged 15 to 44	3.7	5.2	–1.5
Aged 45 to 64	5.1	8.2	–3.1
Aged 65 or older	6.2	10.7	–4.5

Source: National Center for Health Statistics, 1998 Summary: National Hospital Discharge Survey, Advance Data, No. 316, 2000; and National Hospital Discharge Survey: Annual Summary: 1997, Series 13, No. 144, 2000; calculations by New Strategist

Hospital Admissions and Outpatient Visits, 1980 and 1998

(number of hospital admissions and number of outpatient visits by type of hospital and size of community hospital; percent of total surgeries at community hospitals performed on outpatients, 1980 and 1998; percent change in admissions, and percentage point change in surgeries, 1980–98)

	1998	1980	percent change, 1980–98
ADMISSIONS (in 000s)			
Total hospitals	**33,766**	**38,892**	**–13.2%**
Federal	1,133	2,044	–44.6
Nonfederal	32,633	36,848	–11.4
Community	31,812	36,143	–12.0
Nonprofit	23,282	24,179	–3.7
Profit	3,971	3,242	22.5
State/local government	4,559	6,028	–24.4
Total community hospitals	**31,812**	**36,848**	**–13.7**
6 to 24 beds	139	159	–12.6
25 to 49 beds	965	1,254	–23.0
50 to 99 beds	2,265	3,700	–38.8
100 to 199 beds	6,656	7,162	–7.1
200 to 299 beds	6,230	6,596	–5.5
300 to 399 beds	5,021	5,358	–6.3
400 to 499 beds	3,390	4,401	–23.0
500 or more beds	7,146	7,513	–4.9
OUTPATIENT VISITS (in 000s)			
Total hospitals	**545,481**	**262,951**	**107.4**
Federal	63,642	50,566	25.9
Nonfederal	481,838	212,385	126.9
Community	474,193	202,310	134.4
Nonprofit	352,114	142,156	147.7
Profit	42,072	9,696	333.9
State/local government	80,008	50,459	58.6

(continued)

(continued from previous page)

	1998	1980	percent change, 1980–98
Total community hospitals	**474,193**	**202,310**	**134.4%**
6 to 24 beds	4,278	1,155	270.4
25 to 49 beds	22,694	6,227	264.4
50 to 99 beds	42,161	17,976	134.5
100 to 199 beds	107,966	36,453	196.2
200 to 299 beds	85,494	36,073	137.0
300 to 399 beds	67,070	30,495	119.9
400 to 499 beds	49,022	25,501	92.2
500 or more beds	95,508	48,430	97.2

			percentage point change 1980–98
Outpatient surgery (percent of total surgeries)			
Community hospitals	61.6%	16.3%	45.3

Source: 1981 and 2000 Editions of Hospital Statistics™, *Health Forum, LLC, an American Hospital Association company. Copyright 1981 and 2000; calculations by New Strategist*

Hospitals, Hospital Beds, and Occupancy Rates, 1980 and 1998

(number of hospitals, hospital beds, and occupancy rates, by type of ownership and size of community hospital, 1980 and 1998; percent change in number of hospitals and beds and percentage point change in occupancy rates, 1980–98)

	1998	1980	percent change 1980–98
NUMBER OF HOSPITALS			
Total hospitals	**6,021**	**6,965**	**–13.6%**
Federal	275	359	–23.4
Nonfederal	5,746	6,606	–13.0
Community	5,015	5,830	–14.0
Nonprofit	3,026	3,322	–8.9
Profit	771	730	5.6
State/local government	1,218	1,778	–31.5
Total community hospitals	**5,015**	**5,830**	**–14.0**
6 to 24 beds	293	259	13.1
25 to 49 beds	900	1,029	–12.5
50 to 99 beds	1,085	1,462	–25.8
100 to 199 beds	1,304	1,370	–4.8
200 to 299 beds	644	715	–9.9
300 to 399 beds	352	412	–14.6
400 to 499 beds	183	266	–31.2
500 or more beds	254	317	–19.9
NUMBER OF BEDS			
Total hospitals	**1,012,582**	**1,364,516**	**–25.8**
Federal	56,698	117,328	–51.7
Nonfederal	955,884	1,247,188	–23.4
Community	839,988	988,387	–15.0
Nonprofit	587,658	692,459	–15.1
Profit	112,975	87,033	29.8
State/local government	139,355	208,895	–33.3

(continued)

(continued from previous page)

	1998	1980	percent change 1980–98
Total community hospitals	**839,988**	**988,387**	**–15.0%**
6 to 24 beds	5,351	4,932	8.5
25 to 49 beds	33,510	37,478	–10.6
50 to 99 beds	78,035	105,278	–25.9
100 to 199 beds	186,118	192,892	–3.5
200 to 299 beds	156,978	172,390	–8.9
300 to 399 beds	120,512	139,434	–13.6
400 to 499 beds	81,247	117,724	–31.0
500 beds or more	178,237	218,259	–18.3

	1998	1980	percentage point change 1980–98
OCCUPANCY RATE			
Total hospitals	**65.4%**	**77.7%**	**–12.3**
Federal	78.9	80.1	–1.2
Nonfederal	64.6	77.4	–12.8
Community	62.5	75.6	–13.1
Nonprofit	64.2	78.2	–14.0
Profit	53.2	65.2	–12.0
State/local government	62.7	71.1	–8.4
Total community hospitals	**62.5**	**75.6**	**–13.1**
6 to 24 beds	33.2	46.8	–13.6
25 to 49 beds	41.2	52.8	–11.6
50 to 99 beds	54.7	64.2	–9.5
100 to 199 beds	58.4	71.4	–13.0
200 to 299 beds	62.9	77.4	–14.5
300 to 399 beds	64.7	79.7	–15.0
400 to 499 beds	67.3	81.2	–13.9
500 or more beds	70.9	82.1	–11.2

Source: 1981 and 2000 Editions of Hospital Statistics™, *Health Forum, LLC, an American Hospital Association company. Copyright 1981 and 2000; calculations by New Strategist*

Length of Hospital Stay by Diagnosis, 1980 and 1998

(average length of stay in days for discharges from short-stay hospitals by first-listed diagnosis, 1980 and 1998; excludes newborn infants)

	1998	1980	change 1980–98
TOTAL CONDITIONS	**5.1**	**7.3**	**–2.2**
Infectious and parasitic diseases	**6.3**	**6.9**	**–0.6**
Septicemia	7.6	14.3	–6.7
Neoplasms	**6.4**	**10.5**	**–4.1**
Malignant neoplasms	7.2	11.9	–4.7
Malignant neoplasm of large intestine and rectum	8.8	15.7	–6.9
Malignant neoplasm of trachea, bronchus, and lung	8.0	12.8	–4.8
Malignant neoplasm of breast	2.7	10.9	–8.2
Benign neoplasms	3.5	6.2	–2.7
Endocrine, nutritional and metabolic diseases, and immunity disorders	**4.8**	**9.6**	**–4.8**
Diabetes mellitus	5.2	10.5	–5.3
Volume depletion	4.3	8.9	–4.6
Diseases of the blood and blood forming organs	**4.6**	**7.2**	**–2.6**
Mental disorders	**7.6**	**11.6**	**–4.0**
Psychoses	8.7	14.8	–6.1
Alcohol dependence syndrome	5.7	10.1	–4.4
Diseases of the nervous system and sense organs	**5.2**	**5.4**	**–0.2**
Diseases of the circulatory system	**5.2**	**10.0**	**–4.8**
Heart disease	4.9	9.5	–4.6
Acute myocardial infarction	5.9	12.6	–6.7
Coronary atherosclerosis	4.1	10.0	–5.9
Other ischemic heart disease	3.2	7.7	–4.5
Cardiac dysrhythmias	4.0	7.6	–3.6
Congestive heart failure	5.9	10.4	–4.5
Cerebrovascular disease	5.9	12.4	–6.5
Diseases of the respiratory system	**5.6**	**6.3**	**–0.7**
Acute bronchitis and bronchiolitis	3.7	4.7	–1.0
Pneumonia	6.0	8.3	–2.3
Chronic bronchitis	5.8	–	–
Asthma	3.3	6.0	–2.7

(continued)

(continued from previous page)

	1998	1980	change 1980–98
Diseases of the digestive system	**4.8**	**7.0**	**−2.2**
Appendicitis	3.5	5.5	−2.0
Noninfectious enteritis and colitis	4.3	5.6	−1.3
Diverticula of intestine	5.4	−	−
Cholelithiasis	3.7	9.3	−5.6
Diseases of the genitourinary system	**3.8**	**5.6**	**−1.8**
Calculus of kidney and ureter	2.2	5.0	−2.8
Complications of pregnancy, childbirth, and the puerperium	**2.5**	**2.5**	**0.0**
Diseases of the skin and subcutaneous tissue	**5.7**	**8.0**	**−2.3**
Cellulitis and abscess	4.9	8.0	−3.1
Diseases of the musculoskeletal system and connective tissue	**4.3**	**8.3**	**−4.0**
Osteoarthrosis and allied disorders	4.5	−	−
Intervertebral disc disorders	2.9	9.9	−7.0
Congenital anomalies	**4.9**	**6.6**	**−1.7**
Certain conditions originating in the perinatal period	**9.2**	**8.7**	**0.5**
Symptoms, signs, and ill-defined conditions	**2.7**	**4.5**	**−1.8**
Injury and poisoning	**5.4**	**7.7**	**−2.3**
Fractures, all sites	5.8	10.8	−5.0
Fracture of neck of femur	6.8	20.6	−13.8
Poisonings	3.0	−	−
Supplementary classifications	**3.8**	**3.7**	**0.1**
Females with deliveries	2.5	3.8	−1.3

Note: (−) means data not available.
Source: National Center for Health Statistics, Trends in Hospital Utilization: United States, 1988–92, *Vital and Health Statistics, Series 13, No. 124, 1996; and* 1998 Summary: National Hospital Discharge Survey, *Advance Data, No. 316, 2000; calculations by New Strategist*

Discharges from Hospitals by Diagnosis, 1998

(number and percent distribution of hospital discharges and discharge rate per 10,000 population by first-listed diagnosis; excludes newborn infants; numbers in thousands)

	number	percent	rate per 10,000 population
TOTAL CONDITIONS	**31,827**	**100.0%**	**1,165.3**
Infectious and parasitic diseases	**866**	**2.7**	**31.7**
Septicemia	347	1.1	12.7
Neoplasms	**1,706**	**5.4**	**62.5**
Malignant neoplasms	1,266	4.0	46.4
Malignant neoplasm of large intestine and rectum	169	0.5	6.2
Malignant neoplasm of trachea, bronchus, and lung	165	0.5	6.0
Malignant neoplasm of breast	124	0.4	4.5
Benign neoplasms	389	1.2	14.2
Endocrine, nutritional and metabolic diseases, and immunity disorders	**1,332**	**4.2**	**48.8**
Diabetes mellitus	513	1.6	18.8
Volume depletion	448	1.4	16.4
Diseases of the blood and blood forming organs	**358**	**1.1**	**13.1**
Mental disorders	**1,974**	**6.2**	**72.3**
Psychoses	1,253	3.9	45.9
Alcohol dependence syndrome	179	0.6	6.5
Diseases of the nervous system and sense organs	**511**	**1.6**	**18.7**
Diseases of the circulatory system	**6,272**	**19.7**	**229.6**
Heart disease	4,335	13.6	158.7
Acute myocardial infarction	783	2.5	28.7
Coronary atherosclerosis	1,094	3.4	40.1
Other ischemic heart disease	308	1.0	11.3
Cardiac dysrhythmias	670	2.1	24.5
Congestive heart failure	978	3.1	35.8
Cerebrovascular disease	1,010	3.2	37.0
Diseases of the respiratory system	**3,403**	**10.7**	**124.6**
Acute bronchitis and bronchiolitis	219	0.7	8.0
Pneumonia	1,328	4.2	48.6
Chronic bronchitis	498	1.6	18.2
Asthma	423	1.3	15.5

(continued)

(continued from previous page)

	number	percent	rate per 10,000 population
Diseases of the digestive system	**3,046**	**9.6%**	**111.5**
Appendicitis	249	0.8	9.1
Noninfectious enteritis and colitis	275	0.9	10.1
Diverticula of intestine	230	0.7	8.4
Cholelithiasis	358	1.1	13.1
Diseases of the genitourinary system	**1,720**	**5.4**	**63.0**
Calculus of kidney and ureter	177	0.6	6.5
Complications of pregnancy, childbirth, and the puerperium	**512**	**1.6**	**18.8**
Diseases of the skin and subcutaneous tissue	**517**	**1.6**	**18.9**
Cellulitis and abscess	364	1.1	13.3
Diseases of the musculoskeletal system and connective tissue	**1,534**	**4.8**	**56.2**
Osteoarthrosis and allied disorders	435	1.4	15.9
Intervertebral disc disorders	352	1.1	12.9
Congenital anomalies	**197**	**0.6**	**7.2**
Certain conditions originating in the perinatal period	**150**	**0.5**	**5.5**
Symptoms, signs, and ill-defined conditions	**297**	**0.9**	**10.9**
Injury and poisoning	**2,540**	**8.0**	**93.0**
Fractures, all sites	966	3.0	35.4
Fracture of neck of femur	329	1.0	12.0
Poisonings	198	0.6	7.2
Supplementary classifications	**4,892**	**15.4**	**179.1**
Females with deliveries	4,000	12.6	146.5

Source: National Center for Health Statistics, 1998 Summary: National Hospital Discharge Survey, *Advance Data, No. 316, 2000*

Discharges from Hospitals by Procedure, 1998

(number and percent distribution of hospital discharges and discharge rate per 10,000 population by all listed procedures; excludes newborn infants; numbers in thousands)

	number	percent	rate per 10,000 population
TOTAL PROCEDURES	**41,500**	**100.0%**	**1,519.4**
Operations on the nervous system	**1,062**	**2.6**	**38.9**
Spinal tap	321	0.8	11.8
Operations on the endocrine system	**96**	**0.2**	**3.5**
Operations on the eye	**122**	**0.3**	**4.5**
Operations on the ear	**57**	**0.1**	**2.1**
Operations on the nose, mouth, and pharynx	**288**	**0.7**	**10.5**
Operations on the respiratory system	**1,004**	**2.4**	**36.7**
Bronchoscopy with or without biopsy	264	0.6	9.7
Operations on the cardiovascular system	**5,791**	**14.0**	**212.0**
Removal of coronary artery obstruction and insertion of stent(s)	926	2.2	33.9
Coronary artery bypass graft	553	1.3	20.3
Cardiac catheterization	1,202	2.9	44.0
Insertion, replacement, removal, and revision of pacemaker	364	0.9	13.3
Hemodialysis	425	1.0	15.5
Operations on the hemic and lymphatic system	**334**	**0.8**	**12.2**
Operations on the digestive system	**5,116**	**12.3**	**187.3**
Endoscopy of small intestine with or without biopsy	892	2.1	32.7
Endoscopy of large intestine with or without biopsy	531	1.3	19.4
Partial excision of large intestine	242	0.6	8.9
Appendectomy, excluding incidental	278	0.7	10.2
Cholecystectomy	439	1.1	16.1
Lysis of peritoneal adhesions	310	0.7	11.3
Operations on the urinary system	**946**	**2.3**	**34.6**
Cystoscopy with or without biopsy	194	0.5	7.1
Operations on the male genital organs	**298**	**0.7**	**10.9**
Prostatectomy	203	0.5	7.4
Operations on the female genital organs	**2,187**	**5.3**	**80.1**
Oophorectomy and salpingo-oophorectomy	491	1.2	18.0
Bilateral destruction or occlusion of fallopian tubes	364	0.9	13.3
Hysterectomy	645	1.6	23.6

(continued)

(continued from previous page)

	number	percent	rate per 10,000 population
Obstetrical procedures	**6,640**	**16.0%**	**243.1**
Episiotomy with or without forceps or vacuum extraction	1,220	2.9	44.7
Artificial rupture of membranes	815	2.0	29.8
Caesarean section	900	2.2	32.9
Repair of current obstetric laceration	1,093	2.6	40.0
Operations on the musculoskeletal system	**3,257**	**7.8**	**119.3**
Partial excision of bone	260	0.6	9.5
Reduction of fracture	610	1.5	22.3
Open reduction of fracture with internal fixation	416	1.0	15.2
Excision or destruction of intervertebral disc	312	0.8	11.4
Total hip replacement	160	0.4	5.9
Total knee replacement	266	0.6	9.7
Operations on the integumentary system	**1,325**	**3.2**	**48.5**
Debridement of wound, infection, or burn	335	0.8	12.3
Miscellaneous diagnostic and therapeutic procedures	**12,977**	**31.3**	**475.1**
Computerized axial tomography	986	2.4	36.1
Arteriography and angiocardiography using contrast material	1,961	4.7	71.8
Diagnostic ultrasound	1,123	2.7	41.1
Respiratory therapy	1,109	2.7	40.6
Insertion of endotracheal tube	399	1.0	14.6
Injection or infusion of cancer chemotherapeutic substance	254	0.6	9.3

Source: National Center for Health Statistics, 1998 Summary: National Hospital Discharge Survey, Advance Data, No. 316, 2000

Visits to Hospital Outpatient Departments by Sex and Age, 1998

(number, percent distribution, and rate of hospital outpatient department visits by sex and age, 1998; numbers in thousands)

	number	percent	number of visits per 100 people per year
Total visits	**75,412**	**100.0%**	**28.0**
Under age 15	15,894	21.1	26.5
Aged 15 to 24	8,141	10.8	21.8
Aged 25 to 44	20,548	27.2	24.7
Aged 45 to 64	17,980	23.8	31.7
Aged 65 to 74	6,869	9.1	38.2
Aged 75 or older	5,979	7.9	41.6
Total females	**45,424**	**100.0**	**32.9**
Under age 15	7,349	16.2	25.1
Aged 15 to 24	5,889	13.0	31.7
Aged 25 to 44	13,355	29.4	31.6
Aged 45 to 64	11,112	24.5	37.9
Aged 65 to 74	4,062	8.9	41.1
Aged 75 or older	3,656	8.0	41.5
Total males	**29,988**	**100.0**	**22.8**
Under age 15	8,544	28.5	27.9
Aged 15 to 24	2,252	7.5	12.0
Aged 25 to 44	7,193	24.0	17.7
Aged 45 to 64	6,868	22.9	25.0
Aged 65 to 74	2,807	9.4	34.7
Aged 75 or older	2,324	7.7	41.7

Source: National Center for Health Statistics, National Hospital Ambulatory Medical Care Survey: 1998 Outpatient Department Summary, *Advance Data, No. 317, 2000*

Hospital Outpatient Department Visits by Major Reason for Visit, 1998

(number and percent distribution of hospital outpatient department visits by age, sex, race, and major reason for visit, 1998; numbers in thousands)

	total	acute problem	chronic problem, routine	chronic problem, flareup	pre- or post-surgery/injury followup	nonillness care
Total visits	**75,412**	**26,711**	**23,856**	**4,565**	**4,689**	**13,334**
Age						
Under age 5	15,894	7,060	3,303	637	770	3,770
Aged 15 to 24	8,141	3,136	1,486	312	397	2,645
Aged 25 to 44	20,548	7,556	5,854	1,219	1,333	4,013
Aged 45 to 64	17,980	5,318	7,436	1,409	1,376	1,858
Aged 65 to 74	6,869	1,807	3,131	491	482	634
Aged 75 or older	5,979	1,835	2,646	497	332	413
Sex						
Female	45,424	15,660	13,551	2,652	2,390	9,891
Male	29,988	11,052	10,306	1,913	2,299	3,444
Race						
Black	17,974	4,614	6,211	1,099	1,206	4,324
White	54,895	21,258	16,885	3,337	3,396	8,363
Other	2,543	840	760	129	87	648
Total visits	**100.0%**	**35.4%**	**31.6%**	**6.1%**	**6.2%**	**17.7%**
Age						
Under age 5	100.0	44.4	20.8	4.0	4.8	23.7
Aged 15 to 24	100.0	38.5	18.3	3.8	4.9	32.5
Aged 25 to 44	100.0	36.8	28.5	5.9	6.5	19.5
Aged 45 to 64	100.0	29.6	41.4	7.8	7.7	10.3
Aged 65 to 74	100.0	26.3	45.6	7.1	7.0	9.2
Aged 75 or older	100.0	30.7	44.3	8.3	5.6	6.9
Sex						
Female	100.0	34.5	29.8	5.8	5.3	21.8
Male	100.0	36.9	34.4	6.4	7.7	11.5
Race						
Black	100.0	25.7	34.6	6.1	6.7	24.1
White	100.0	38.7	30.8	6.1	6.2	15.2
Other	100.0	33.0	29.9	5.1	3.4	25.5

Note: Numbers will not add to total because blank and unknown are not shown.
Source: National Center for Health Statistics, National Hospital Ambulatory Medical Care Survey: 1998 Outpatient Department Summary, *Advance Data, No. 317, 2000*

Visits to Hospital Outpatient Departments by Detailed Reason for Visit, 1998

(number and percent distribution of hospital outpatient department visits by the 20 principal reasons most frequently mentioned by patients for visit, 1998; numbers in thousands)

	number	percent
Total visits	**75,412**	**100.0%**
Progress visit	6,848	9.1
General medical examination	4,628	6.1
Routine prenatal examination	2,478	3.3
Cough	2,136	2.8
Throat symptoms	1,521	2.0
Medication, other and unspecified	1,422	1.9
Well-baby examination	1,264	1.7
Postoperative visit	1,231	1.6
Stomach and abdominal pain, cramps, spasms	1,226	1.6
Fever	1,189	1.6
Counseling, not otherwise stated	1,101	1.5
Earache or ear infection	1,072	1.4
Skin rash	1,061	1.4
Hypertension	949	1.3
Depression	911	1.2
Headache	908	1.2
Diabetes mellitus	836	1.1
Back symptoms	763	1.0
Chest pain and related symptoms	745	1.0
Nasal congestion	700	0.9
All other reasons	42,421	56.3

Source: National Center for Health Statistics, National Hospital Ambulatory Medical Care Survey: 1998 Outpatient Department Summary, *Advance Data, No. 317, 2000*

Visits to Hospital Outpatient Departments by Providers Seen, 1998

(number and percent distribution of hospital outpatient department visits by providers seen, 1998; numbers in thousands)

	number	percent
Total visits	**75,412**	**100.0%**
Staff physician	52,028	69.0
Registered nurse	32,190	42.7
Resident/intern	10,547	14.0
Medical/nursing assistant	10,523	14.0
Licensed practical nurse	10,355	13.7
Nurse practitioner	4,751	6.3
Physician assistant	3,825	5.1
Other physician	1,808	2.4
Nurse midwife	422	0.6
Other	10,401	13.8

Source: National Center for Health Statistics, National Hospital Ambulatory Medical Care Survey: 1998 Outpatient Department Summary, *Advance Data, No. 317, 2000*

Visits to Hospital Outpatient Departments by Services Provided, 1998

(number and percent distribution of hospital outpatient department visits by services ordered or provided, 1998; numbers in thousands)

	number	percent
Total visits	**75,412**	**100.0%**
Examinations		
Skin	6,132	8.1
Pelvic	4,989	6.6
Breast	3,959	5.2
Visual	3,109	4.1
Rectal	2,009	2.7
Glaucoma	1,041	1.4
Hearing	1,021	1.4
Tests		
Blood pressure	42,581	56.5
Urinalysis	7,452	9.9
Hematocrit/hemoglobin	3,902	5.2
Pap test	2,810	3.7
Cholesterol	2,039	2.7
EKG	1,862	2.5
Strep test	949	1.3
Pregnancy test	889	1.2
HIV serology	790	1.0
Blood lead level	694	0.9
PSA	378	0.5
Other STD test	897	1.2
Other blood test	12,781	16.9
Imaging		
X-ray	5,398	7.2
Ultrasound	2,088	2.8
Mammography	1,543	2.0
CAT scan/MRI	1,106	1.5

(continued)

(continued from previous page)

	number	percent
Counseling/education		
Diet/nutrition	10,519	13.9%
Exercise	5,793	7.7
Growth/development	2,087	2.8
Prenatal instructions	1,957	2.6
Tobacco use/exposure	1,931	2.6
Injury prevention	1,871	2.5
Mental health	1,847	2.4
Family planning/contraception	1,768	2.3
Stress management	1,433	1.9
Breast self-exam	1,404	1.9
HIV/STD transmission	1,254	1.7
Skin cancer prevention	415	0.6
Other therapy		
Physiotherapy	3,897	5.2
Psychotherapy	1,317	1.7
Psychopharmacotherapy	1,322	1.8
Other	8,564	11.4

Source: National Center for Health Statistics, National Hospital Ambulatory Medical Care Survey: 1998 Outpatient Department Summary, *Advance Data, No. 317, 2000*

Visits to Hospital Emergency Departments by Sex and Age, 1998

(number, percent distribution, and rate of hospital emergency department visits by sex and age, 1998; numbers in thousands)

	number	percent	number of visits per 100 people per year
Total visits	**100,385**	**100.0%**	**37.3**
Under age 15	22,328	22.2	37.3
Aged 15 to 24	15,959	15.9	42.7
Aged 25 to 44	30,192	30.1	36.4
Aged 45 to 64	16,425	16.4	29.0
Aged 65 to 74	6,350	6.3	35.3
Aged 75 or older	9,132	9.1	63.5
Total females	**52,798**	**100.0**	**38.2**
Under age 15	10,174	19.3	34.8
Aged 15 to 24	8,791	16.7	47.3
Aged 25 to 44	15,723	29.8	37.2
Aged 45 to 64	8,686	16.5	29.6
Aged 65 to 74	3,484	6.6	35.3
Aged 75 or older	5,940	11.3	67.4
Total males	**47,587**	**100.0**	**36.3**
Under age 15	12,154	25.5	39.7
Aged 15 to 24	7,167	15.1	38.1
Aged 25 to 44	14,469	30.4	35.5
Aged 45 to 64	7,738	16.3	28.2
Aged 65 to 74	2,866	6.0	35.4
Aged 75 or older	3,192	6.7	57.3

Source: National Center for Health Statistics, National Hospital Ambulatory Medical Care Survey: 1998 Emergency Department Summary, *Advance Data, No. 313, 2000*

Visits to Hospital Emergency Departments by Reason for Visit, 1998

(number and percent distribution of hospital emergency department visits by the 20 principal reasons most frequently mentioned by patients for visit, 1998; numbers in thousands)

	number	percent
Total visits	**100,385**	**100.0%**
Stomach and abdominal pain, cramps, and spasms	5,958	5.9
Chest pain and related symptoms	5,329	5.3
Fever	4,419	4.4
Headache, pain in head	2,867	2.9
Cough	2,471	2.5
Laceration and cuts—upper extremity	2,293	2.3
Back symptoms	2,284	2.3
Shortness of breath	2,283	2.3
Symptoms referable to throat	2,205	2.2
Pain, site not referable to specific body system	1,990	2.0
Vomiting	1,985	2.0
Earache or ear infection	1,947	1.9
Labored or difficult breathing (dyspnea)	1,690	1.7
Laceration and cuts—facial area	1,623	1.6
Accident, not otherwise specified	1,560	1.6
Injury, other and unspecified type— head, neck, and face	1,465	1.5
Skin rash	1,369	1.4
Neck symptoms	1,346	1.3
Low back symptoms	1,298	1.3
Other	46,382	46.2

Source: National Center for Health Statistics, National Hospital Ambulatory Medical Care Survey: 1998 Emergency Department Summary, *Advance Data, No. 313, 2000*

Visits to Hospital Emergency Departments by Providers Seen, 1998

(number and percent distribution of hospital emergency department visits by providers seen, 1998; numbers in thousands)

	number	percent
Total visits	**100,385**	**100.0%**
Registered nurse	89,273	88.9
Staff physician	87,404	87.1
Resident/intern	8,989	9.0
Other physician	7,889	7.9
Emergency medical technician	6,277	6.3
Medical/nursing assistant	5,579	5.6
Licensed practical nurse	4,212	4.2
Physician assistant	4,073	4.1
Nurse practitioner	956	1.0
Other	9,849	9.8

Source: National Center for Health Statistics, National Hospital Ambulatory Medical Care Survey: 1998 Emergency Department Summary, *Advance Data, No. 313, 2000*

Visits to Hospital Emergency Departments by Services Provided, 1998

(number and percent distribution of hospital emergency department visits by services ordered or provided, 1998; numbers in thousands)

	number	percent
Total visits	**100,385**	**100.0%**
Diagnostic screening services		
Blood pressure	73,338	73.1
CBC (complete blood count)	24,818	24.7
Other blood test	22,377	22.3
Pulse oximetry	20,270	20.2
Chest X-ray	16,647	16.6
Urinalysis	15,626	15.6
EKG	14,565	14.5
Mental status exam	13,682	13.6
Extremity X-ray	11,297	11.3
Other X-ray	10,647	10.6
Cardiac monitor	8,400	8.4
CAT scan	4,096	4.1
Pregnancy test	2,854	2.8
Ultrasound	1,555	1.5
Blood alcohol concentration	1,647	1.6
Other diagnostic image	1,321	1.3
Other sexually transmitted disease test	712	0.7
HIV serology	200	0.2
MRI imaging	138	0.1
Other test	7,176	7.1
None	12,126	12.1
Procedures		
IV fluids	16,617	16.6
Wound care	12,034	12.0
Orthopedic care	7,370	7.3
Eye, ear, nose, throat care	3,313	3.3
Bladder catheter	1,884	1.9
OB/GYN care	2,071	2.1
Nasogastric tube/gastric lavage	517	0.5
Endotracheal intubation	386	0.4
Lumbar puncture	215	0.2
Cardiopulmonary resuscitation	233	0.2
Other	2,884	2.9
None	58,390	58.2

Source: National Center for Health Statistics, National Hospital Ambulatory Medical Care Survey: 1998 Emergency Department Summary, *Advance Data, No. 313, 2000*

Visits to Hospital Emergency Departments by Urgency Status, 1998

(number and percent distribution of visits to hospital emergency departments by immediacy with which patient should be seen, by sex and age, 1998; numbers in thousands)

| | number | percent distribution by immediacy with which patient should be seen | | | | |
		total	emergent	urgent	semiurgent	nonurgent
Total visits	**100,385**	**100.0%**	**19.2%**	**31.2%**	**13.7%**	**9.0%**
Under age 15	22,328	100.0	15.3	32.0	14.4	11.4
Aged 15 to 24	15,959	100.0	15.7	31.0	15.3	10.1
Aged 25 to 44	30,192	100.0	16.7	30.9	14.9	9.1
Aged 45 to 64	16,425	100.0	22.2	31.3	12.9	7.6
Aged 65 to 74	6,350	100.0	28.2	30.6	11.0	6.7
Aged 75 or older	9,132	100.0	31.2	30.5	9.0	4.8
Total females	**52,798**	**100.0**	**19.1**	**32.0**	**13.4**	**8.8**
Under age 15	10,174	100.0	14.6	31.6	14.1	11.5
Aged 15 to 24	8,791	100.0	15.3	32.3	15.5	10.3
Aged 25 to 44	15,723	100.0	16.8	32.9	14.1	8.6
Aged 45 to 64	8,686	100.0	21.4	31.0	14.1	7.8
Aged 65 to 74	3,484	100.0	27.1	33.6	10.3	7.0
Aged 75 or older	5,940	100.0	30.5	30.9	8.5	4.9
Total males	**47,587**	**100.0**	**19.3**	**30.2**	**14.1**	**9.2**
Under age 15	12,154	100.0	15.9	32.4	14.7	11.3
Aged 15 to 24	7,167	100.0	16.3	29.4	15.0	10.0
Aged 25 to 44	14,469	100.0	16.6	28.7	15.7	9.6
Aged 45 to 64	7,738	100.0	23.1	31.7	11.7	7.4
Aged 65 to 74	2,866	100.0	29.5	26.9	11.8	6.4
Aged 75 or older	3,192	100.0	32.6	29.6	9.8	4.7

Note: Emergent, *a patient should be seen in less than 15 minutes;* urgent, *a patient should be seen in 15 to 60 minutes;* semiurgent, *a patient should be seen in 60 to 120 minutes;* nonurgent, *a patient should be seen within 24 hours. Numbers will not add to total because unknown is not shown.*
Source: National Center for Health Statistics, National Hospital Ambulatory Medical Care Survey: 1998 Emergency Department Summary, *Advance Data, No. 313, 2000*

Home Health Care Patients by Age, Sex, and Race, 1996

(number and percent distribution of current home health care patients by age at admission, sex, race, and marital status, 1996)

	number	percent distribution
Total patients	2,427,500	100.0%
Age		
Under age 45	347,400	14.3
Aged 45 to 54	130,200	5.4
Aged 55 to 64	187,600	7.7
Aged 65 or older	1,753,400	72.2
Aged 65 to 69	213,600	8.8
Aged 70 to 74	314,300	12.9
Aged 75 to 79	416,200	17.1
Aged 80 to 84	404,300	16.7
Aged 85 or older	404,900	16.7
Sex		
Male	798,700	32.9
Female	1,628,500	67.1
Race		
White	1,579,300	65.1
Black	292,400	12.0
Other	44,900	1.9
Unknown	511,500	21.1
Marital status		
Never married	455,100	18.7
Married	703,000	29.0
Divorced or separated	100,100	4.1
Widowed	857,600	35.3
Unknown	311,600	12.8

Source: National Center for Health Statistics, An Overview of Home Health and Hospice Care Patients: 1996 National Home and Hospice Care Survey, *Advance Data, No. 297, 1998*

Home Health Care Patients by Diagnosis, 1996

(number and percent distribution of current home health care patients by first-listed and all listed diagnoses at admission, 1996)

	primary diagnosis		all listed diagnoses	
	number	*percent*	*number*	*percent*
Total patients	**2,427,500**	**100.0%**	**7,171,500**	**100.0%**
Infectious and parasitic diseases	17,100	0.7	48,300	0.7
Neoplasms	126,800	5.2	221,800	3.1
Malignant neoplasms	115,000	4.7	203,700	2.8
Endocrine, nutritional, and metabolic diseases and immunity disorders	247,200	10.2	795,100	11.1
Diabetes mellitus	203,600	8.4	545,200	7.6
Diseases of the blood and blood-forming organs	58,500	2.4	188,000	2.6
Mental disorders	82,500	3.4	298,800	4.2
Diseases of the nervous system and sense organs	139,300	5.7	453,700	6.3
Diseases of the circulatory system	615,700	25.4	2,071,000	28.9
Essential hypertension	107,500	4.4	599,800	8.4
Heart disease	262,800	10.8	868,400	12.1
Diseases of the respiratory system	186,200	7.7	453,700	6.3
Diseases of the digestive system	68,400	2.8	258,600	3.6
Diseases of the genitourinary system	56,600	2.3	188,100	2.6
Diseases of the skin and subcutaneous tissue	85,900	3.5	169,400	2.4
Diseases of the musculoskeletal system and connective tissue	211,800	8.7	645,500	9.0
Symptoms, signs, and ill-defined conditions	194,800	8.0	684,800	9.5
Injury and poisoning	166,800	6.9	291,800	4.1
Supplementary classification	88,400	3.6	280,700	3.9
All other diagnoses	62,800	2.6	122,300	1.7

Source: National Center for Health Statistics, An Overview of Home Health and Hospice Care Patients: 1996 National Home and Hospice Care Survey, *Advance Data, No. 297, 1998*

Home Health Care Patients by Procedure, 1996

(number of current home health care patients with a surgical or diagnostic procedure related to admission for home health care, and percent distribution by type of procedure, 1996)

Total patients with a procedure, number	**744,300**
Total patients with a procedure, percent	**100.0%**
Operations on the respiratory system	1.8
Operations on the cardiovascular system	22.4
Operations on the heart and pericardium	10.2
Operations on the digestive system	15.1
Operations on the intestines	4.8
Operations on the musculoskeletal system	26.6
Reduction of fracture	7.3
Repair or replacement of hip	4.4
Repair or replacement of knee	6.2
Operations on the integumentary system	6.6
Miscellaneous diagnostic and therapeutic procedures	20.6
Diagnostic radiology and related techniques and radioisotope scan and function study	6.2
Microscopic examination (laboratory tests)	6.2
Therapeutic radiology and chemotherapy	–
All other procedures	19.0

Note: (–) means sample is too small to make a reliable estimate.
Source: National Center for Health Statistics, An Overview of Home Health and Hospice Care Patients: 1996 National Home and Hospice Care Survey, *Advance Data, No. 297, 1998*

Home Health Care Discharges, 1996

(number and percent distribution of home health care discharges by age, sex, race, and marital status, 1996)

	number	percent distribution
Total discharges	**7,775,700**	**100.0%**
Age		
Under age 45	1,518,100	19.5
Aged 45 to 54	462,600	5.9
Aged 55 to 64	652,400	8.4
Aged 65 or older	5,137,500	66.1
Aged 65 to 69	840,400	10.8
Aged 70 to 74	1,024,600	13.2
Aged 75 to 70	967,400	12.4
Aged 80 to 84	1,104,300	14.2
Aged 85 or older	1,200,900	15.4
Sex		
Male	2,840,300	36.5
Female	4,935,400	63.5
Race		
White	4,880,500	62.8
Black	576,300	7.4
Other	200,600	2.6
Unknown	2,118,300	27.2
Marital status		
Never married	1,433,900	18.4
Married	2,874,400	37.0
Divorced or separated	385,900	5.0
Widowed	1,914,100	24.6
Unknown	1,167,300	15.0

Source: National Center for Health Statistics, An Overview of Home Health and Hospice Care Patients: 1996 National Home and Hospice Care Survey, *Advance Data, No. 297, 1998*

Elderly Home Health Care Patients by Demographic Characteristic, 1996

(number and percent distribution of current home health care patients aged 65 or older by age, race, Hispanic origin, marital status, living arrangement, and sex, 1996)

	number			percent distribution		
	total	men	women	total	men	women
Total, aged 65 or older	**1,753,400**	**528,300**	**1,224,800**	**100.0%**	**100.0%**	**100.0%**
Aged 65 to 74	527,900	180,400	347,500	30.1	34.1	28.4
Aged 75 to 84	820,500	253,500	566,800	46.8	48.0	46.3
Aged 85 or older	404,900	94,400	310,600	23.1	17.9	25.4
Race						
Black	190,900	56,200	134,700	10.9	10.6	11.0
White	1,215,300	353,900	861,400	69.3	67.0	70.3
Other	23,100	8,800	14,400	1.3	1.7	1.2
Unknown	324,000	109,400	214,400	18.5	20.7	17.5
Hispanic origin						
Hispanic	47,300	17,200	30,100	2.7	3.3	2.5
Non-Hispanic	1,134,800	320,000	814,800	64.7	60.6	66.5
Unknown	571,200	191,000	379,900	32.6	36.2	31.0
Marital status						
Married	510,600	268,200	242,200	29.1	50.8	19.8
Widowed	820,200	102,600	717,700	46.8	19.4	58.6
Divorced/separated	49,700	18,800	31,000	2.8	3.6	2.5
Never married	144,100	49,000	95,100	8.2	9.3	7.8
Unknown	228,700	89,800	138,900	13.0	17.0	11.3
Living quarters						
Private residence	1,616,600	496,800	1,119,500	92.2	94.0	91.4
Other	116,500	31,500	105,300	6.6	6.0	8.6
Living arrangement						
With family members	881,700	317,100	564,400	50.3	60.0	46.1
With nonfamily members	9,270	24,100	68,700	0.5	4.6	5.6
Alone	685,600	143,100	542,400	39.1	27.1	44.3
Other or unknown	93,400	44,000	49,300	5.3	8.3	4.0

Source: National Center for Health Statistics, Characteristics of Elderly Home Health Care Users: Data from the 1996 National Home and Hospice Care Survey, *Advance Data, No. 309, 1999*

Elderly Home Health Care Patients by Diagnosis, 1996

(total number of current home health care patients aged 65 or older and percent distribution by primary diagnosis at admission, by sex, 1996)

	total	*men*	*women*
Number aged 65 or older	**1,753,400**	**528,300**	**1,224,800**
Percent aged 65 or older	**100.0%**	**100.0%**	**100.0%**
Diagnosis			
Neoplasms	4.9	5.5	4.6
Malignant neoplasms	4.5	5.0	4.2
Endocrine, nutritional and metabolic diseases, and immmunity disorders	10.4	10.1	10.6
Diabetes mellitus	9.0	9.3	8.9
Diseases of the blood and blood-forming organs	2.6	–	2.9
Diseases of the nervous system and sense organs	3.5	4.5	3.1
Diseases of the circulatory system	30.8	30.4	30.9
Essential hypertension	5.7	–	7.0
Heart disease	13.8	14.5	13.5
Cerebrovascular disease	9.0	10.0	8.5
Diseases of the respiratory system	9.3	14.6	7.0
Chronic obstructive pulmonary disease	5.7	7.2	5.0
Diseases of the digestive system	2.4	–	2.4
Diseases of the genitourinary system	2.3	–	2.3
Diseases of the skin and subcutaneous tissue	3.5	4.2	3.2
Diseases of the musculoskeletal system and connective tissue	10.2	6.2	11.9
Symptoms, signs, and ill-defined conditions	8.2	7.7	8.5
Injury and poisonings	6.5	4.7	7.2
Supplementary classification and unknown	4.7	3.8	5.1

Source: National Center for Health Statistics, Characteristics of Elderly Home Health Care Users: Data from the 1996 National Home and Hospice Care Survey, *Advance Data, No. 309, 1999*

Elderly Home Health Care Patients Receiving Help with Daily Activities, 1996

(total number of current home health care patients aged 65 or older, percent receiving help with activities by type of activity, and percent with continence problems, by sex, 1996)

	total	men	women
Number aged 65 or older	1,753,400	528,300	1,224,800
Percent aged 65 or older	100.0%	100.0%	100.0%
Received assistance with ADLs			
Bathing or showering	53.2	50.9	54.2
Dressing	45.8	43.0	47.1
Eating	9.3	9.4	9.2
Transferring in or out of bed/chair	29.6	30.2	29.3
Using toilet	22.6	19.7	23.9
Help with walking	30.6	28.4	31.6
Received assistance with IADLs			
Doing light housework	38.9	34.1	41.0
Managing money	2.8	–	2.8
Shopping for groceries or clothes	84.3	79.5	85.8
Using telephone	2.7	–	3.1
Preparing meals	23.0	20.1	24.3
Taking medications	23.4	20.7	24.6
Continence status			
Difficulty controlling bowels	15.0	14.6	15.1
Difficulty controlling bladder	27.4	23.5	29.1
Difficulty controlling both bowels and bladder	11.8	10.7	12.3
Have an ostomy or an indwelling catheter	5.9	7.8	5.1
Received help in caring for this device	5.8	7.8	4.9

Note: An ADL is an activity of daily living and an IADL is an instrumental activity of daily living. (–) means sample is too small for a reliable estimate.
Source: National Center for Health Statistics, Characteristics of Elderly Home Health Care Users: Data from the 1996 National Home and Hospice Care Survey, *Advance Data, No. 309, 1999*

Elderly Home Health Care Patients by Services Received, 1996

(total number of current home health care patients aged 65 or older, and percent receiving services during the last 30 days, by type of service and sex, 1996)

	total	men	women
Number aged 65 or older	1,753,400	528,300	1,224,800
Percent aged 65 or older	100.0%	100.0%	100.0%
Services received			
Continuous home care	5.7	4.5	6.3
Counseling	2.3	2.5	2.1
Homemaker-household services	28.1	23.0	30.3
Mental health services	9.8	7.5	10.8
Nursing services	1.7	9.6	2.0
Nutritional services	84.2	84.8	83.9
Occupational therapy	3.3	9.6	3.4
Physical therapy	4.9	6.4	4.2
Physician services	19.8	22.0	18.9
Social services	3.7	4.5	3.3
Speech therapy and/or audiology	10.6	10.1	10.8
Transportation	1.6	–	–
Other services	10.7	11.8	10.2

Note: (–) means sample is too small to make a reliable estimate.
Source: National Center for Health Statistics, Characteristics of Elderly Home Health Care Users: Data from the 1996 National Home and Hospice Care Survey, *Advance Data, No. 309, 1999*

Elderly Home Health Care Patients by Length of Service, 1996

(total number of current home health care patients aged 65 or older, average length of service in days, and percent distribution by length of service, by sex, 1996)

	total	men	women
Number aged 65 or older	**1,753,400**	**528,300**	**1,224,800**
Average length of service (in days)	**336**	**331**	**338**
Percent aged 65 or older	**100.0%**	**100.0%**	**100.0%**
0 to 14 days	8.8	10.3	8.2
15 to 30 days	9.4	9.6	9.3
31 to 60 days	14.0	15.7	13.3
61 to 90 days	8.2	9.6	7.7
91 to 180 days	15.4	13.2	16.3
181 or more days	44.1	41.5	45.2

Source: National Center for Health Statistics, Characteristics of Elderly Home Health Care Users: Data from the 1996 National Home and Hospice Care Survey, *Advance Data, No. 309, 1999*

Discharges of Elderly Home Health Care Patients by Length of Service, 1996

(total number of discharges of people aged 65 or older from home health care, average length of service in days, and percent distribution by length of service, by sex, 1996)

	total	men	women
Discharges of people aged 65 or older, number	5,137,500	1,716,000	3,421,500
Average length of service (in days)	107	104	109
Discharges of people aged 65 or older, percent	100.0%	100.0%	100.0%
0 to 14 days	20.2	22.2	19.2
15 to 30 days	20.6	24.3	18.7
31 to 60 days	28.7	27.0	29.6
61 to 90 days	8.6	10.0	7.9
91 to 180 days	9.2	7.9	9.8
181 or more days	12.7	8.7	14.8

Source: National Center for Health Statistics, Characteristics of Elderly Home Health Care Users: Data from the 1996 National Home and Hospice Care Survey, *Advance Data, No. 309, 1999*

Nursing Home Residents by Sex and Age, 1973–74 and 1997

(number of nursing home residents aged 65 or older, and number of residents per 1,000 people in age group, by sex and age, 1973–74 and 1997; percent change 1973–74 to 1997)

	1997	1973–74	percent change 1973–74 to 1997
Total aged 65 or older	**1,465,000**	**961,500**	**52.4%**
Aged 65 to 74	198,400	163,100	21.6
Aged 75 to 84	528,300	384,900	37.3
Aged 85 or older	738,300	413,600	78.5
Female residents	**1,092,900**	**695,800**	**57.1**
Aged 65 to 74	117,700	98,000	20.1
Aged 75 to 84	368,900	282,600	30.5
Aged 85 or older	606,300	315,300	92.3
Male residents	**372,100**	**265,700**	**40.0**
Aged 65 to 74	80,800	65,100	24.1
Aged 75 to 84	159,300	102,300	55.7
Aged 85 or older	132,000	98,300	34.3
Rate (per 1,000 people)			
Total aged 65 or older	**43.4**	**44.7**	**–2.9**
Aged 65 to 74	10.8	12.3	–12.2
Aged 75 to 84	45.5	57.7	–21.1
Aged 85 or older	192.0	257.3	–25.4
Female residents	**55.1**	**54.9**	**0.4**
Aged 65 to 74	11.6	13.1	–11.5
Aged 75 to 84	52.7	68.9	–23.5
Aged 85 or older	221.6	294.9	–24.9
Male residents	**26.7**	**30.0**	**–11.0**
Aged 65 to 74	9.8	11.3	–13.3
Aged 75 to 84	34.6	39.9	–13.3
Aged 85 or older	119.0	182.7	–34.9

Source: National Center for Health Statistics, Health, United States, 2000*; calculations by New Strategist*

Nursing Home Residents by Selected Characteristics, 1997

(number and percent distribution of current nursing home residents aged 65 or older by age at admission, race, Hispanic origin, marital status, living arrangement prior to admission, and sex, 1997)

	number			percent distribution		
	total	*men*	*women*	*total*	*men*	*women*
Total, aged 65 or older	**1,465,000**	**372,100**	**1,092,900**	**100.0%**	**100.0%**	**100.0%**
Aged 65 to 74	198,400	80,800	117,700	13.5	21.7	10.8
Aged 75 to 84	528,300	159,300	368,900	36.1	42.8	33.8
Aged 85 or older	738,300	132,000	606,300	50.4	35.5	55.5
Race						
Black	137,400	44,800	92,500	9.4	12.0	8.5
White	1,294,900	315,800	979,100	88.4	84.9	89.6
Other	18,000	7,400	10,600	1.2	2.0	1.0
Unknown	14,700	4,100	10,600	1.0	1.1	1.0
Hispanic origin						
Hispanic	32,100	11,100	20,900	2.2	3.0	1.9
Non-Hispanic	1,339,900	338,900	1,001,000	91.5	91.1	91.6
Unknown	93,000	22,100	71,000	6.3	5.9	6.5
Marital status						
Married	248,800	140,200	108,600	17.0	37.7	9.9
Widowed	924,400	131,000	793,400	63.1	35.2	72.6
Divorced/separated	98,200	34,600	63,600	6.7	9.3	5.8
Never married	173,800	61,300	112,500	11.9	16.5	10.3
Unknown	19,800	4,900	14,800	1.4	1.3	1.4
Living arrangement prior to admission						
Private residence	472,100	114,600	357,500	32.2	30.8	32.7
Retirement home	33,900	5,300	28,600	2.3	1.4	2.6
Residential facility	67,300	15,300	51,900	4.6	4.1	4.7
Nursing home	179,000	47,600	131,400	12.2	12.8	12.0
Hospital	651,300	172,400	478,900	44.5	46.3	43.8
Mental health facility	19,000	5,900	13,100	1.3	1.6	1.2
Other/unknown	42,400	11,000	31,500	2.9	3.0	2.9

Source: National Center for Health Statistics, Characteristics of Elderly Nursing Home Current Residents and Discharges: Data from the 1997 National Nursing Home Survey, *Advance Data, No. 312, 2000*

Nursing Home Residents Receiving Assistance with Daily Activities, 1997

(number and percent distribution of current nursing home residents aged 65 or older by services received and continence status, by sex, 1997)

	number			percent distribution		
	total	*men*	*women*	*total*	*men*	*women*
Total, aged 65 or older	**1,465,000**	**372,100**	**1,092,900**	**100.0%**	**100.0%**	**100.0%**
Received assistance with ADLs						
Bathing or showering	1,409,300	351,400	1,057,900	96.2	94.4	96.8
Dressing	1,277,600	318,900	958,700	87.2	85.7	87.7
Eating	658,800	159,300	499,500	45.0	42.8	45.7
Transferring in or out of bed/chair	372,100	87,300	284,800	25.4	23.5	26.1
Using toilet room	822,600	196,300	626,300	56.2	52.8	57.3
Received assistance with IADLs						
Care of personal possessions	1,130,100	287,200	842,900	77.1	77.2	77.1
Managing money	1,057,900	266,500	791,400	72.2	71.6	72.4
Securing personal items	1,115,800	278,100	837,700	76.2	74.7	76.6
Using telephone	910,500	233,500	677,000	62.2	62.8	61.9
Continence status						
Difficulty controlling both bowels and bladder	647,200	156,400	490,900	44.2	42.0	44.9
Difficulty controlling bowels	18,900	6,600	12,200	1.3	1.8	1.1
Difficulty controlling bladder	189,700	44,600	145,100	12.9	12.0	13.3

Note: An ADL is an activity of daily living and an IADL is an instrumental activity of daily living.
Source: National Center for Health Statistics, Characteristics of Elderly Nursing Home Current Residents and Discharges: Data from the 1997 National Nursing Home Survey, *Advance Data, No. 312, 2000*

Nursing Home Residents by Functional Status, 1997

(percent distribution of nursing home residents aged 65 or older by functional status, sex, and age, 1997)

	total residents	dependent mobility	incontinent	dependent eating	dependent mobility, eating, and incontinent
Total aged 65 or older	**100.0%**	**79.4%**	**64.9%**	**45.1%**	**35.6%**
Aged 65 to 74	100.0	73.1	59.2	42.1	30.7
Aged 75 to 84	100.0	77.1	64.3	44.8	34.5
Aged 85 or older	100.0	82.6	66.9	46.1	37.8
Female residents	**100.0**	**80.6**	**65.1**	**45.8**	**36.3**
Aged 65 to 74	100.0	73.7	58.6	41.6	29.2
Aged 75 to 84	100.0	78.0	63.6	45.3	34.4
Aged 85 or older	100.0	83.5	67.2	46.9	38.8
Male residents	**100.0**	**75.6**	**64.5**	**42.9**	**33.7**
Aged 65 to 74	100.0	72.3	60.1	42.7	32.9
Aged 75 to 84	100.0	75.1	65.9	43.7	34.6
Aged 85 or older	100.0	78.3	65.6	42.1	33.0

Note: Nursing home residents who are dependent in mobility and eating require the assistance of a person or special equipment. Nursing home residents who are incontinent have difficulty in controlling bowels and/or bladder or have an ostomy or indwelling catheter.
Source: National Center for Health Statistics, Health, United States, 2000

Nursing Home Residents by Type of Aids Used, 1997

(number and percent distribution of current nursing home residents aged 65 or older by type of aids used, vision and hearing status, by sex, 1997)

	number			percent distribution		
	total	*men*	*women*	*total*	*men*	*women*
Total, aged 65 or older	**1,465,000**	**372,100**	**1,092,900**	**100.0%**	**100.0%**	**100.0%**
Aids used						
Glasses	973,400	230,100	743,200	66.4	61.8	68.0
Hearing aid	155,600	39,400	116,200	10.6	10.6	10.6
Transfer equipment	185,000	52,000	133,000	12.6	14.0	12.2
Wheelchair	913,300	227,500	685,800	62.3	61.1	62.8
Cane	95,400	34,000	61,300	6.5	9.1	5.6
Walker	369,100	82,600	286,500	25.2	22.2	26.2
Oxygen	84,500	28,100	56,500	5.8	7.6	5.2
Brace (any type)	46,200	12,200	34,100	3.2	3.3	3.1
Commode	121,600	25,400	96,200	8.3	6.8	8.8
Other aids or devices	250,100	69,800	180,300	17.1	18.8	16.5
Vision						
Not impaired	959,200	254,200	705,000	65.5	68.3	64.5
Impaired	396,700	93,000	303,700	27.1	25.0	27.8
Unknown	109,100	24,900	84,100	7.4	6.7	7.7
Hearing						
Not impaired	1,005,800	256,500	749,300	68.7	68.9	68.6
Impaired	347,600	90,800	256,800	23.7	24.4	23.5
Unknown	111,600	24,800	86,800	7.6	6.7	7.9

Source: National Center for Health Statistics, Characteristics of Elderly Nursing Home Current Residents and Discharges: Data from the 1997 National Nursing Home Survey, *Advance Data, No. 312, 2000*

Nursing Home Residents by Services Received, 1997

(number and percent distribution of nursing home residents aged 65 or older by services received and sex, 1997)

	number			percent distribution		
	total	*men*	*women*	*total*	*men*	*women*
Total, aged 65 or older	**1,465,000**	**372,100**	**1,092,900**	**100.0%**	**100.0%**	**100.0%**
Dental care	267,200	73,300	193,900	18.2	19.7	17.7
Equipment or devices	743,100	188,700	554,400	50.7	50.7	50.7
Medical services	1,334,400	340,700	993,800	91.1	91.6	90.9
Mental health services	242,200	69,200	173,000	16.5	18.6	15.8
Nursing services	1,425,600	362,700	1,062,900	97.3	97.5	97.3
Nutritional services	1,084,700	278,900	805,800	74.0	75.0	73.7
Occupational therapy	277,500	75,800	201,600	18.9	20.4	18.4
Personal care	1,333,600	339,000	994,500	91.0	91.1	91.0
Physical therapy	399,100	110,400	288,700	27.2	29.7	26.4
Medicines	1,371,800	348,400	1,023,400	93.6	93.6	93.6
Social services	1,029,200	258,900	770,400	70.3	69.6	70.5
Speech or hearing therapy	118,700	37,000	81,700	8.1	9.9	7.5
Transportation	282,400	79,900	202,600	19.3	21.5	18.5
Other services	202,700	50,500	152,100	13.8	13.6	13.9

Source: National Center for Health Statistics, Characteristics of Elderly Nursing Home Current Residents and Discharges: Data from the 1997 National Nursing Home Survey, *Advance Data, No. 312, 2000*

Nursing Home Residents by Method of Payment, 1997

(number and percent distribution of current nursing home residents aged 65 or older by primary method of payment upon admission, by sex, 1997)

	total	men	women
Total, aged 65 or older	**1,465,000**	**372,100**	**1,092,900**
Private insurance, own income, family support	413,600	97,000	316,600
Medicare	435,600	107,000	328,600
Medicaid	560,000	144,100	415,900
Government assistance, charity, and other	25,200	14,500	10,800
Unknown	30,500	9,500	21,000
Total, aged 65 or older	**100.0%**	**100.0%**	**100.0%**
Private insurance, own income, family support	28.2	26.1	29.0
Medicare	29.7	28.8	30.1
Medicaid	38.2	38.7	38.1
Government assistance, charity, and other	1.7	3.9	1.0
Unknown	2.1	2.6	1.9

Source: National Center for Health Statistics, Characteristics of Elderly Nursing Home Current Residents and Discharges: Data from the 1997 National Nursing Home Survey, *Advance Data, No. 312, 2000*

Nursing Home Residents by Average Length of Stay, 1997

(number of nursing home residents aged 65 or older and average length of stay in days, by age, marital status, and sex, 1997)

	total	*men*	*women*
Total, aged 65 or older	**1,465,000**	**372,100**	**1,092,900**
Average length of stay (in days)	870	761	907
Age			
Aged 65 to 74	857	823	881
Aged 75 to 84	789	759	801
Aged 85 or older	932	725	977
Marital status			
Married	596	531	681
Widowed	852	677	881
Divorced/separated	911	867	936
Never married	1,318	1,325	1,314

Source: National Center for Health Statistics, Characteristics of Elderly Nursing Home Current Residents and Discharges: Data from the 1997 National Nursing Home Survey, *Advance Data, No. 312, 2000*

7

Staying Fit and Eating Right

American lifestyles have changed significantly over the past few decades. Today's generations of young and middle-aged adults are more physically active than their parents and grandparents were at the same age. An increasingly educated population is more aware of the link between behavior and physical well-being. The passage of Title IX, which mandated equal opportunity for females in public school sports programs, boosted the participation of girls and women in a variety of individual and team sports.

The growing affluence of Americans has allowed more of them to take advantage of recreational activities and to afford better diets. And thanks to media coverage of scientific research, the public is becoming better informed each year about the benefits of exercise and proper nutrition. The largest hurdle may be making sense of ever-changing nutrition information. For nearly 20 years, for example, saccharine was listed as a possible human carcinogen. In May 2000, its name was cleared.[1] Such changes in nutritional advice make it more difficult to figure out what a healthy diet should—and should not—contain.

Despite the changing nature of nutritional information, the baby-boom generation is the first to benefit fully from an enhanced awareness of the individual's role in maintaining a healthy lifestyle. As boomers push through their fifties, the participation of middle-aged Americans in a variety of activities is rising. The smoking rate has dropped over the past few decades, and consumption of fruits and vegetables has soared. Surprisingly, however, the number of people who say that they are "very concerned" about nutrition is declining. Today, only 46 percent of shoppers say they are very concerned about nutrition, down from a peak of 62 percent in 1994.[2] A possible explanation, according to Kai Robertson, senior research manager at the Food Marketing Institute, is that consumers have integrated healthy living into their life so much that eating well no longer requires conscious effort.[3]

Staying fit

Unlike many topics in the field of health, there is consensus among experts about the benefits of physical activity. Exercise reduces the risk of heart disease, colon cancer, diabetes, and high blood pressure. It helps maintain healthy bones, muscles, and joints. It can relieve symptoms of anxiety and depression. There is controversy, however, over how much and what type of exercise is necessary to achieve those benefits.

Despite the increase in Americans' physical activity over the past few decades, most Americans are not physically active on a regular basis, according to the 1997 National Health Interview Survey. Forty percent of Americans lead a sedentary lifestyle—that is, they do not engage in any exercise, sport, or other physical activity for at least 20 minutes during their leisure time. Most likely to be couch potatoes are Americans aged 65 or older—fully 57 percent are sedentary.[4]

Women are more likely than men to be sedentary, 43 versus 37 percent. More than half of Hispanics and blacks are sedentary, compared with 36 percent of non-Hispanic whites.

These numbers may not improve in the future. The Centers for Disease Control's 1997 Youth Risk Behavior Surveillance System found that about one-third of high school students are not participating in vigorous physical activity, and the number of overweight and sedentary young adults is on the rise. The percentage of children who are overweight has increased from 7 to 9 percent between 1989 and 1997.[5] Genetics play a factor in some children's weight problems, but lifestyle factors, like watching too much television and spending too much time sitting in front of a computer—combined with the relentless marketing of junk food and its increased availability at school—have contributed to the

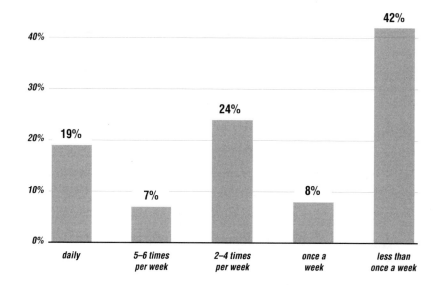

Many Americans do not exercise regularly

(percent distribution of people aged 20 or older by frequency of vigorous exercise, 1994–96)

problem. The American Academy of Pediatrics has suggested that parents limit their children's TV viewing to one or two hours a day. TV also affects children's diets. "Children eat the foods they see advertised on TV. If you've seen any children's shows, you know that these foods tend to be fast foods, sugared breakfast cereals and snacks. TV is a behavioral health hazard," says William H. Dietz, Director of the National Center for Chronic Disease Prevention and Health Promotion's Division of Nutrition and Physical Activity.[6] Sixty percent of overweight 5- to 10-year-olds have at least one risk factor for heart disease. Obese children will also find it more difficult to lose weight as they age because their metabolism changes due to the excess pounds. Nutrition experts like Michael Jacobson and Kelly Brownell have proposed a national tax on soda, the proceeds of which would be used to promote healthful alternatives.[7] Expect more attention to this issue as children's weight increases.

While many Americans are sedentary, millions of others are not. The most popular recreational activity in the U.S. is walking. Thirty-six million Americans walk at least once a year for fitness. During the past 12 years, the number of fitness walkers increased 32 percent, according to the Sporting Goods Manufacturers Association. Many other fitness activities saw declines during the same period, however. The number of participants in high-impact aerobics, for example, fell 55 percent over the past 12 years. Fitness swimming was down 16 percent, while participation in skiing (both downhill and cross-country) fell even more sharply.[8]

By far the most popular and rapidly growing fitness activity is exercise on gym equipment. Nearly 8 million people use home gym equipment, up 103 percent since 1987. More than 50 million use a treadmill or stair climber machine, up more that 600 percent during the past 12 years.[9]

Given the benefits of exercise, why don't more people participate? There are a variety of reasons, according to researcher Bess H. Marcus writing in *Research Quarterly for Exercise and Sport*. A person's ability to set goals and an understanding of how the benefits of exercise outweigh the costs play a large part in the decision to exercise. Another important factor is readiness to become physically active. Most programs are designed for those eager to participate, but many people aren't ready to commit themselves to regular physical activity, which may account for the high dropout rate from exercise programs. Marcus also notes that family or spousal support is an important determinant, especially for women. Less-strenuous programs, conveniently located, are more likely to keep people coming back for more.[10]

There has been no shortage of efforts to get Americans involved in physical fitness, but most have shown only modest success. The Centers for Disease Control recommends a comprehensive public health effort, including individual outreach, mass media efforts, and environmental and policy goals aimed at increasing the opportunities for physical activity. It recommends brisk walking, using stairs rather than elevators, bicycling, swimming, and playing sports.

Eating well

The quality of the American diet is subject to endless analysis, with oft-conflicting conclusions. Few studies, however, bother to ask consumers what they think about their own diet. Yet those attitudes are the key to consumer behavior in the grocery store, the health club, and the doctor's office.

Most people think they eat about right, according to a USDA study which asked Americans what they thought about their diet. Two-thirds of both men and women say they consume the right amount of vitamin C, for example. Most also think they consume the right amount of calcium, iron, and fiber. But they are less confident about their fat intake, and 50 percent of men and 48 percent of women say they eat too much fat. Forty percent of women think they consume too many calories, as do 38 percent of men.

Americans are eating more fruits and vegetables, but also consuming more soft drinks, fats, and oils

(percent increase in per capita consumption of selected items, 1970–97)

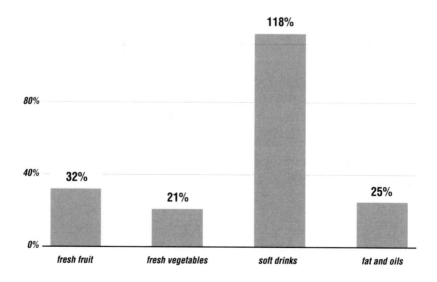

Most consumers use food labels to determine the nutritional content of food. Forty-one percent of women "often" or "always" check the saturated fat content on food labels. Forty-four percent check calories, and 37 percent check cholesterol. Men are much less likely than women to pay attention to food labels.

The public is well versed in nutritional information. Both men and women take dietary guidelines seriously. The majority regard it as very important to eat a diet rich in fruits and vegetables. Most men and women also think it is very important to maintain a healthy weight, eat a variety of food, and choose a low-fat, low-cholesterol diet. But only 28 percent of the public is willing to give up convenience for health benefits when buying food, according to surveys by HealthFocus, a market research company in Des Moines, Iowa. Just 39 percent avoid some of their favorite food to eat healthier. That's why a larger share of Americans drink carbonated soft drinks on an average day (50 percent) than citrus juice (27 percent). It explains why only 25 percent eat salad daily versus the 41 percent who eat cakes, cookies, pastries, and pies.

Many Americans depend on vitamin pills to make up for shortcomings in their diet, although demand for vitamins appears to be leveling off. During the mid-1990s, sales of dietary supplements increased at double-digit rates. Growth slowed to 8 percent between 1998 and 1999 and is expected to increase another 7 percent between 1999 and 2000.[11] Overall, 47 percent of people take vitamin/mineral supplements, with vitamin consumption peaking in the older age groups. Women are more likely to be vitamin users than men, and many take a multivitamin as well as single vitamin/mineral supplements such as calcium or vitamin C, according to a USDA survey.

Although millions of Americans do not have an optimal diet, over the past 25 years there has been a remarkable shift toward healthy eating. Per capita consumption of fresh vegetables increased more than 21 percent between 1970 and 1997. Consumption of broccoli was ten times greater in 1997 than in 1970. Fresh fruit consumption rose 32 percent during those years, with grape and strawberry consumption more than doubling. Americans consume less red meat and more poultry than they once did, fewer eggs and more yogurt, less whole milk and more low-fat milk. But they also drink more soft drinks and eat more high-fat snack foods, which probably accounts for the growing bulk of the American population.

As a drive down any highway will illustrate, on an average day most people (57 percent) eat away from home. Men are more likely than women to eat out. Among adults, those aged 20 to 29 are most likely to eat away from home on an average day, and 72 percent of men and 63 percent of women do so.

While restaurants and fast-food places are where most people go to eat away from home, other locations are also popular. Among children, for example, one-third of those eating away from home are eating food supplied by someone else such as a baby-sitter or friend. Twenty percent of children under age 6 eat food from a day care center each day. Nearly half of children aged 6 to 11 eat food from a school cafeteria on an average day. One-fourth of those eating away from home eat at a store, a figure that should climb in the years ahead as supermarkets continue to turn themselves into take-out restaurants. Even at home, many people consume food prepared at restaurants and supermarkets. According to the FMI 2000 report, 34 percent of Americans most often get their take-out food from fast-food restaurants, 22 percent from sit-down restaurants, and 18 percent from supermarkets.[12]

With all this eating going on, it is no surprise that most Americans are overweight—and increasingly so. The share of men and women who are overweight rose from 45 to 54 percent between the early 1960s and 1997, reports the National Center for Health Statistics. According to the 1997 National Health Interview Survey, 19 percent of adults are obese—meaning their body mass index is 30 or higher. Weight problems increase with age, peaking at ages 45 to 64 for both men and women.[13]

According to the International Food Information Council, 54 million Americans are currently on a diet.[14] Overweight consumers have spawned a diet industry with sales of $33 billion in 1999, according to MarketData in Tampa, Florida. This figure includes spending on everything from diet soda to drugs and weight-loss clubs. Paying money to lose weight is not a new concept. During the 1920s, affluent women took pills to help them lose pounds. The pills turned out to be tapeworm eggs, which may have been as effective and as dangerous as many of the cures available today.

The Centers for Disease Control's 1998 Behavior Risk Factor Surveillance System quizzed Americans about their weight-loss behavior. Although most Americans are over-weight, 64 percent said they were not trying to lose weight. This may be because their doctors don't tell them to do so. Only 11 percent had been told by a doctor, nurse, or other medical professional to lose weight.

Consumers may be more interested in maintaining their weight than reducing it—56 percent said they were trying to maintain their current weight. The CDC also asked Americans if they were cutting back on calories or fat to either lose or maintain their weight. More than one-quarter said they were doing neither. Eleven percent were eating fewer calories, 32 percent were eating less fat, and 32 percent said they were cutting back on both calories and fat.

Although weight loss programs abound, customers are hard to satisfy. A 1993 *Consumer Reports* survey of readers who had joined commercial diet programs found the level of dissatisfaction with weight loss programs "higher than that for all other consumer services we have evaluated in reader surveys over the years."[15] In 1999, weight loss programs like Weight Watchers and Jenny Craig agreed to abide by provisions that will allow dieters to comparison-shop between programs.[16]

For the severely obese, there are radical options such as surgery or diet drugs. In the past few years, a growing number of only slightly overweight consumers have turned to these methods, some of which have proven dangerous, such as the diet drug Phen/Fen which had to be removed from the market when it was shown to cause heart damage. The Phen/Fen fiasco did not kill the diet pill industry, however. Pharmaceutical companies are already working on new concoctions because there will always be millions of consumers willing to spend big to shed pounds. In fact, new drugs like Xenical and Meredia have already entered the market, and they have not appeared to face any significant market backlash. Datamonitor, a market research firm, projects that Xenical's global sales will rise from $82 million in 1998 to a whopping $2 billion in 2005.[17]

The future of fitness

In the future, Americans will be more fit and eat better than today. Reasons for this optimistic forecast include the rising educational level of the public, the aging of the baby-boom generation, and the rapid gains in our understanding of the benefits of proper diet and nutrition. At the same time, there's likely to be a backlash as well—consumers who have tried for years to make sense of mixed messages will simply give up.

TREND 1: MORE AND BETTER

Today's active older Americans are becoming role models of healthy aging. The baby-boom generation is likely to be even more active in old age. From the baby-boom's example, today's children and young adults will learn that getting old does not necessarily mean becoming a couch potato. They will have plenty of help in getting fit and eating right as businesses vie for their dollars.

To appeal to aging Americans, health clubs will reinvent themselves as social hubs, becoming more like country clubs or spas by offering on-site restaurants, a variety of therapists, hobby rooms, and regular social activities. Some health clubs will boost their business by opening satellite gyms near work areas and shopping centers. According to the Society of Human Resource Managers, 19 percent of companies provide on-site fitness centers.[18] As employers realize productivity gains from encouraging physical fitness on the job, more companies will provide exercise options. For employees who don't have a regular office, enterprising programs will fill the gap. An example of this is the Rolling Strong Gym, located at a truck stop along a highway in Texas.[19] Truck drivers have more difficulty participating in regular physical activity than most people. The Texas program provides 500 truckers with free gym memberships for one year, tracking their use of the facility. Rolling Strong Gym could spawn more clubs in other unusual locations.

Trend 2: Functional foods

Nutrition will improve in the future thanks to the rapidly growing functional foods industry. Functional foods, defined as food providing health benefits such as through added calcium, vitamin C, or cold-fighting ingredients, will be a common fixture in tomorrow's supermarkets. In the future, consumers who feel a cold coming on might choose a breakfast cereal infused with echinacea, an herb said to boost the immune system. Or they may drink a vitamin C–enhanced soda at lunch. Entire diets will be designed and marketed to combat specific diseases or to achieve certain goals such as stress reduction. Fully 95 percent of Americans believe that certain foods have benefits that go beyond basic nutrition, according to a 1998 International Food Information Council study.

Some companies have already attempted to market such products, although not all have met with success. Campbell Soup tested "Intelligent Quisine," a meal program designed for people with high blood pressure, high cholesterol, or Type II diabetes. The company had planned to deliver complete, microwave-ready meals proven to alleviate these medical problems. The test program failed to meet Campbell's sales goals, however, and the product was pulled from the market in 1998. More than likely this failure was due to poor product design or marketing rather than consumer resistance to the functional foods concept itself. Similar problems plagued a Kellogg's launch. In 1999, the company's Ensemble line of foods fortified by the dietary fiber psyllium experienced a rapid demise. The company pulled the plug on the program before it left the test market.

Despite these failures, more companies are experimenting with foods that prevent or treat health problems. Some are certain to become staples in kitchen cupboards across the country. In the success column is Viactiv, a line of calcium-enriched nutraceuticals aimed at older women. Starbucks offers a "power" concoction of vitamins and minerals which customers can add to its Frappucinos. Gingko Bilboa and Kava Kava are added ingredients in beverages made by SoBe. Tropicana is about to get into the smoothie game with the forthcoming Tropicana Ultimate Smoothie—soy based, low in fat, and lactose free. And don't forget the tortilla chips infused with mood-elevating St. John's Wort from Robert's American Gourmet, or the BetaSweet carrot—super-fortified with betacarotene—that's being test marketed in Texas.

Nutraceutical offerings in the not-so-distant future will be coming from Heinz, best known for its ketchup. Heinz is repositioning ketchup as a functional food by emphasizing the nutritional value of lycopene, commonly found in tomatoes. Novartis plans to launch Aviva, a line of foods that promise to reduce cholesterol, strengthen bones, and improve digestion. Functional foods may even go prenatal: Novartis is researching products that may provide prenatal benefits in vision and nervous system development.

In a strange twist, Johnson and Johnson recently ended its consumer advertising for the cholesterol-lowering margarine, Benecol. The company will market its product to physicians instead, which is an odd choice since much of the demand for functional foods is the trend toward self health care. Also, "many physicians in family practice and in specialty practice do not quite understand where these products fit in," says Walter Glinsmann, M.D., a Washington, D.C.–based doctor who has worked with the FDA in clinical nutrition research.[20]

TREND 3: LIFESTYLE GURUS

No other industry in our society is as prone to fads as health care. All it takes is a book about a new concept for staying healthy, eating well, or losing pounds and there's a new guru of the week. Examples are Depak Chopra's *Perfect Health*, Andrew Wiel's *Spontaneous Healing*, Dean Ornish's *Eat More, Weigh Less*, and Robert C. Atkins' *The New Diet Revolution*.

A battle has been brewing between Ornish and Atkins in recent years. Whereas Ornish recommends a low-protein, high-fruit and vegetable regimen, Atkins promotes a high-protein, low-carbohydrate diet. Each camp has ardent followers. In an effort to make sense of the competing diets, the USDA sponsored a nutritional summit, inviting both Ornish and Atkins to the event, where each attacked the scientific merits of the other's diet in an entertaining and spirited debate.[21] The result: The USDA's Behavioral Nutrition Initiative will examine a variety of eating plans and draw up recommendations for the healthiest type of diet.[22]

While many popular health advisors provide sound advice, the credibility of others is questionable. Nevertheless, health gurus will continue to emerge as Americans search for nirvana. The most popular gurus of the future will be those with a holistic approach, offering improvement to body, mind, and spirit, thanks to the aging of the baby-boom generation.

TREND 4: SELF-ACCEPTANCE

Expect healthy living to become the goal of a growing number of Americans as aging boomers give up on achieving the ideal weight or perfect muscle tone. Moderation will become the goal of fitness and nutrition programs. This perspective will encourage more people to live a healthy lifestyle.

Too many of today's exercise programs make participants feel like failures because they are unable to achieve perfection. When exercising is promoted with unattainable goals, many people shrug their shoulders and say, "Why bother?" But this perspective is changing, and moderation is becoming more important in exercise programs and promotions. Expect to see growing participation in moderate physical activities like walking, hiking, swimming, tennis, and golf. Also, expect to see more interest in holistic activities. Already, participation in yoga and Tai Chi is on the rise—up 12 percent between 1998 and 1999, according to the Sporting Goods Manufacturers Association.[23] Many more activities connecting spirituality and fitness will emerge in the years ahead. One example is JoSand, a new type of exercise that involves putting a stick into the sand while doing various jumps and squats.[24]

Increasingly, exercise will be promoted as a way to live well longer rather than as a means to get a date. The same tone of moderation is creeping into the weight-loss industry as well, with many weight-loss products and services replacing the harsh word "diet" with the softer terms "lifestyle change" and "wellness."

TREND 5: FOOD SAFETY

Food safety is an issue of growing concern to Americans. In fact, food safety was the number one nutrition news topic of 1997, according to the International Food Information Council's *Food for Thought* survey. Food safety was narrowly bumped into the number two spot in 1999.[25] The Food Marketing Institute has found consumers to have become less confident in the safety of supermarket food. In 1996, 84 percent of consumers said that they were "completely" or "mostly" confident that the food in their supermarket was safe. By 2000, the figure had fallen to 74 percent.[26] Americans are increasingly alarmed about pesticides, bacteria, mad cow disease, and other health threats to the food supply.

Food-borne diseases cause an estimated 76 million illnesses and 5,000 deaths in the United States each year. These figures are probably underestimates, since many cases of food-borne illness are not reported to authorities. Most often, the cause of food-borne disease is careless food preparation or the personal hygiene of the food preparer—not an unsafe food source, according to the CDC.[27] The public's heightened awareness of food safety problems will lead to greater demand for food quality regulations in restaurants—and hopefully to better food safety practices in the home.

The politics surrounding the issue of food irradiation shows just how much public attitudes have changed over the past few years. Most Americans once resisted irradiation, associating it with the dangers of nuclear energy. Today irradiation has strong public acceptance because it is one way to ensure food safety. Food biotechnology will be the next frontier in food safety. In Europe, biotech-engineered foods have met with great consumer resistance. In the United States, a movement to label foods that have been engineered by science is underway. One organization, Alliance for Bio-Integrity, is suing the Food and Drug Administration, asking for mandatory safety testing and labeling.[28] "Labeling is inevitable," said Congressman Dennis Kucinich of Ohio in an interview with *Business Week*.[29] And although consumers haven't been overly concerned about biotech food just yet, a study by IFIC shows consumer support for engineered foods is on the decline. In surveys from 1997 to 1999, the organization asked consumers whether they felt that biotechnology would provide benefits for themselves or their families over the next five years. In 1997, 78 percent said yes. By 2000, the figure had declined to 59 percent. The number of people answering the question negatively climbed from 14 percent in 1997 to 25 percent in 2000.[30]

Concerns over pesticides are behind the phenomenal growth of organic foods, which have made the transition from health food stores to supermarket shelves. Organic food accounts for only 1 percent of national food sales, but revenues have grown more than 20 percent annually since 1990 and are expected to reach $6.6 billion by 2000, according to Packaged Facts.[31] Twenty-eight percent of consumers currently purchase organically grown produce, according to the Food Marketing Institute.[32] Nearly six in ten shoppers purchase organic food at the supermarket.

Another safety issue revolves around food allergies. A growing number of Americans are complaining of allergic reactions to certain foods or food additives. According to the International Food Information Council, the most common food allergies are to peanuts, tree nuts, dairy, soy, wheat, eggs, fish, and shellfish. Americans who suffer from food allergies are another driving force in the robust market for organic and additive-free foods. They are also an important pressure group in demanding stricter standards for food labeling. Expect their demands to escalate in the future.

Notes

1. National Institute of Environmental Health Sciences, "Fact Sheet: The Report on Carcinogens–9th Edition" (May 15, 2000). <www.niehs.nih.gov>.

2. Food Marketing Institute, *Trends in the United States—Consumer Attitudes and the Supermarket, 2000* (2000).

3. Interview with Kai Robertson (June 14, 2000).

4. National Center for Health Statistics, "The Prevalence of Sedentary Leisure-Time Behavior Among Adults in the United States," Health E-Stats (July 2, 2000). <www.cdc.gov/nchs>.

5. "CDC Finds Low Breastfeeding Rates, More Children Overweight," *Public Health Reports* 3, no. 2 (May 1999): 209.

6. *Chronic Disease Notes and Reports Newsletter* 13, no. 1 (Winter 2000): 1.

7. "Generation XXL: Childhood Obesity Now Threatens One in Three Kids with Long Term Health Problems, and the Problem Is Growing," *Newsweek* (July 3, 2000): 40.

8. Sporting Goods Manufacturers Association, *Sports Participation Trends 1999, Statistical Highlights from the Superstudy of Sports Participation* (April 2000). <www.sportlink.com>.

9. Ibid.

10. Bess H. Marcus, "Exercise Behavior and Strategies for Intervention," *Research Quarterly for Exercise and Sport* 66, no. 4 (December 1995): 319–326.

11. Carolyn Wilhelm, "Leveling Demand for Dietary Supplements," *Chemical Market Reporter* 257, no. 22 (May 29, 2000): 8.

12. Food Marketing Institute.

13. National Center for Health Statistics.

14. International Food Information Council, "Diets: Look Before You Leap" (July 1, 2000). <www.ific.org>.

15. "Rating the Diets," *Consumer Reports* (June 1993): 353-355.

16. "Guaranteed: Lose 1 Pound in 90 Days," *US News and World Report* 126, no. 7 (February 22, 1999): 67.

17. Jenny Coe, *Blockbuster Lifestyle Drugs* (2000).

18. "Workouts at Work Can Sweeten Long Days, But Don't Cut Loose on the Boss," *US News and World Report* 128, no. 24 (June 19, 2000): 57.

19. Ira Dreyfuss, "Health Club Targets Truckers," The Associated Press via America Online News (December 14, 1997).

20. Interview with Walter Glinsman (March 2, 2000).

21. Robert Hager, "Weight-Loss Gurus Debate Fad Diets," MSNBC (February 24, 2000). <www.msnbc.com>.

22. Third Age News Service, "Feds Eye Dueling Diets" (June 1, 2000). <www.thirdage.com>.

23. Sporting goods Manufacturers Association.

24. Marlene Rentmeester, "Balancing Act," *Women's Sports and Fitness* 2, no. 4 (May 1999): 31.

25. International Food Information Council Foundation, *Food for Thought II—Reporting of Diet, Nutrition and Food Safety, Executive Summary* (February 1998): 20.

26. Food Marketing Institute.

27. Sonja J. Olsen, Linda C. MacKinon, Joy S. Goulding, Nancy H. Bean, and Laurence Slutsker, "Surveillance for Foodborne Disease Outbreaks—United States, 1993–1997," *MMWR* 49, no. 10 (March 17, 2000): 201–205.

28. "The Judge Has Not Yet Ruled in a Suit Challenging FDA's Policy on Biotech Food," *Food Chemical News* 42, no. 9 (April 17, 2000): 38.

29. "The Frankenfood Monster Stalks Capitol Hill," *Business Week* (December 13, 1999): 55.

30. The International Food Information Council, *U.S. Attitudes Toward Food Biotechnology*, (2000).

31. "Panel Sees Sharp Upturn for Organics," *Food Processing* 60, no. 10 (October 1999): 16.

32. Food Marketing Institute, *Shopping for Health 1997* (1997).

Prevalence of a Sedentary Lifestyle, 1997

(percent of people aged 18 or older who never engage in vigorous, moderate, or light physical activity for at least 20 minutes during their leisure time, by age, sex, race, Hispanic origin, and education, 1997)

	percent sedentary
Total people	**39.8%**
Aged 18 to 24	31.5
Aged 25 to 44	34.2
Aged 45 to 64	42.1
Aged 65 or older	56.9
Total men	**35.9**
Aged 18 to 24	25.8
Aged 25 to 44	31.8
Aged 45 to 64	39.6
Aged 65 or older	50.5
Total women	**43.3**
Aged 18 to 24	37.1
Aged 25 to 44	36.5
Aged 45 to 64	44.4
Aged 65 or older	61.4
Race and Hispanic origin	
White, non-Hispanic	36.3
Black, non-Hispanic	52.2
Asian, non-Hispanic	43.0
Hispanic	53.5
Education	
Less than 9th grade	71.6
Grades 9 to 11	57.3
GED	47.4
High school graduate	44.5
Some college, no degree	34.0
Bachelor's degree	23.8
Graduate degree	23.5

Source: National Center for Health Statistics, "Prevalence of Sedentary Leisure-time Behavior Among Adults in the United States," NCHS Health E-Stats, Internet site <www.cdc/nchs/products/pubs/pubd/hestats/3and4/sedentary.htm>

Vigorous Exercise by Sex and Age, 1996

(percent of people aged 20 or older who exercise vigorously by sex, age, and frequency of vigorous exercise, 1996)

	daily	5 to 6 times per week	2 to 4 times per week	once a week	less than once a week*
Total people	**18.6%**	**7.1%**	**23.7%**	**8.0%**	**42.1%**
Total men	**24.6**	**8.2**	**24.4**	**7.7**	**34.5**
Aged 20 to 29	27.8	9.7	27.1	9.2	25.9
Aged 30 to 39	23.3	8.1	31.4	7.9	29.0
Aged 40 to 49	19.9	1.0	24.7	9.5	35.7
Aged 50 to 59	26.5	6.9	23.7	8.0	34.1
Aged 60 to 69	29.3	5.6	14.2	4.6	45.5
Aged 70 or older	23.7	6.1	13.0	3.1	53.1
Total women	**13.1**	**6.2**	**23.0**	**8.2**	**49.2**
Aged 20 to 29	12.1	7.0	25.6	10.2	44.4
Aged 30 to 39	15.4	5.4	23.6	10.1	45.5
Aged 40 to 49	9.2	7.6	29.8	8.8	44.4
Aged 50 to 59	14.9	7.8	24.0	7.9	44.0
Aged 60 to 69	18.5	4.9	18.4	5.4	52.5
Aged 70 or older	9.8	3.6	11.0	3.9	71.2

* Includes rarely or never.
Note: Numbers will not add to total because "don't know" and no answer are not shown.
Source: USDA, ARS Food Surveys Research Group, Data Tables: Results from USDA's 1994–96 Continuing Survey of Food Intakes by Individuals and 1994–96 Diet and Health Knowledge Survey, 1999; Internet web site <http://www.barc.usda.gov/bhnrc/foodsurvey/home.htm>; calculations by New Strategist

Sports Participation Trends, 1987 to 1999

(number of people aged 6 or older participating at least once per year in selected sports and fitness activities, 1987 and 1999; percent change in participation, 1987–99; numbers in thousands)

	1999	1987	percent change 1987–99
Fitness activities			
Aerobics (high impact)	6,249	13,961	–55.2%
Aerobics (low impact)	11,585	11,888	–2.5
Aerobics (step)	9,503	–	–
Aquatic exercise	5,557	–	–
Fitness bicycling	12,307	–	–
Fitness walking	35,976	27,164	32.4
Running/jogging	34,047	37,136	–8.3
Fitness swimming	14,194	16,912	–16.1
Yoga/Tai Chi	6,404	–	–
Equipment exercise			
Free weights	42,810	22,553	89.8
Weight/resistance machines	22,961	15,261	50.5
Home gym exercise	7,918	3,905	102.8
Rowing machine	6,269	14,481	–56.7
Stationary cycling	30,942	30,765	0.6
Treadmill	37,463	4,396	752.2
Stair-climbing machine	16,288	2,121	667.9
Team sports			
Baseball	12,069	15,098	–20.1
Basketball	39,368	35,737	10.2
Ice hockey	2,385	2,393	–0.3
Football (touch)	16,729	20,292	–17.6
Soccer	17,582	15,388	14.3
Softball	19,766	30,995	–36.2
Volleyball	24,176	35,984	–32.8
Racquet sports			
Badminton	8,884	14,793	–39.9
Racquetball	5,633	10,395	–45.8
Tennis	16,817	21,147	–20.5

(continued)

(continued from previous page)

	1999	1987	percent change 1987–99
Indoor sports			
Billiards/pool	36,425	35,297	3.2%
Bowling	52,577	47,823	9.9
Skating sports			
Roller skating (inline wheels)	27,865	–	–
Skateboarding	7,807	10,888	–28.3
Ice skating	17,499	–	
Other recreational activities			
Bicycling (recreational)	56,227	–	–
Golf	28,216	26,261	7.4
Gymnastics	5,254	–	–
Walking (recreational)	84,096	–	–
Outdoor activities			
Camping (tent)	40,803	35,232	15.8
Camping (RV)	17,577	22,655	–22.4
Hiking	40,639	–	–
Horseback riding	16,906	–	–
Mountain biking	7,849	1,512	419.1
Mountain/rock climbing	2,103	–	–
Artificial wall climbing	4,817	–	–
Shooting sports			
Archery	6,937	8,558	–18.9
Hunting (shotgun/rifle)	16,779	25,241	–33.5
Shooting (trap/skeet)	4,745	5,073	–6.5
Target shooting	18,312	18,947	–3.4
Fishing			
Fishing (fly)	6,134	11,359	–46.0
Fishing (freshwater)	44,452	50,500	–12.0
Fishing (saltwater)	14,807	19,646	–24.6
Snow sports			
Skiing (cross-country)	3,988	8,344	–52.2
Skiing (downhill)	13,865	17,676	–21.6
Snowboarding	4,729	–	–
Snowmobiling	5,490	–	–

(continued)

(continued from previous page)

	1999	1987	percent change 1987–99
Water sports			
Boardsailing/windsurfing	624	1,145	–45.5%
Canoeing	12,785	–	–
Kayaking	4,012	–	–
Jet skiing	9,981	–	–
Sailing	5,327	6,368	–16.3
Scuba diving	3,095	2,433	27.2
Snorkeling	10,694	–	–
Surfing	1,736	1,459	19.0
Swimming (recreational)	95,094	–	–
Water skiing	9,961	19,902	–49.9

Note: (–) means data not available.
Source: Sporting Goods Manufacturers Association, Sports Participation Trends 1999—Statistical Highlights from the Superstudy of Sports Participation, *Internet site <http://www.sgma.com> 2000*

Quality of Diet by Sex, 1996

(percent distribution of people aged 20 or older by self-assessed quality of diet, by sex, 1996)

	too low		about right		too high	
	men	women	men	women	men	women
Calories	5.0%	6.7%	54.4%	50.6%	38.1%	39.9%
Calcium	26.3	43.6	61.7	51.5	4.7	1.9
Iron	22.6	35.2	65.3	58.1	3.2	1.1
Vitamin C	28.0	30.4	64.4	65.8	4.2	1.4
Protein	10.7	16.1	72.0	73.2	13.9	8.4
Fat	6.6	5.8	40.9	44.9	50.1	48.0
Saturated fat	9.3	5.7	40.8	52.5	42.6	36.1
Cholesterol	5.8	5.5	54.7	59.1	34.0	30.7
Salt or sodium	10.8	9.0	62.6	68.2	24.4	21.9
Fiber	33.6	37.3	58.6	59.1	3.0	1.5
Sugar and sweets	9.4	6.2	53.6	56.3	36.0	36.2

Note: Numbers will not add to 100 percent because "don't know" and no answer are not shown.
Source: USDA, Food Surveys Research Group, Data Tables: Results from USDA's 1996 Continuing Survey of Food Intakes by Individuals and 1996 Diet and Health Knowledge Survey, 1999; Internet site <http://www.barc.usda.gov/ bhnrc/foodsurvey/home>

Importance of Dietary Guidelines by Sex, 1996

(percent of people saying dietary guidelines are very important, by sex, 1996)

	men	women
Maintain a healthy weight	70.7%	76.0%
Choose a diet with plenty of fruits and vegetables	60.2	74.7
Eat a variety of foods	58.3	65.9
Choose a diet low in cholesterol	54.5	59.5
Choose a diet low in fat	52.3	63.3
Choose a diet with adequate fiber	47.7	54.9
Choose a diet low in saturated fat	46.7	60.1
Use salt or sodium only in moderation	45.8	53.1
Use sugars only in moderation	45.2	54.0
Choose a diet with plenty of breads, cereals, rice, and pasta	31.2	34.8
Eat at least two servings of dairy products daily	30.8	43.1

Source: USDA, Food Surveys Research Group, Data Tables: Results from USDA's 1996 Continuing Survey of Food Intakes by Individuals and 1996 Diet and Health Knowledge Survey, 1999; Internet site <http://www.barc.usda.gov/bhnrc/foodsurvey/home>

Knowledge of Health Problems Associated with Nutrition, 1994–95

(percent of people aged 20 or older who are aware of health problems associated with selected eating behaviors, and associated health problems mentioned by at least 10 percent of respondents, by sex, 1994–95)

	men	women
Eating too much fat	**85.7%**	**89.3%**
Heart disease/high blood cholesterol	71.7	75.4
Obesity	24.7	26.8
Not eating enough fiber	**58.4**	**70.7**
Bowel problems	42.7	56.1
Cancer	12.0	16.6
Eating too much salt or sodium	**86.0**	**90.8**
Hypertension	54.6	57.8
Heart disease/high blood cholesterol	30.7	32.4
Not eating enough calcium	**75.1**	**86.6**
Bone problems/osteoporosis	68.2	79.0
Dental problems	12.1	13.9
Eating too much cholesterol	**88.7**	**90.1**
Heart disease/high blood cholesterol	79.3	80.9
Hypertension	10.5	11.6
Eating too much sugar	**77.5**	**82.0**
Diabetes	46.3	55.3
Obesity	19.0	27.8
Dental problems	14.2	11.3
Being overweight	**94.4**	**94.7**
Heart disease/high blood cholesterol	74.7	76.2
Hypertension	21.9	21.6
Diabetes	12.7	19.0
Obesity	11.2	10.7

Source: USDA, Diet and Health Knowledge Survey, 1994–95, ARS, Beltsville Human Nutrition Research Center, Food Surveys Research Group, 1997

Use of Nutrition Information on Food Labels, 1994–95

(percent of people aged 20 or older who use nutritional information on food labels, by frequency of use and sex, 1994–95)

	men	women
Calories		
Often or always	25.0%	44.2%
Sometimes	26.5	27.4
Rarely or never	25.9	19.2
Salt or sodium		
Often or always	24.6	34.2
Sometimes	22.7	29.1
Rarely or never	30.0	27.4
Total fat		
Often or always	32.2	50.5
Sometimes	22.3	23.6
Rarely or never	22.9	16.9
Saturated fat		
Often or always	26.4	40.7
Sometimes	22.5	25.4
Rarely or never	28.6	24.7
Cholesterol		
Often or always	26.0	37.1
Sometimes	23.6	28.2
Rarely or never	27.9	25.4
Vitamins or minerals		
Often or always	16.4	25.1
Sometimes	30.3	36.5
Rarely or never	30.8	29.1
Fiber		
Often or always	13.6	20.4
Sometimes	24.8	33.1
Rarely or never	38.8	37.2
Sugars		
Often or always	18.6	30.7
Sometimes	25.8	31.0
Rarely or never	33.1	29.1

Source: USDA, Diet and Health Knowledge Survey, 1994–95, *ARS, Beltsville Human Nutrition Research Center, Food Surveys Research Group, 1997*

Vitamin Use by Age and Sex, 1994–96

(percent of people taking vitamin/mineral supplements by age, sex, and type of supplement, 1994–96)

		type of supplement			
	any supplement	multivitamin	multivitamin with iron or other minerals	combination of vitamin C and iron	single vitamins or minerals
Total people	**46.8%**	**20.7%**	**16.8%**	**2.9%**	**15.3%**
Under age 5	47.1	22.6	20.1	2.0	4.6
Under age 1	15.3	5.6	5.6	0.2	4.3
Aged 1 to 2	44.9	21.3	19.0	1.6	4.3
Aged 3 to 5	56.1	27.6	24.3	2.7	4.9
Males					
Aged 6 to 11	46.1	23.9	17.1	2.4	5.6
Aged 12 to 19	29.2	14.6	7.6	3.0	8.8
Aged 20 or older	41.9	20.2	13.2	2.5	14.6
Aged 20 to 29	36.4	18.1	9.7	3.2	9.6
Aged 30 to 39	39.7	20.6	14.1	3.1	10.2
Aged 40 to 49	43.8	20.6	14.1	1.5	15.6
Aged 50 to 59	43.8	21.6	12.0	2.3	19.2
Aged 60 to 69	47.6	20.5	15.4	1.5	22.7
Aged 70 or older	47.1	19.2	15.7	2.4	20.1
Females					
Aged 6 to 11	41.7	20.1	15.7	2.2	6.3
Aged 12 to 19	39.3	15.7	12.5	4.0	11.8
Aged 20 or older	55.8	22.1	21.5	3.6	22.4
Aged 20 to 29	52.0	22.7	21.9	3.9	13.7
Aged 30 to 39	54.4	19.8	25.6	3.5	17.5
Aged 40 to 49	56.7	21.9	21.8	3.7	23.8
Aged 50 to 59	62.6	24.5	20.7	4.7	32.7
Aged 60 to 69	57.3	21.5	19.4	2.6	30.9
Aged 70 or older	53.6	23.1	15.7	2.7	23.2

Source: USDA, ARS Food Surveys Research Group, Supplementary Data Tables: USDA's 1994–96 Continuing Survey of Food Intakes by Individuals, Internet web site <http://www.barc.usda.gov/bhnrc/foodsurvey/home.htm>; calculations by New Strategist

Food and Beverage Consumption, 1970 and 1997

(number of pounds of selected foods and gallons of selected beverages consumed per person, 1970 and 1997; percent change in consumption, 1970–97)

	1997	1970	percent change 1970–97
Red meat	**111.0**	**131.7**	**–15.7%**
Beef	63.8	79.6	–19.8
Pork	45.6	48.0	–5.0
Poultry	**64.8**	**33.8**	**91.7**
Chicken	50.9	27.4	85.8
Turkey	13.9	6.4	117.2
Fish and shellfish	**14.5**	**11.7**	**23.9**
Canned tuna	3.1	2.5	24.0
Fresh and frozen fish	6.1	4.5	35.6
Fresh and frozen shellfish	3.8	2.4	58.3
Eggs (number)	**238.7**	**308.9**	**–22.7**
Processed	65.5	33.0	98.5
Shell	173.1	275.9	–37.3
Cheese	**28.0**	**11.4**	**145.6**
Cheddar	9.6	5.8	65.5
Mozzarella	8.4	1.2	600.0
Swiss	1.0	0.9	11.1
Beverage milk	**206.9**	**269.1**	**–23.1**
Plain whole milk	70.2	213.5	–67.1
2% milk	66.7	28.0	138.2
Skim milk	34.4	11.6	196.6
Yogurt	5.1	0.8	537.5
Frozen dairy products	**28.7**	**28.5**	**0.7**
Ice cream	16.2	17.8	–9.0
Fats and oils	**65.6**	**52.6**	**24.7**
Butter	4.2	5.4	–22.2
Margarine	8.6	10.8	–20.4
Salad and cooking oils	28.7	15.4	86.4
Fresh fruits	**133.2**	**101.2**	**31.6**
Apples	18.5	17.0	8.8
Bananas	27.7	17.4	59.2
Cantaloupe	11.7	7.2	62.5
Grapefruit	6.3	8.2	–23.2
Grapes	8.0	2.9	175.9
Oranges	14.1	16.2	–13.0
Peaches and nectarines	5.7	5.8	–1.7

(continued)

(continued from previous page)

	1997	1970	percent change 1970–97
Pears	3.5	1.9	84.2%
Strawberries	4.2	1.7	147.1
Watermelon	16.1	13.5	19.3
Canned fruits	**18.0**	**23.3**	**−22.7**
Frozen fruits	**3.3**	**3.3**	**0.0**
Fruit juices	**9.2**	**5.7**	**61.4**
Apple juice	1.6	0.5	220.0
Orange juice	5.9	3.8	55.3
Fresh vegetables	**185.6**	**152.9**	**21.4**
Bell peppers	7.2	2.2	227.3
Broccoli	5.2	0.5	940.0
Cabbage	10.2	8.8	15.9
Carrots	12.5	6.0	108.3
Celery	6.0	7.3	−17.8
Corn	8.1	7.8	3.8
Cucumbers	6.3	2.8	125.0
Garlic	2.1	0.4	425.0
Head lettuce	24.3	22.4	8.5
Onions	17.9	10.1	77.2
Potatoes	47.9	61.8	−22.5
Tomatoes	18.9	12.1	56.2
Peanuts	**5.8**	**5.5**	**5.5**
Peanut butter	2.8	2.7	3.7
Flour and cereal products	**200.1**	**135.6**	**47.6**
Ready-to-eat cereals	14.3	8.9	60.7
Ready-to-cook cereals	2.6	1.7	52.9
Caloric sweeteners	**154.1**	**122.3**	**26.0**
Sugar	66.5	101.8	−34.7
Corn sweeteners	86.2	19.1	351.3
Candy	**24.8**	**19.9**	**24.6**
Bottled water	**13.1**	**1.2***	**383.3**
Coffee	**23.5**	**33.4**	**−29.6**
Tea	**7.4**	**6.8**	**8.8**
Soft drinks	**53.0**	**24.3**	**118.1**
Diet	11.6	2.1	452.4
Regular	41.4	22.2	86.5
Alcoholic beverages**	**38.9**	**35.7**	**9.0**
Beer	33.9	30.6	10.8
Wine	3.0	2.2	36.4
Distilled spirits	1.9	3.0	−36.7

* Data for 1976.
** Per person aged 21 or older.
Source: USDA, Economic Research Service, Food Consumption, Prices, and Expenditures, 1970–1997; calculations by New Strategist

Food Consumption of Males by Type of Food and Age, 1994–96

(percent of total persons and males aged 6 or older consuming selected types of foods on an average day, by age, 1994-96)

	total, both sexes	males							
		6 to 11	12 to 19	20 to 29	30 to 39	40 to 49	50 to 59	60 to 69	70 or older
Grain products	96.9%	98.8%	98.2%	94.4%	96.6%	96.4%	97.1%	97.4%	98.6%
Yeast breads and rolls	66.3	68.3	62.7	62.3	67.5	68.5	69.7	78.2	76.3
Cereals and pastas	46.8	65.0	44.6	34.1	37.6	40.2	42.0	49.6	60.4
Ready-to-eat cereals	28.5	53.3	33.2	17.5	20.1	19.1	22.6	28.2	38.2
Rice	11.0	10.0	10.0	11.8	13.0	13.1	12.6	11.1	7.5
Pasta	7.4	7.9	5.9	8.5	6.8	9.9	6.4	7.7	5.1
Quick breads, pancakes, french toast	22.7	26.0	24.5	18.6	22.7	23.4	25.9	24.4	21.9
Cakes, cookies, pastries, pies	41.2	52.1	41.3	32.2	37.8	39.6	41.0	41.8	47.9
Crackers, popcorn, pretzels, corn chips	27.8	33.8	27.2	27.7	25.4	24.2	27.0	24.8	24.3
Mixtures, mainly grain	35.9	44.8	46.1	41.6	39.4	32.4	26.7	21.2	19.7
Vegetables	82.8	79.6	78.2	83.7	87.9	86.7	86.9	87.2	84.2
White potatoes, total	44.3	48.8	49.6	49.7	49.9	43.7	45.5	44.2	44.2
Fried	27.0	38.4	38.7	37.0	33.0	26.3	22.3	19.7	14.0
Dark-green vegetables	9.8	6.1	3.6	6.7	11.5	9.9	12.7	13.4	12.5
Deep-yellow vegetables	12.9	12.0	8.1	7.2	11.2	12.4	14.4	17.7	18.6
Tomatoes	38.8	38.0	43.0	45.5	42.2	42.6	40.0	41.9	37.3
Lettuce, lettuce-based salads	24.9	14.2	23.8	26.0	27.0	29.2	30.3	29.3	25.4
Green beans	7.7	6.8	3.5	4.6	6.1	7.2	8.1	10.5	12.6
Corn, green peas, lima beans	11.7	14.0	7.4	8.4	9.9	14.1	14.9	12.1	16.0
Other vegetables	42.5	30.1	33.3	41.1	50.4	50.8	49.8	52.7	52.6

(continued)

(continued from previous page)

	total, both sexes	males							
		6 to 11	12 to 19	20 to 29	30 to 39	40 to 49	50 to 59	60 to 69	70 or older
Fruits	53.7%	55.9%	44.5%	41.6%	40.0%	47.6%	56.8%	62.4%	69.6%
Citrus fruits and juices	26.5	24.1	24.8	23.8	21.3	24.1	29.5	31.2	37.9
Juices	20.4	20.6	21.7	21.0	16.1	17.6	22.6	23.3	27.7
Other fruits, mixtures, and juices	39.3	43.8	27.0	25.2	26.5	32.6	42.7	47.2	55.4
Apples	12.2	18.9	8.2	7.4	8.3	8.7	12.9	13.7	16.1
Bananas	13.4	8.1	6.0	7.3	11.2	13.3	16.7	24.4	29.0
Melons and berries	7.8	6.2	4.1	4.7	4.6	7.3	10.0	11.0	12.3
Other fruits and mixtures, mainly fruit	13.7	15.1	7.1	7.2	10.0	12.1	14.2	16.1	19.2
Noncitrus juices and nectars	8.5	11.3	8.1	5.0	3.8	4.9	5.5	4.0	7.1
Milk and milk products	78.9	92.1	81.3	67.9	74.3	74.2	72.7	80.0	85.5
Milk, milk drinks, yogurt	60.5	84.9	65.8	42.7	51.2	51.7	51.1	62.8	71.0
Fluid milk	55.6	79.4	59.5	39.6	47.5	48.5	48.7	59.8	68.2
Whole	19.4	31.3	22.7	13.2	17.0	17.0	11.8	15.0	17.5
Low fat	26.3	43.1	30.5	19.4	23.5	20.7	25.5	28.0	36.3
Skim	11.0	9.8	7.1	7.0	6.8	12.6	11.7	15.2	15.7
Yogurt	4.0	3.5	1.7	1.9	3.6	3.6	2.7	2.2	2.1
Milk desserts	17.4	25.5	13.6	12.4	16.7	16.9	17.7	21.1	25.5
Cheese	32.6	30.0	37.1	37.7	36.7	32.2	27.9	27.8	28.5
Meat, poultry, and fish	86.2	87.1	86.9	89.1	90.0	89.2	92.7	92.0	92.2
Beef	20.9	22.5	24.2	22.8	27.9	26.9	23.4	24.6	19.6
Pork	15.8	12.5	15.8	13.3	15.4	18.4	22.1	21.7	24.9

(continued)

(continued from previous page)

	total, both sexes	males							
		6 to 11	12 to 19	20 to 29	30 to 39	40 to 49	50 to 59	60 to 69	70 or older
Frankfurters, sausages, luncheon meats	28.6%	35.0%	31.8%	30.9%	31.9%	32.9%	31.3%	32.5%	32.4%
Poultry	22.6	22.2	20.6	24.1	23.0	23.1	22.7	22.1	19.6
Chicken	19.2	19.6	17.7	19.6	20.3	19.1	17.4	17.1	16.9
Fish and shellfish	8.0	5.6	5.1	6.6	10.8	7.5	13.6	11.6	11.5
Mixtures, mainly meat, poultry, fish	36.2	35.6	38.4	44.9	39.8	38.3	38.4	38.7	35.7
Eggs	19.1	15.4	17.0	18.7	19.6	21.3	23.0	26.8	27.8
Legumes	13.6	9.8	11.0	12.0	16.9	15.7	13.0	15.2	15.1
Nuts and seeds	9.6	15.4	8.7	7.0	7.6	8.2	10.7	9.7	11.2
Fats and oils	54.5	46.5	43.2	46.3	56.7	58.5	63.1	69.8	67.3
Table fats	30.4	27.7	20.8	18.8	28.7	32.3	35.8	44.8	47.0
Salad dressings	29.3	25.2	27.7	29.7	30.6	33.7	32.5	35.1	30.9
Sugars and sweets, total	53.2	58.5	46.6	39.4	49.9	53.1	58.2	61.5	65.2
Sugars	28.1	12.1	13.4	18.7	32.4	35.0	41.1	45.1	44.8
Candy	15.4	29.1	21.0	14.9	12.1	11.7	11.9	12.1	7.4
Beverages	**86.9**	**74.9**	**87.4**	**91.5**	**94.0**	**95.5**	**95.3**	**95.4**	**91.8**
Alcoholic	12.5	0.0	2.9	27.8	23.4	24.0	22.9	19.2	14.8
Wine	3.5	0.0	0.3	3.1	3.5	5.8	5.8	6.1	5.5
Beer and ale	7.6	0.0	2.3	24.3	19.1	17.1	14.5	10.3	5.7

(continued)

(continued from previous page)

	total, both sexes	males							
		6 to 11	12 to 19	20 to 29	30 to 39	40 to 49	50 to 59	60 to 69	70 or older
Nonalcoholic	85.8%	74.9%	86.8%	87.1%	92.5%	94.0%	93.5%	94.7%	90.6%
Coffee	39.5	1.0	6.1	24.6	51.9	63.4	70.3	78.0	75.0
Tea	22.8	9.3	16.3	17.6	26.9	25.6	25.7	26.2	25.7
Fruit drinks and ades, total	19.7	38.8	28.5	20.5	13.2	14.8	14.4	10.0	10.7
Carbonated soft drinks, total	50.4	47.6	69.1	68.3	62.9	53.8	50.7	37.7	25.7
Regular	39.3	43.7	66.1	62.9	51.0	41.0	33.3	22.6	16.1
Low calorie	12.8	5.8	5.2	6.7	14.2	15.3	19.0	16.4	9.7

Source: USDA, ARS Food Surveys Research Group, Supplementary Data Tables: USDA's 1994–96 Continuing Survey of Food Intakes by Individuals, Internet web site <http://www.barc.usda.gov/bhnrc/foodsurvey/home.htm>

Food Consumption of Females by Type of Food and Age, 1994–96

(percent of total persons and females aged 6 or older consuming selected types of foods on an average day, by age, 1994–96)

	both sexes		females							
		6 to 11	12 to 19	20 to 29	30 to 39	40 to 49	50 to 59	60 to 69	70 or older	
Grain products	96.9%	99.3%	97.6%	95.6%	96.1%	96.6%	97.9%	98.0%	98.8%	
Yeast breads and rolls	66.3	70.7	60.8	59.7	64.6	66.1	72.6	73.2	74.8	
Cereals and pastas	46.8	59.1	45.9	41.7	38.8	40.2	41.7	46.8	56.2	
Ready-to-eat cereals	28.5	45.3	30.2	23.6	20.5	19.6	22.0	26.9	35.3	
Rice	11.0	9.5	8.6	13.5	11.5	12.9	10.2	8.9	6.5	
Pasta	7.4	7.3	9.3	6.8	8.2	8.2	6.6	6.9	4.4	
Quick breads, pancakes, french toast	22.7	27.0	19.9	19.7	21.3	23.3	23.4	21.6	22.0	
Cakes, cookies, pastries, pies	41.2	54.8	40.7	35.9	38.1	40.3	38.2	42.4	46.9	
Crackers, popcorn, pretzels, corn chips	27.8	35.6	30.9	24.6	29.8	27.5	26.5	29.3	22.5	
Mixtures, mainly grain	35.9	45.5	46.1	40.2	38.0	30.8	28.0	21.1	19.7	
Vegetables	**82.8**	**81.9**	**79.5**	**81.2**	**82.6**	**83.6**	**85.1**	**86.1**	**85.7**	
White potatoes	44.3	49.8	46.4	42.3	41.9	39.4	40.0	39.2	38.5	
Fried	27.0	38.4	34.6	28.1	23.5	21.4	16.9	13.3	9.5	
Dark-green vegetables	9.8	5.5	7.0	9.2	10.8	12.1	15.4	13.8	15.5	
Deep-yellow vegetables	12.9	12.2	10.6	11.3	15.3	15.9	17.4	15.6	15.0	
Tomatoes	38.8	33.5	35.3	40.6	40.4	39.1	38.9	39.7	36.2	
Lettuce, lettuce-based salads	24.9	17.4	25.1	25.5	28.8	31.1	31.6	32.2	24.0	
Green beans	7.7	7.8	4.4	7.1	7.4	7.4	7.7	11.4	11.7	
Corn, green peas, lima beans	11.7	15.5	7.4	7.6	12.4	10.9	11.4	11.4	15.7	
Other vegetables	42.5	30.2	34.5	40.9	42.8	47.5	51.5	55.3	51.3	

(continued)

(continued from previous page)

	both sexes	females							
		6 to 11	12 to 19	20 to 29	30 to 39	40 to 49	50 to 59	60 to 69	70 or older
Fruits	53.7%	61.5%	45.6%	46.5%	47.2%	51.6%	59.3%	66.7%	71.1%
Citrus fruits and juices	26.5	27.2	22.4	24.3	21.4	24.8	32.4	35.7	40.3
Juices	20.4	21.3	18.1	18.9	15.5	18.0	23.5	25.3	31.2
Other fruits, mixtures, and juices	39.3	46.9	30.2	28.9	34.3	39.2	45.2	52.2	54.1
Apples	12.2	16.0	8.2	6.8	9.9	12.8	13.2	17.4	14.3
Bananas	13.4	6.8	4.4	9.0	12.5	13.2	18.6	20.4	26.3
Melons and berries	7.8	7.4	5.9	4.5	8.1	11.6	12.9	15.0	9.7
Other fruits and mixtures, mainly fruit	13.7	18.5	11.4	10.7	10.8	13.6	15.5	18.6	21.7
Noncitrus juices and nectars	8.5	15.0	9.7	6.0	5.4	4.7	2.6	5.2	6.2
Milk and milk products	78.9	90.6	75.4	73.1	75.9	76.5	77.7	79.0	83.1
Milk, milk drinks, yogurt	60.5	82.2	53.9	51.2	53.3	51.4	57.5	60.9	66.6
Fluid milk	55.6	77.0	49.6	46.1	49.0	47.9	50.9	57.5	63.7
Whole	19.4	33.4	17.5	17.7	14.2	14.0	11.2	13.6	16.6
Low fat	26.3	39.1	23.8	16.3	24.0	21.5	21.3	25.4	30.8
Skim	11.0	8.1	9.4	12.1	11.2	13.3	18.0	18.9	17.2
Yogurt	4.0	2.9	2.2	3.5	6.7	5.0	8.8	5.1	3.4
Milk desserts	17.4	22.7	17.0	11.2	14.0	15.7	18.6	20.0	22.4
Cheese	32.6	31.0	36.1	34.4	35.9	34.7	30.7	29.1	23.8
Meat, poultry, and fish	86.2	85.8	80.2	79.7	84.4	86.1	86.5	89.1	87.8
Beef	20.9	19.4	22.2	16.3	20.4	18.9	18.1	19.2	15.9
Pork	15.8	10.8	11.3	12.8	15.2	17.0	18.4	19.2	20.6

(continued)

(continued from previous page)

					females				
	both sexes	6 to 11	12 to 19	20 to 29	30 to 39	40 to 49	50 to 59	60 to 69	70 or older
Frankfurters, sausages, luncheon meats	28.6%	31.7%	24.5%	22.5%	26.9%	23.6%	22.0%	27.4%	23.0%
Poultry	22.6	22.4	21.6	23.4	19.3	23.3	26.5	21.6	23.4
Chicken	19.2	19.4	19.0	20.6	16.8	18.6	20.4	18.5	20.4
Fish and shellfish	8.0	5.9	5.8	6.2	7.1	8.1	10.9	10.4	10.0
Mixtures, mainly meat, poultry, fish	36.2	33.3	33.9	36.9	36.1	34.0	32.6	34.1	33.1
Eggs	19.1	13.8	15.1	17.7	17.2	19.3	17.7	23.8	19.4
Legumes	13.6	11.1	10.7	15.0	15.9	15.4	14.3	15.1	11.7
Nuts and seeds	9.6	16.6	7.8	7.0	7.1	7.5	7.8	8.7	10.3
Fats and oils	54.5	48.3	45.6	48.5	59.1	63.7	66.3	67.5	65.5
Table fats	30.4	30.0	23.9	23.0	29.2	33.4	39.3	41.5	44.5
Salad dressings	29.3	23.0	28.6	27.9	32.0	36.0	37.2	34.8	28.0
Sugars and sweets	53.2	60.8	46.3	47.0	56.5	58.6	60.2	56.1	60.8
Sugars	28.1	13.3	11.9	26.7	36.7	37.9	40.7	38.5	38.3
Candy	15.4	28.5	23.8	13.2	12.2	15.1	13.8	8.3	8.5
Beverages	**86.9**	**72.0**	**86.9**	**90.3**	**90.0**	**93.5**	**94.4**	**92.7**	**88.3**
Alcoholic	12.5	0.2	1.7	13.0	12.8	12.5	13.2	13.6	5.3
Wine	3.5	0.0	0.4	2.9	4.8	6.4	6.6	7.9	3.4
Beer and ale	7.6	0.0	0.9	8.1	5.7	4.6	3.4	1.7	0.7

(continued)

(continued from previous page)

	both sexes	females							
		6 to 11	12 to 19	20 to 29	30 to 39	40 to 49	50 to 59	60 to 69	70 or older
Nonalcoholic	85.8%	72.0%	86.7%	88.4%	89.3%	92.9%	93.6%	92.0%	87.9%
Coffee	39.5	0.8	3.7	24.7	45.9	61.1	68.6	71.1	70.8
Tea	22.8	11.0	19.2	25.8	29.3	31.5	33.1	32.8	29.4
Fruit drinks and ades	19.7	35.3	27.2	20.3	15.6	12.6	12.1	10.9	11.8
Carbonated soft drinks	50.4	44.4	62.2	63.2	56.0	54.6	45.1	36.9	21.2
Regular	39.3	40.3	56.2	50.3	39.2	31.1	26.1	20.6	12.4
Low calorie	12.8	6.0	8.5	15.7	18.6	25.5	20.8	17.3	8.9

Source: USDA, ARS Food Surveys Research Group, Supplementary Data Tables: USDA's 1994–96 Continuing Survey of Food Intakes by Individuals, Internet web site <http://www.barc.usda.gov/bhnrc/foodsurvey/home.htm>

People Eating away from Home by Sex, Age, and Source of Food, 1994–96

(percent of people obtaining and eating food away from home on an average day, by sex, age, and source of food, 1994–96)

	total eating away from home	sit-down restaurant	fast-food restaurant	someone else or gift	store	school cafeteria	other cafeteria	daycare	other
					source				
Total people	57.1%	26.9%	32.2%	22.7%	23.7%	12.0%	6.7%	2.2%	23.0%
Under age 5	43.3	12.5	25.6	33.1	19.6	10.7	1.1	19.5	7.4
Under age 1	16.2	1.0	12.4	43.0	42.7	0.0	0.0	4.5	1.4
Aged 1 to 2	36.7	12.1	27.9	35.1	20.8	1.4	1.5	19.4	5.7
Aged 3 to 5	54.0	13.4	25.6	31.5	17.4	15.6	0.9	20.6	8.5
Males									
Aged 6 to 11	67.5	11.5	23.2	25.5	14.4	49.6	1.4	3.6	9.6
Aged 12 to 19	72.0	12.5	40.2	20.4	24.8	33.8	1.7	0.4	17.7
Aged 20 or older	71.2	29.7	43.7	19.0	31.9	2.3	6.8	0.3	30.6
Aged 20 to 29	66.9	26.5	35.5	19.1	31.7	1.1	9.5	0.0	32.9
Aged 30 to 39	66.2	30.7	35.9	15.4	28.3	2.3	10.2	0.0	28.3
Aged 40 to 49	59.1	39.1	30.9	12.3	25.4	1.7	8.2	0.0	28.4
Aged 50 to 59	47.9	42.4	27.3	18.1	13.5	0.9	7.2	0.7	22.1
Aged 60 to 69	31.3	46.7	21.0	20.1	11.4	0.0	7.4	0.2	17.1
Aged 70 or older	61.2	32.2	35.6	17.3	27.7	1.7	8.5	0.1	29.1

(continued)

(continued from previous page)

	total eating away from home	sit-down restaurant	fast-food restaurant	someone else or gift	source store	school cafeteria	other cafeteria	daycare	other
Females									
Aged 6 to 11	66.2%	8.9%	25.9%	31.5%	16.2%	49.9%	1.1%	5.2%	9.1%
Aged 12 to 19	64.3	19.5	33.0	31.4	24.6	33.6	1.0	0.4	19.6
Aged 20 or older	63.0	35.6	37.5	22.5	25.8	2.6	10.0	1.2	27.3
Aged 20 to 29	56.5	27.3	35.7	22.4	23.8	2.3	11.4	1.3	27.5
Aged 30 to 39	54.6	36.0	31.2	22.5	24.1	3.1	9.7	0.1	28.9
Aged 40 to 49	52.0	34.6	22.5	23.7	20.9	2.8	10.4	0.3	24.0
Aged 50 to 59	39.9	40.4	19.5	29.1	15.9	1.4	7.7	0.9	16.9
Aged 60 to 69	26.9	40.4	12.7	26.6	10.4	1.8	6.4	1.6	17.8
Aged 70 or older	51.0	34.1	30.3	23.5	22.3	2.5	9.9	0.9	25.6

Note: Numbers will not add to 100 because food may be eaten at more than one location during the day.
Source: USDA, ARS Food Surveys Research Group, Supplementary Data Tables: USDA's 1994–96 Continuing Survey of Food Intakes by Individuals,
Internet web site <http://www.barc.usda.gov/bhnrc/foodsurvey/home.htm>

Overweight and Obese People, 1994–96

(percent of people aged 18 or older who are overweight or obese by sex, age, and education, 1994–96)

	overweight	obese
Total people	**54.1%**	**19.0%**
Aged 18 to 24	37.4	13.0
Aged 25 to 44	53.3	18.7
Aged 45 to 64	62.7	23.8
Aged 65 or older	54.5	16.5
Total men	**62.2**	**18.9**
Aged 18 to 24	41.5	13.9
Aged 25 to 44	63.7	19.2
Aged 45 to 64	70.7	23.0
Aged 65 or older	59.8	14.4
Total women	**46.4**	**19.2**
Aged 18 to 24	33.3	12.1
Aged 25 to 44	42.9	18.2
Aged 45 to 64	55.0	24.6
Aged 65 or older	50.5	18.0
Education		
Less than 9th grade	61.8	24.1
Grades 9 to 11	59.0	24.3
GED	60.1	23.8
High school graduate	56.6	20.8
Some college, no degree	54.9	19.1
Bachelor's degree	46.8	12.9
Graduate degree	42.5	10.5

Note: Overweight is defined as a body mass index of 25 or more. Obesity is defined as a body mass index of 30 or more. BMI is calculated by dividing weight in kilograms by the square of height in meters.
Source: National Center for Health Statistics, data from the 1997 National Health Interview Survey, NCHS Health E-Stats, July 1, 2000, Internet site <http://www.cdc.gov/nchs>

8

Managing Diseases

In the past, most people died of acute illnesses—infectious diseases for which there was no cure. Because many of those diseases struck in childhood, mortality rates among the young were high, limiting life expectancy.

The introduction of sanitary practices and the development of vaccines and antibiotics tamed many once-fatal illnesses, leaving chronic conditions as the primary killers of Americans. Consequently, life expectancy rose. In 1900, life expectancy was only 47 years. This does not mean people lived until their mid-forties and then dropped dead. It meant many people died in childhood—so many, in fact, that the chance of living until adulthood was far smaller than it is today. Many of those who did survive childhood, however, lived to old age.

Today, the life expectancy of Americans is a much higher 77 years because the great majority now survive childhood. The young are still the ones most susceptible to acute conditions such as colds, flu, parasites, and other illnesses. The young are also more likely

Fewer Americans have high blood pressure

(percent of people aged 20 or older with hypertension, 1960–62 and 1988–94)

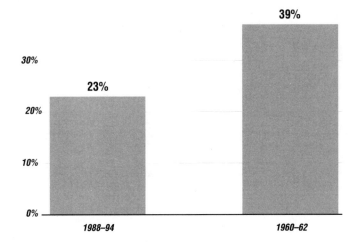

to be injured, and the injury rate peaks among 18-to-24-year-olds. The incidence of acute conditions declines with age. In their place come chronic conditions such as high blood pressure, diabetes, arthritis, and hearing problems.

Most, but not all, chronic illnesses become more prevalent with age. For people under age 18, the most common chronic conditions are sinusitis, asthma, and hay fever. Acne and dermatitis are also common in this age group. Adults aged 18 to 44 are the ones most likely to suffer from migraine headaches and, among women, diseases of the female genital organs. The largest number of AIDS cases have been diagnosed in the 30-to-49 age group.

In the 45-to-64 age group, the prevalence of many serious chronic conditions—such as diabetes and high blood pressure—rises steeply. Chronic conditions become even more common in older age groups. Among people aged 75 or older, more than one-half have arthritis and more than one-third suffer from hearing impairments and high blood pressure.

In the past few decades, Americans have made major strides in combating chronic disease. Many conditions that once killed are now managed with drugs and lifestyle changes. AIDS is perhaps the most dramatic example of this shift. Once a certain death sentence, AIDS is becoming a manageable chronic disease—at least for now—thanks to new drug cocktails.

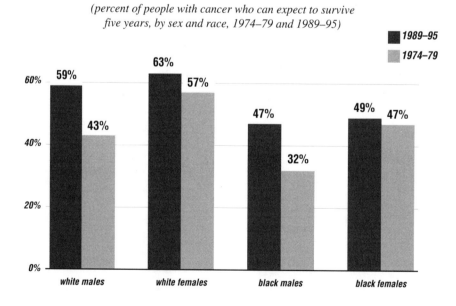

More Americans are surviving cancer

(percent of people with cancer who can expect to survive five years, by sex and race, 1974–79 and 1989–95)

■ 1989–95
▨ 1974–79

As the nation's new health care consumers learn more about chronic diseases, they are taking better care of themselves. In the past few decades the percentages of Americans with high blood pressure and high serum cholesterol have fallen sharply. Survival rates are rising for many types of cancer, although the incidence of cancer is also on the rise.

Few Americans allow chronic conditions to limit them. Only 13 percent report being limited in their activities because of a chronic condition, including just 50 percent of those aged 75 or older. While most people with chronic conditions see doctors regularly to help them manage their disease, few end up in the hospital—especially as hospitals shift care from inpatient procedures to outpatient services. According to an analysis of 1990-92 data (the latest available), among the 20 million Americans with heart disease at that time, 89 percent had seen a doctor in the past year, but only 45 percent had been hospitalized for the condition. Similarly, while virtually all of those with diabetes saw a doctor for their condition in the past year, only 27 percent were hospitalized because of it.

The nation's new health care consumers are learning how to live well despite their problems. While improved quality of life is a great benefit to the individuals suffering from chronic conditions, new therapy options also create a problem for society because they greatly increase the costs of treating disease. When heart disease was the silent killer, medical expenses were few—limited to emergency medical care following a heart attack. Now, heart disease is a noisy companion rather than a silent killer. It can begin in middle age and require decades of medication and monitoring, followed by procedures such as angioplasty and heart bypass surgery. Managing heart disease has become extraordinarily expensive.

As the cost of managing diseases increases, the solution lies in preventing chronic conditions before they occur. But preventing disease requires lifestyle changes decades before problems appear. While many new health care consumers are interested in doing just that, there will always be millions who are unwilling to change their lifestyle until they have a serious problem.

The future of managing disease

As the baby-boom generation ages into its fifties and sixties, when chronic conditions become common, the cost of treating those diseases is likely to soar. For many boomers, it's already too late for prevention. The only way to control the costs of disease management will be to develop less expensive medications and more efficient procedures for treating chronic problems.

TREND 1: GENETIC RESEARCH INTO CAUSES AND CURES

Now that the human genome has been mapped, the potential for understanding and curing disease has expanded enormously. "Under the disease management approach, drugs will be packaged with sophisticated diagnostic tests—and ultimately, detailed maps of a patient's genetic inheritance—to transform today's wasteful, hit and miss system of prescribing medicines," says Dr. Victor McKusick, a founder of modern medical genetics and one of the creators of the Human Genome Project.[1] McKusick identified several trends in genetic research:

♦ A shift in the focus of research from genetic defects to how defective genes cause disease. McKusick explains: "If you know the steps that connect an abnormal gene to a disorder … then you can often intervene along the way with appropriate drugs and essentially cure the condition." This research is likely to lead to more effective treatment of a variety of diseases.

♦ More research into complex disorders involving more than one gene. Major diseases involve multiple genetic defects, but today's research focuses on rarer, single-gene disorders. Expanded research will make genetic discoveries more relevant to health care consumers.

♦ More genetic research into segments of the population such as racial and ethnic minorities. The detailed genetic information forthcoming will add to the knowledge base and produce more effective disease treatments.

TREND 2: LIFESTYLE MANAGEMENT

Genetics are only one risk factor in disease. Environmental factors are also important. As we pay more attention to how environment affects chronic conditions, doctors will be able to better target high-risk groups. Studies published in *The New England Journal of Medicine* in 1996, for example, found that diet, smoking, lifestyle, poverty, and racism are more important in determining the risk of heart disease among blacks than any inherent racial factors.[2,3,4]

Increased knowledge of environmental risks will lead to a more inclusive definition of health, encompassing emotional as well as physical factors. Extreme anger, for example, can increase the chance of heart disease, according to a Harvard Medical School study.[5] High blood pressure appears to take its greatest toll on people with few social contacts. Two separate studies appearing in the journal *Epidemiology* link social isolation to higher death rates among the elderly and higher blood pressure among blacks.[6] In the future, doctors may prescribe attendance at anger management seminars or order their patients to make more friends.

Children's diseases also have an environmental ink. About half the cases of asthma and chronic bronchitis among children are caused by secondhand smoke, according to a 1998 study by the Agency for Health Care Policy and Research.[7] Compared with children in nonsmoking homes, children aged two months to five years who lived in a home where an adult smoked at least one pack per day were twice as likely to have asthma and 2.5 times as likely to have chronic bronchitis. As Americans learn more about these risk factors, parents, schools, and other concerned parties are likely to take steps to eliminate or alleviate them, thus improving the health of the next generation.

Notes

1. Laura Van Dan, "The Gene Doctor Is In," Massachusetts Institute of Technology's *Technology Review* (July 1997): 46–52.

2. Jing Gang, Shantha Madhavan, and Michael H. Alderman, "The Association between Birthplace and Mortality from Cardiovascular Causes among Black and White Residents of New York City," *The New England Journal of Medicine* 335, no. 21 (November 21, 1996): 1545–1552.

3. Arline T. Geronimus, John Bound, Timothy A. Waidmann, Marianne H. Hillemeier, and Patricia B. Burns, "Excess Mortality among Blacks and Whites in the United States," *The New England Journal of Medicine* 335, no. 21 (November 21, 1996): 1552–1559.

4. Barry M. Poplin, Anna Maria Siega-Riz, and Pamela S. Haines, "A Comparison of Dietary Trends among Racial and Socioeconomic Groups in the U.S.," *The New England Journal of Medicine* 335, no. 21 (November 21, 1996): 716–721.

5. "Anger Doubles Risk of Attack for Heart Disease Patients," *The New York Times* (March 19, 1994): 7.

6. Bruce Bower, "Social Links May Counter Health Risks," *Science News* 152 (August 30, 1997): 135.

7. Marilyn Elias, "Half of Kids' Ailments Tied to Adults' Smoking," *USA Today* (February 3, 1998). Report available at <www.pediatrics.org>.

Number of Acute Health Conditions by Age, 1996

(number of acute conditions by type and age, 1996; numbers in thousands)

	total	under 5	5 to 17	18 to 24	25 to 44	45 to 64	65 or older
Total acute conditions	**432,001**	**63,866**	**104,842**	**45,272**	**120,332**	**60,442**	**37,247**
Infective & parasitic diseases	54,192	11,447	19,018	5,695	10,138	5,843	2,050
Common childhood diseases	3,118	1,369	1,203	221	325	–	–
Intestinal virus	15,980	2,861	5,313	1,530	3,932	1,497	847
Viral infections	15,067	4,533	4,929	688	2,183	2,396	337
Other	20,027	2,684	7,573	3,256	3,698	1,951	865
Respiratory conditions	**208,623**	**25,991**	**52,088**	**21,150**	**64,114**	**29,725**	**15,557**
Common cold	62,251	9,756	17,318	5,839	15,630	8,719	4,990
Other acute upper respiratory infections	29,866	2,635	7,690	3,961	9,642	4,012	1,925
Influenza	95,049	10,780	22,744	9,946	31,803	13,882	5,895
Acute bronchitis	12,116	1,446	2,214	947	4,270	1,842	1,398
Pneumonia	4,791	783	883	347	1,084	491	1,203
Other respiratory conditions	4,550	590	1,238	110	1,685	780	147
Digestive system conditions	**17,646**	**1,931**	**5,030**	**1,584**	**4,212**	**2,799**	**2,090**
Dental conditions	2,970	720	537	274	714	459	265
Indigestion, nausea, vomiting	7,963	457	3,786	617	1,796	924	383
Other digestive conditions	6,713	754	706	693	1,702	1,417	1,441
Injuries	**57,279**	**4,597**	**10,952**	**7,736**	**20,742**	**7,775**	**5,476**
Fractures and dislocations	8,465	246	3,019	736	1,506	1,836	1,122
Sprains and strains	12,977	100	1,794	1,790	6,907	2,020	367
Open wounds and lacerations	9,027	1,375	1,008	1,634	3,635	884	490
Contusions and superficial injuries	9,979	715	2,004	1,433	3,691	1,435	701
Other current injuries	16,832	2,161	3,127	2,143	5,004	1,599	2,797
Selected other acute conditions	**63,090**	**16,055**	**12,521**	**6,243**	**13,994**	**8,169**	**6,109**
Eye conditions	3,478	760	339	384	334	929	732
Acute ear infections	21,766	11,038	6,385	937	2,397	599	411
Other ear conditions	3,833	596	1,151	185	986	685	230
Acute urinary conditions	8,405	477	1,013	707	2,523	1,737	1,948
Disorders of menstruation	839	–	133	169	537	–	–

(continued)

(continued from previous page)

	total	under 5	5 to 17	18 to 24	25 to 44	45 to 64	65 or older
Other disorders of female genital tract	1,597	–	38	446	613	357	143
Delivery and other conditions of pregnancy	3,279	–	311	1,096	1,871	–	–
Skin conditions	4,986	572	739	493	1,182	1,207	793
Acute musculoskeletal conditions	8,461	603	419	1,321	2,514	1,855	1,749
Headache, excl. migraine	1,738	–	395	282	586	372	102
Fever, unspecified	4,708	2,009	1,597	224	451	428	–
Other acute conditions	**31,170**	**3,846**	**5,233**	**2,863**	**7,131**	**6,131**	**5,965**

Note: The acute conditions shown here are those that caused people to seek medical attention or to restrict their activity for at least half a day. (–) means not applicable or sample is too small to make a reliable estimate.
Source: National Center for Health Statistics, Current Estimates from the National Health Interview Survey, 1996, *Series 10, No. 200, 1999*

Rate of Acute Health Conditions by Age, 1996

(number of acute conditions per 100 people by type of condition and age, 1996)

	total	*under 5*	*5 to 17*	*18 to 24*	*25 to 44*	*45 to 64*	*65 or older*
Total acute conditions	**163.5**	**317.9**	**204.4**	**184.2**	**144.3**	**113.7**	**117.3**
Infective and parasitic diseases	20.5	57.0	37.1	23.2	12.2	11.0	6.5
Common childhood diseases	1.2	6.8	2.3	0.9	0.4	–	–
Intestinal virus	6.0	14.2	10.4	6.2	4.7	2.8	2.7
Viral infections	5.7	22.6	9.6	2.8	2.6	4.5	1.1
Other	7.6	13.4	14.8	13.2	4.4	3.7	2.7
Respiratory conditions	**78.9**	**129.4**	**101.5**	**86.0**	**76.9**	**55.9**	**49.0**
Common cold	23.6	48.6	33.8	23.8	18.7	16.4	15.7
Other acute upper respiratory infections	11.3	13.1	15.0	16.1	11.6	7.5	6.1
Influenza	36.0	53.7	44.3	40.5	38.1	26.1	18.6
Acute bronchitis	4.6	7.2	4.3	3.9	5.1	3.5	4.4
Pneumonia	1.8	3.9	1.7	1.4	1.3	0.9	3.8
Other respiratory conditions	1.7	2.9	2.4	0.4	2.0	1.5	0.5
Digestive system conditions	**6.7**	**9.6**	**9.8**	**6.4**	**5.1**	**5.3**	**6.6**
Dental conditions	1.1	3.6	1.0	1.1	0.9	0.9	0.8
Indigestion, nausea, vomiting	3.0	2.3	7.4	2.5	2.2	1.7	1.2
Other digestive conditions	2.5	3.8	1.4	2.8	2.0	2.7	4.5
Injuries	**21.7**	**22.9**	**21.4**	**31.5**	**24.9**	**14.6**	**17.2**
Fractures and dislocations	3.2	1.2	5.9	3.0	1.8	3.5	3.5
Sprains and strains	4.9	0.5	3.5	7.3	8.3	3.8	1.2
Open wounds and lacerations	3.4	6.8	2.0	6.6	4.4	1.7	1.5
Contusions and superficial injuries	3.8	3.6	3.9	5.8	4.4	2.7	2.2
Other current injuries	6.4	10.8	6.1	8.7	6.0	3.0	8.8
Selected other acute conditions	**23.9**	**79.9**	**24.4**	**25.4**	**16.8**	**15.4**	**19.2**
Eye conditions	1.3	3.8	0.7	1.6	0.4	1.7	2.3
Acute ear infections	8.2	55.0	12.4	3.8	2.9	1.1	1.3
Other ear conditions	1.5	3.0	2.2	0.8	1.2	1.3	0.7
Acute urinary conditions	3.2	2.4	2.0	2.9	3.0	3.3	6.1
Disorders of menstruation	0.3	–	0.3	0.7	0.6	–	–

(continued)

(continued from previous page)

	total	under 5	5 to 17	18 to 24	25 to 44	45 to 64	65 or older
Other disorders of female genital tract	0.6	–	0.1	1.8	0.7	0.7	0.5
Delivery and other conditions of pregnancy	1.2	–	0.6	4.5	2.2	–	–
Skin conditions	1.9	2.8	1.4	2.0	1.4	2.3	2.5
Acute musculoskeletal conditions	3.2	3.0	0.8	5.4	3.0	3.5	5.5
Headache, excluding migraine	0.7	–	0.8	1.1	0.7	0.7	0.3
Fever, unspecified	1.8	10.0	3.1	0.9	0.5	0.8	–
Other acute conditions	**11.8**	**19.1**	**10.2**	**11.6**	**8.6**	**11.5**	**18.8**

Note: The acute conditions shown here are those that caused people to seek medical attention or to restrict their activity for at least half a day. (–) means not applicable or sample is too small to make a reliable estimate.
Source: National Center for Health Statistics, Current Estimates from the National Health Interview Survey, 1996, *Series 10, No. 200, 1999*

Distribution of Acute Health Conditions by Age, 1996

(percent distribution of acute conditions by type and age, 1996; numbers in thousands)

	total	under 5	5 to 17	18 to 24	25 to 44	45 to 64	65 or older
Total acute conditions	**100.0%**	**14.8%**	**24.3%**	**10.5%**	**27.9%**	**14.0%**	**8.6%**
Infective & parasitic diseases	100.0	21.1	35.1	10.5	18.7	10.8	3.8
Common childhood diseases	100.0	43.9	38.6	7.1	10.4	–	–
Intestinal virus	100.0	17.9	33.2	9.6	24.6	9.4	5.3
Viral infections	100.0	30.1	32.7	4.6	14.5	15.9	2.2
Other	100.0	13.4	37.8	16.3	18.5	9.7	4.3
Respiratory conditions	**100.0**	**12.5**	**25.0**	**10.1**	**30.7**	**14.2**	**7.5**
Common cold	100.0	15.7	27.8	9.4	25.1	14.0	8.0
Other acute upper respiratory infections	100.0	8.8	25.7	13.3	32.3	13.4	6.4
Influenza	100.0	11.3	23.9	10.5	33.5	14.6	6.2
Acute bronchitis	100.0	11.9	18.3	7.8	35.2	15.2	11.5
Pneumonia	100.0	16.3	18.4	7.2	22.6	10.2	25.1
Other respiratory conditions	100.0	13.0	27.2	2.4	37.0	17.1	3.2
Digestive system conditions	**100.0**	**10.9**	**28.5**	**9.0**	**23.9**	**15.9**	**11.8**
Dental conditions	100.0	24.2	18.1	9.2	24.0	15.5	8.9
Indigestion, nausea, vomiting	100.0	5.7	47.5	7.7	22.6	11.6	4.8
Other digestive conditions	100.0	11.2	10.5	10.3	25.4	21.1	21.5
Injuries	**100.0**	**8.0**	**19.1**	**13.5**	**36.2**	**13.6**	**9.6**
Fractures and dislocations	100.0	2.9	35.7	8.7	17.8	21.7	13.3
Sprains and strains	100.0	0.8	13.8	13.8	53.2	15.6	2.8
Open wounds and lacerations	100.0	15.2	11.2	18.1	40.3	9.8	5.4
Contusions and superficial injuries	100.0	7.2	20.1	14.4	37.0	14.4	7.0
Other current injuries	100.0	12.8	18.6	12.7	29.7	9.5	16.6
Selected other acute conditions	**100.0**	**25.4**	**19.8**	**9.9**	**22.2**	**12.9**	**9.7**
Eye conditions	100.0	21.9	9.7	11.0	9.6	26.7	21.0
Acute ear infections	100.0	50.7	29.3	4.3	11.0	2.8	1.9
Other ear conditions	100.0	15.5	30.0	4.8	25.7	17.9	6.0
Acute urinary conditions	100.0	5.7	12.1	8.4	30.0	20.7	23.2
Disorders of menstruation	100.0	–	15.9	20.1	64.0	–	–

(continued)

(continued from previous page)

	total	under 5	5 to 17	18 to 24	25 to 44	45 to 64	65 or older
Other disorders of female genital tract	100.0%	–	2.4%	27.9%	38.4%	22.4%	9.0%
Delivery and other conditions of pregnancy	100.0	–	9.5	33.4	57.1	–	–
Skin conditions	100.0	11.5%	14.8	9.9	23.7	24.2	15.9
Acute musculoskeletal conditions	100.0	7.1	5.0	15.6	29.7	21.9	20.7
Headache, excluding migraine	100.0	–	22.7	16.2	33.7	21.4	5.9
Fever, unspecified	100.0	42.7	33.9	4.8	9.6	9.1	–
Other acute conditions	**100.0**	**12.3**	**16.8**	**9.2**	**22.9**	**19.7**	**19.1**

Note: The acute conditions shown here are those that caused people to seek medical attention or to restrict their activity for at least half a day. (–) means not applicable or sample is too small to make a reliable estimate.
Source: National Center for Health Statistics, Current Estimates from the National Health Interview Survey, 1996, *Series 10, No. 200, 1999; calculations by New Strategist*

Most Prevalent Chronic Conditions by Sex, 1990–92

(most common chronic conditions in rank order, by sex, 1990–92)

	total	males	females
Deformities or orthopedic impairments	1	1	3
Chronic sinusitis	2	2	2
Arthritis	3	5	1
High blood pressure	4	4	4
Hay fever or allergic rhinitis without asthma	5	6	5
Deafness and other hearing impairments	6	3	7
Heart disease	7	7	6
Chronic bronchitis	8	9	8
Asthma	9	8	–
Other headache (excludes tension headache)	10	–	10
Blindness and other visual impairments	–	10	–

Note: (–) means rank is not in top 10.
Source: National Center for Health Statistics, Prevalence of Selected Chronic Conditions: United States, 1990–92, *Vital and Health Statistics, Series 10, No. 194, 1997*

Most Prevalent Chronic Conditions by Age, 1990–92

(most common chronic conditions in rank order, by age, 1990–92)

	total	< age 18	18 to 44	45 to 64	65 to 74	75+
Deformities or orthopedic impairments	1	6	1	3	5	5
Chronic sinusitis	2	2	2	4	6	7
Arthritis	3	–	8	1	1	1
High blood pressure	4	–	6	2	2	3
Hay fever or allergic rhinitis without asthma	5	1	3	7	10	–
Deafness and other hearing impairments	6	10	7	5	3	2
Heart disease	7	9	–	6	4	4
Chronic bronchitis	8	4	9	9	–	–
Asthma	9	3	10	–	–	–
Other headache (excl. tension headache)	10	–	4	–	–	–
Blindness and other visual impairments	–	–	–	–	–	8
Migraine headache	–	–	5	–	–	–
Dermatitis	–	5	–	–	–	–
Acne	–	7	–	–	–	–
Chronic disease of tonsils and adenoids	–	8	–	–	–	–
Speech impairments	–	10	–	–	–	–
Hemorrhoids	–	–	–	8	–	–
Diabetes	–	–	–	10	8	9
Cataracts	–	–	–	–	7	6
Tinnitus	–	–	–	–	9	10

Note: (–) means rank is not in top 10.
Source: National Center for Health Statistics, Prevalence of Selected Chronic Conditions: United States, 1990–92, *Vital and Health Statistics, Series 10, No. 194, 1997*

Number of Chronic Health Conditions by Age, 1996

(number of chronic conditions by type and age, 1996; numbers in thousands)

	total	<18	18 to 44	45 to 64	aged 65 or older total	65 to 74	75 or older
Skin and musculoskeletal conditions							
Arthritis	33,638	136	5,409	12,759	15,335	8,339	6,996
Gout, incl. gouty arthritis	2,487	–	320	1,190	977	584	393
Intervertebral disc disorders	6,700	69	2,275	3,334	1,022	703	320
Bonespur or tendinitis	2,934	–	1,181	1,233	520	269	251
Disorders of bone or cartilage	1,730	34	334	532	831	287	543
Bunions	2,360	96	704	862	698	390	307
Bursitis	5,006	55	1,410	2,334	1,207	792	415
Sebaceous skin cyst	1,190	32	616	481	62	62	–
Acne	4,952	1,743	2,968	241	–	–	–
Psoriasis	2,940	228	1,134	1,102	475	300	176
Dermatitis	8,249	2,175	3,251	2,023	799	490	309
Dry, itching skin	6,627	903	2,636	1,535	1,552	691	861
Ingrown nails	5,807	374	2,810	1,426	1,197	626	571
Corns and calluses	3,778	80	1,404	1,351	942	499	443
Impairments							
Visual impairment	8,280	448	2,592	2,567	2,674	1,281	1,393
Color blindness	2,811	283	1,075	855	598	380	219
Cataracts	7,022	33	299	1,240	5,449	2,796	2,653
Glaucoma	2,595	–	214	546	1,835	859	977
Hearing impairment	22,044	897	4,522	6,987	9,638	4,697	4,941
Tinnitus	7,866	186	1,728	3,167	2,785	1,767	1,018
Speech impairment	2,720	1,160	839	349	372	184	188
Absence of extremities	1,285	70	293	305	617	395	223
Paralysis of extremities	2,138	274	550	715	599	228	371
Deformity or orthopedic impairment	29,499	1,830	13,216	9,447	5,007	3,222	1,784
Back	16,905	552	8,705	5,465	2,182	1,473	709
Upper extremities	4,170	189	1,438	1,562	981	717	264
Lower extremities	12,696	1,339	4,669	4,383	2,305	1,433	872

(continued)

(continued from previous page)

| | total | <18 | 18 to 44 | 45 to 64 | aged 65 or older | | |
					total	65 to 74	75 or older
Digestive conditions							
Ulcer	3,709	96	1,270	1,386	957	680	277
Hernia of abdominal cavity	4,470	122	1,166	1,644	1,539	705	834
Gastritis or duodenitis	3,729	218	1,461	1,173	877	626	251
Frequent indigestion	6,420	238	2,882	2,238	1,063	710	353
Enteritis or colitis	1,686	119	745	529	293	154	140
Spastic colon	2,083	48	849	730	455	311	145
Diverticula of intestines	2,529	–	263	935	1,331	663	668
Frequent constipation	3,149	380	913	783	1,073	439	634
Genitourinary, nervous, endocrine, metabolic, and blood conditions							
Goiter or other thyroid disorders	4,598	71	1,405	1,594	1,528	925	603
Diabetes	7,627	89	1,270	3,091	3,178	1,811	1,367
Anemias	3,457	359	1,798	569	731	253	479
Epilepsy	1,335	351	478	308	198	99	99
Migraine headache	11,546	1,084	6,477	3,079	906	527	380
Neuralgia or neuritis, unspecified	353	15	30	129	178	47	131
Kidney trouble	2,553	168	1,272	678	435	253	182
Bladder disorders	3,139	239	1,215	832	853	367	486
Diseases of prostate	2,803	–	241	780	1,781	899	882
Diseases of female genital organs	4,420	242	2,615	1,099	464	304	161
Circulatory conditions							
Rheumatic fever	1,759	83	745	553	378	144	234
Heart disease	20,653	1,688	4,246	6,184	8,535	4,384	4,151
Ischemic heart disease	7,672	–	453	2,743	4,476	2,411	2,065
Heart rhythm disorders	8,716	1,217	3,140	2,164	2,195	1,218	977
Tachycardia or rapid heart	2,310	–	687	642	980	571	410
Heart murmurs	4,783	1,188	2,034	937	624	393	231
Other heart rhythm disorders	1,624	29	420	584	591	255	336
Other selected diseases of heart	4,265	471	653	1,278	1,864	755	1,110
High blood pressure (hypertension)	28,314	36	5,355	11,376	11,547	6,553	4,994
Cerebrovascular disease	2,999	29	221	682	2,067	739	1,328

(continued)

(continued from previous page)

	total	<18	18 to 44	45 to 64	aged 65 or older total	65 to 74	75 or older
Hardening of the arteries	1,556	–	–	354	1,202	522	680
Varicose veins of lower extremities	7,399	–	2,397	2,488	2,514	1,362	1,152
Hemorrhoids	8,231	20	3,716	2,850	1,945	1,339	607
Respiratory conditions							
Chronic bronchitis	14,150	4,087	4,904	3,142	2,017	1,118	899
Asthma	14,598	4,429	6,141	2,581	1,445	804	641
Hay fever or allergic rhinitis	23,721	4,190	11,809	5,572	2,150	1,139	1,011
Chronic sinusitis	33,161	4,559	15,628	9,253	3,721	2,337	1,383
Deviated nasal septum	1,985	122	868	796	198	59	139
Chronic disease of tonsils and adenoids	2,513	1,444	885	159	26	26	–
Emphysema	1,821	–	90	701	1,030	595	435

Note: Chronic conditions are those that last at least three months or belong to a group of conditions that are considered to be chronic regardless of when they begin. (–) means sample is too small to make a reliable estimate.
Source: National Center for Health Statistics, Current Estimates from the National Health Interview Survey, 1996, *Series 10, No. 200, 1999*

Rate of Chronic Health Conditions by Age, 1996

(number of chronic conditions per 1,000 people by type of condition and age, 1996)

	total	<18	18 to 44	45 to 64	aged 65 or older total	65 to 74	75 or older
Skin and musculoskeletal conditions							
Arthritis	127.3	1.9	50.1	240.1	482.7	453.1	523.6
Gout, including gouty arthritis	9.4	–	3.0	22.4	30.8	31.7	29.4
Intervertebral disc disorders	25.4	1.0	21.1	62.7	32.2	38.2	24.0
Bonespur or tendinitis	11.1	–	10.9	23.2	16.4	14.6	18.8
Disorders of bone or cartilage	6.5	0.5	3.1	10.0	26.2	15.6	40.6
Bunions	8.9	1.3	6.5	16.2	22.0	21.2	23.0
Bursitis	18.9	0.8	13.1	43.9	38.0	43.0	31.1
Sebaceous skin cyst	4.5	0.4	5.7	9.1	2.0	3.4	–
Acne	18.7	24.4	27.5	4.5	–	–	–
Psoriasis	11.1	3.2	10.5	20.7	15.0	16.3	13.2
Dermatitis	31.2	30.5	30.1	38.1	25.2	26.6	23.1
Dry, itching skin	25.1	12.7	24.4	28.9	48.9	37.5	64.4
Ingrown nails	22.0	5.2	26.0	26.8	37.7	34.0	42.7
Corns and calluses	14.3	1.1	13.0	25.4	29.7	27.1	33.2
Impairments							
Visual impairment	31.3	6.3	24.0	48.3	84.2	69.6	104.3
Color blindness	10.6	4.0	10.0	16.1	18.8	20.6	16.4
Cataracts	26.6	0.5	2.8	23.3	171.5	151.9	198.6
Glaucoma	9.8	–	2.0	10.3	57.8	46.7	73.1
Hearing impairment	83.4	12.6	41.9	131.5	303.4	255.2	369.8
Tinnitus	29.8	2.6	16.0	59.6	87.7	96.0	76.2
Speech impairment	10.3	16.3	7.8	6.6	11.7	10.0	14.1
Absence of extremities	4.9	1.0	2.7	5.7	19.4	21.5	16.7
Paralysis of extremities	8.1	3.8	5.1	13.5	18.9	12.4	27.8
Deformity or orthopedic impairment	111.6	25.6	122.4	177.8	157.6	175.1	133.5
Back	64.0	7.7	80.6	102.8	68.7	80.0	53.1
Upper extremities	15.8	2.6	13.3	29.4	30.9	39.0	19.8
Lower extremities	48.0	18.8	43.2	82.5	72.6	77.9	65.3

(continued)

(continued from previous page)

	total	<18	18 to 44	45 to 64	aged 65 or older total	65 to 74	75 or older
Digestive conditions							
Ulcer	14.0	1.3	11.8	26.1	30.1	36.9	20.7
Hernia of abdominal cavity	16.9	1.7	10.8	30.9	48.4	38.3	62.4
Gastritis or duodenitis	14.1	3.1	13.5	22.1	27.6	34.0	18.8
Frequent indigestion	24.3	3.3	26.7	42.1	33.5	38.6	26.4
Enteritis or colitis	6.4	1.7	6.9	10.0	9.2	8.4	10.5
Spastic colon	7.9	0.7	7.9	13.7	14.3	16.9	10.9
Diverticula of intestines	9.6	–	2.4	17.6	41.9	36.0	50.0
Frequent constipation	11.9	5.3	8.5	14.7	33.8	23.9	47.5
Genitourinary, nervous, endocrine, metabolic, and blood conditions							
Goiter or other thyroid disorders	17.4	1.0	13.0	30.0	48.1	50.3	45.1
Diabetes	28.9	1.2	11.8	58.2	100.0	98.4	102.3
Anemias	13.1	5.0	16.7	10.7	23.0	13.7	35.9
Epilepsy	5.1	4.9	4.4	5.8	6.2	5.4	7.4
Migraine headache	43.7	15.2	60.0	57.9	28.5	28.6	28.4
Neuralgia or neuritis, unspecified	1.3	0.2	0.3	2.4	5.6	2.6	9.8
Kidney trouble	9.7	2.4	11.8	12.8	13.7	13.7	13.6
Bladder disorders	11.9	3.3	11.3	15.7	26.9	19.9	36.4
Diseases of prostate	10.6	–	2.2	14.7	56.1	48.8	66.0
Diseases of female genital organs	16.7	3.4	24.2	20.7	14.6	16.5	12.0
Circulatory conditions							
Rheumatic fever	6.7	1.2	6.9	10.4	11.9	7.8	17.5
Heart disease	78.2	23.6	39.3	116.4	268.7	238.2	310.7
Ischemic heart disease	29.0	–	4.2	51.6	140.9	131.0	154.6
Heart rhythm disorders	33.0	17.0	29.1	40.7	69.1	66.2	73.1
Tachycardia or rapid heart	8.7	–	6.4	12.1	30.9	31.0	30.7
Heart murmurs	18.1	16.6	18.8	17.6	19.6	21.4	17.3
Other heart rhythm disorders	6.1	0.4	3.9	11.0	18.6	13.9	25.1
Other selected diseases of heart	16.1	6.6	6.0	24.0	58.7	41.0	83.1
High blood pressure (hypertension)	107.1	0.5	49.6	214.1	363.5	356.0	373.8
Cerebrovascular disease	11.3	0.4	2.0	12.8	65.1	40.2	99.4

(continued)

(continued from previous page)

	total	<18	18 to 44	45 to 64	aged 65 or older total	65 to 74	75 or older
Hardening of the arteries	5.9	–	–	6.7	37.8	28.4	50.9
Varicose veins of lower extremities	28.0	–	22.2	46.8	79.1	74.0	86.2
Hemorrhoids	32.3	0.3	34.4	53.6	61.2	72.8	45.4
Respiratory conditions							
Chronic bronchitis	53.5	57.3	45.4	59.1	63.5	60.7	67.3
Asthma	55.2	62.0	56.9	48.6	45.5	43.7	48.0
Hay fever or allergic rhinitis	89.8	58.7	109.4	104.8	67.7	61.9	75.7
Chronic sinusitis	125.5	63.9	144.7	174.1	117.1	127.0	103.5
Deviated nasal septum	7.5	1.7	8.0	15.0	6.2	3.2	10.4
Chronic disease of tonsils and adenoids	9.5	20.2	8.2	3.0	0.8	1.4	–
Emphysema	6.9	–	0.8	13.2	32.4	32.3	32.6

Note: Chronic conditions are those that last at least three months or belong to a group of conditions that are considered to be chronic regardless of when they begin. (–) means sample is too small to make a reliable estimate. Source: National Center for Health Statistics, Current Estimates from the National Health Interview Survey, 1996, *Series 10, No. 200, 1999*

Distribution of Chronic Health Conditions by Age, 1996

(percent distribution of chronic conditions by type and age, 1996)

	total	<18	18 to 44	45 to 64	aged 65 or older		
					total	65 to 74	75 or older
Skin and musculoskeletal conditions							
Arthritis	100.0%	0.4%	16.1%	37.9%	45.6%	24.8%	20.8%
Gout, including gouty arthritis	100.0	–	12.9	47.8	39.3	23.5	15.8
Intervertebral disc disorders	100.0	1.0	34.0	49.8	15.3	10.5	4.8
Bonespur or tendinitis	100.0	–	40.3	42.0	17.7	9.2	8.6
Disorders of bone or cartilage	100.0	2.0	19.3	30.8	48.0	16.6	31.4
Bunions	100.0	4.1	29.8	36.5	29.6	16.5	13.0
Bursitis	100.0	1.1	28.2	46.6	24.1	15.8	8.3
Sebaceous skin cyst	100.0	2.7	51.8	40.4	5.2	5.2	–
Acne	100.0	35.2	59.9	4.9	–	–	–
Psoriasis	100.0	7.8	38.6	37.5	16.2	10.2	6.0
Dermatitis	100.0	26.4	39.4	24.5	9.7	5.9	3.7
Dry, itching skin	100.0	13.6	39.8	23.2	23.4	10.4	13.0
Ingrown nails	100.0	6.4	48.4	24.6	20.6	10.8	9.8
Corns and calluses	100.0	2.1	37.2	35.8	24.9	13.2	11.7
Impairments							
Visual impairment	100.0	5.4	31.3	31.0	32.3	15.5	16.8
Color blindness	100.0	10.1	38.2	30.4	21.3	13.5	7.8
Cataracts	100.0	0.5	4.3	17.7	77.6	39.8	37.8
Glaucoma	100.0	–	8.2	21.0	70.7	33.1	37.6
Hearing impairment	100.0	4.1	20.5	31.7	43.7	21.3	22.4
Tinnitus	100.0	2.4	22.0	40.3	35.4	22.5	12.9
Speech impairment	100.0	42.6	30.8	12.8	13.7	6.8	6.9
Absence of extremities	100.0	5.4	22.8	23.7	48.0	30.7	17.4
Paralysis of extremities	100.0	12.8	25.7	33.4	28.0	10.7	17.4
Deformity or orthopedic impairment	100.0	6.2	44.8	32.0	17.0	10.9	6.0
Back	100.0	3.3	51.5	32.3	12.9	8.7	4.2
Upper extremities	100.0	4.5	34.5	37.5	23.5	17.2	6.3
Lower extremities	100.0	10.5	36.8	34.5	18.2	11.3	6.9

(continued)

(continued from previous page)

	total	<18	18 to 44	45 to 64	aged 65 or older total	65 to 74	75 or older
Digestive conditions							
Ulcer	100.0%	2.6%	34.2%	37.4%	25.8%	18.3%	7.5%
Hernia of abdominal cavity	100.0	2.7	26.1	36.8	34.4	15.8	18.7
Gastritis or duodenitis	100.0	5.8	39.2	31.5	23.5	16.8	6.7
Frequent indigestion	100.0	3.7	44.9	34.9	16.6	11.1	5.5
Enteritis or colitis	100.0	7.1	44.2	31.4	17.4	9.1	8.3
Spastic colon	100.0	2.3	40.8	35.0	21.8	14.9	7.0
Diverticula of intestines	100.0	–	10.4	37.0	52.6	26.2	26.4
Frequent constipation	100.0	12.1	29.0	24.9	34.1	13.9	20.1
Genitourinary, nervous, endocrine, metabolic, and blood conditions							
Goiter or other thyroid disorders	100.0	1.5	30.6	34.7	33.2	20.1	13.1
Diabetes	100.0	1.2	16.7	40.5	41.7	23.7	17.9
Anemias	100.0	10.4	52.0	16.5	21.1	7.3	13.9
Epilepsy	100.0	26.3	35.8	23.1	14.8	7.4	7.4
Migraine headache	100.0	9.4	56.1	26.7	7.8	4.6	3.3
Neuralgia or neuritis, unspecified	100.0	4.2	8.5	36.5	50.4	13.3	37.1
Kidney trouble	100.0	6.6	49.8	26.6	17.0	9.9	7.1
Bladder disorders	100.0	7.6	38.7	26.5	27.2	11.7	15.5
Diseases of prostate	100.0	–	8.6	27.8	63.5	32.1	31.5
Diseases of female genital organs	100.0	5.5	59.2	24.9	10.5	6.9	3.6
Circulatory conditions							
Rheumatic fever	100.0	4.7	42.4	31.4	21.5	8.2	13.3
Heart disease	100.0	8.2	20.6	29.9	41.3	21.2	20.1
Ischemic heart disease	100.0	–	5.9	35.8	58.3	31.4	26.9
Heart rhythm disorders	100.0	14.0	36.0	24.8	25.2	14.0	11.2
Tachycardia or rapid heart	100.0	–	29.7	27.8	42.4	24.7	17.7
Heart murmurs	100.0	24.8	42.5	19.6	13.0	8.2	4.8
Other heart rhythm disorders	100.0	1.8	25.9	36.0	36.4	15.7	20.7
Other selected diseases of heart	100.0	11.0	15.3	30.0	43.7	17.7	26.0
High blood pressure (hypertension)	100.0	0.1	18.9	40.2	40.8	23.1	17.6
Cerebrovascular disease	100.0	1.0	7.4	22.7	68.9	24.6	44.3

(continued)

(continued from previous page)

	total	<18	18 to 44	45 to 64	aged 65 or older total	65 to 74	75 or older
Hardening of the arteries	100.0%	–	–	22.8%	77.2%	33.5%	43.7%
Varicose veins of lower extremities	100.0	–	32.4%	33.6	34.0	18.4	15.6
Hemorrhoids	100.0	0.2%	45.1	34.6	23.6	16.3	7.4
Respiratory conditions							
Chronic bronchitis	100.0	28.9	34.7	22.2	14.3	7.9	6.4
Asthma	100.0	30.3	42.1	17.7	9.9	5.5	4.4
Hay fever or allergic rhinitis	100.0	17.7	49.8	23.5	9.1	4.8	4.3
Chronic sinusitis	100.0	13.7	47.1	27.9	11.2	7.0	4.2
Deviated nasal septum	100.0	6.1	43.7	40.1	10.0	3.0	7.0
Chronic disease of tonsils and adenoids	100.0	57.5	35.2	6.3	1.0	1.0	–
Emphysema	100.0	–	4.9	38.5	56.6	32.7	23.9

Note: Chronic conditions are those that last at least three months or belong to a group of conditions that are considered to be chronic regardless of when they begin. (–) means sample is too small to make a reliable estimate. Source: National Center for Health Statistics, Current Estimates from the National Health Interview Survey, 1996, *Series 10, No. 200, 1999; calculations by New Strategist*

Limitations Caused by Chronic Conditions by Age, 1997

(percent of people with any activity limitation caused by chronic conditions by age, 1997)

	with activity limitation
Total people	**13.3%**
Under age 5	3.5
Aged 5 to 17	7.8
Aged 18 to 24	5.1
Aged 25 to 44	7.6
Aged 45 to 54	14.2
Aged 55 to 64	22.2
Aged 65 or older	38.7
Aged 65 to 74	30.0
Aged 75 or older	50.2

Source: National Center for Health Statistics, Health, United States, 2000

Hypertension by Sex and Age, 1960–62 and 1988–94

(percent of people aged 20 to 74 with hypertension by sex and age, 1960–62 and 1988–94; and percentage point change, 1960–62 to 1988–94)

	1988–94	*1960–62*	*percentage point change*
Total people	**23.1%**	**39.0%**	**–15.9**
Total men	**24.7**	**41.7**	**–17.0**
Aged 20 to 34	8.6	22.8	–14.2
Aged 35 to 44	20.9	37.7	–16.8
Aged 45 to 54	34.1	47.6	–13.5
Aged 55 to 64	42.9	60.3	–17.4
Aged 65 to 74	57.3	68.8	–11.5
Aged 75 or older	64.2	–	–
Total women	**21.5**	**36.6**	**–15.1**
Aged 20 to 34	3.4	9.3	–5.9
Aged 35 to 44	12.7	24.0	–11.3
Aged 45 to 54	25.1	43.4	–18.3
Aged 55 to 64	44.2	66.4	–22.2
Aged 65 to 74	60.8	81.5	–20.7
Aged 75 or older	77.3	–	–

Note: A person with hypertension is defined someone who has systolic pressure of at least 140 mmHg or diastolic pressure of at least 90 mmHg, or who takes antiphypertensive medication. (–) means data not available.
Source: National Center for Health Statistics, Health, United States, 2000*; calculations by New Strategist*

High Cholesterol by Sex and Age, 1960–62 and 1988–94

(percent of people aged 20 to 74 with high serum cholesterol by sex and age, 1960–62 and 1988–94; and percentage point change, 1960–62 to 1988–94)

	1988–94	1960–62	percentage point change
Total people	**18.7%**	**33.6%**	**–14.9**
Total men	**17.6**	**30.7**	**–13.1**
Aged 20 to 34	8.2	15.1	–6.9
Aged 35 to 44	19.4	33.9	–14.5
Aged 45 to 54	26.6	39.2	–12.6
Aged 55 to 64	28.0	41.6	–13.6
Aged 65 to 74	21.9	38.0	–16.1
Aged 75 or older	20.4	–	–
Total women	**19.9**	**36.3**	**–16.4**
Aged 20 to 34	7.3	12.4	–5.1
Aged 35 to 44	12.3	23.1	–10.8
Aged 45 to 54	26.7	46.9	–20.2
Aged 55 to 64	40.9	70.1	–29.2
Aged 65 to 74	41.3	68.5	–27.2
Aged 75 or older	38.2	–	–

Note: High cholesterol is defined as 240 mg/dL or more. (–) means data not available.
Source: National Center for Health Statistics, Health, United States, 2000; *calculations by New Strategist*

Cancer Incidence Rates by Sex and Race, 1973 and 1996

(number of new cases of cancer per 100,000 age-adjusted population by sex, selected cancer site, and race, 1973 and 1996; percent change in rate, 1973–96)

	white			black		
	1996	1973	percent change 1973–96	1996	1973	percent change 1973–96
Male, total	**445.8**	**364.3**	**22.4%**	**563.1**	**441.4**	**27.6%**
Prostate gland	127.8	62.6	104.2	211.3	106.3	98.8
Lung and bronchus	68.4	72.4	–5.5	101.4	104.8	–3.2
Colon	34.9	34.8	0.3	36.7	31.7	15.8
Urinary bladder	29.9	27.3	9.5	14.0	10.6	32.1
Non-Hodgkin's lymphoma	19.7	10.3	91.3	15.0	8.8	70.5
Rectum	15.8	19.5	–19.0	14.2	11.1	27.9
Oral cavity and pharynx	14.0	17.6	–20.5	21.9	16.6	31.9
Leukemia	12.4	14.3	–13.3	10.1	12.0	–15.8
Pancreas	9.5	12.8	–25.8	15.9	15.9	0.0
Stomach	8.4	14.0	–40.0	17.6	25.9	–32.0
Esophagus	6.2	4.8	29.2	14.0	13.3	5.3
Female, total	**347.1**	**295.1**	**17.6**	**336.1**	**283.7**	**18.5**
Breast	113.3	84.4	34.2	100.3	69.0	45.4
Lung and bronchus	43.7	17.8	145.5	47.2	20.9	125.8
Colon	25.9	30.3	–14.5	32.9	30.0	9.7
Corpus uteri	21.8	29.5	–26.1	15.7	15.0	4.7
Ovary	15.3	14.6	4.8	8.5	10.5	–19.0
Melanoma of skin	13.2	5.9	123.7	–	–	–
Non-Hodgkin's lymphoma	12.7	7.6	67.1	9.5	5.5	72.7
Rectum	9.6	11.5	–16.5	8.9	11.8	–24.6
Pancreas	7.1	7.5	–5.3	10.8	11.6	–6.9
Cervix uteri	7.0	12.8	–45.3	10.6	29.9	–64.5

Note: Age adjusted incidence rates are calculated by applying age specific incidence rates in each year to a standard population with a fixed age distribution. They should be viewed as an index rather than an actual measure of cancer risk. (–) means data not available.
Source: National Center for Health Statistics, Health, United States, 2000; calculations by New Strategist

Cancer Survival Rates by Sex and Race, 1974–79 and 1989–95

(five-year survival rate for the patient group as a percent of the expected five-year survival rate for people of that age, sex, and race, 1974–79 and 1989–95; percentage point change in rate, 1974–79 to 1989–95)

	white			black		
	1989–95	*1974–79*	*percentage point change*	*1989–95*	*1974–79*	*percentage point change*
Male, total	**59.2%**	**43.4%**	**15.8**	**46.5%**	**32.0%**	**14.5**
Prostate gland	93.0	70.0	23.0	83.6	60.6	23.0
Colon	63.0	50.9	12.1	51.5	45.1	6.4
Rectum	60.0	49.0	11.0	52.0	36.7	15.3
Leukemia	45.5	35.6	9.9	29.7	30.9	–1.2
Urinary bladder	83.9	75.9	8.0	66.6	58.9	7.7
Esophagus	13.2	5.0	8.2	8.0	2.3	5.7
Stomach	16.7	13.9	2.8	20.6	15.2	5.4
Lung and bronchus	12.7	11.6	1.1	9.9	10.0	0.1
Pancreas	3.8	2.7	1.1	3.2	2.4	0.8
Non-Hodgkin's lymphoma	47.7	47.2	0.5	37.6	44.2	–6.6
Oral cavity and pharynx	51.7	54.2	–2.5	28.4	31.2	–2.8
Female, total	**62.6**	**57.3**	**5.3**	**49.1**	**46.8**	**2.3**
Ovary	49.9	37.1	12.8	47.1	40.4	6.7
Breast	86.0	75.3	10.7	71.0	63.2	7.8
Rectum	60.6	50.8	9.8	50.3	43.7	6.6
Colon	61.9	52.6	9.3	52.1	48.7	3.4
Non-Hodgkin's lymphoma	57.3	49.2	8.1	47.5	57.3	–9.8
Melanoma of skin	91.0	85.8	5.2	75.2	69.9	5.3
Pancreas	4.4	2.1	2.3	3.9	4.1	–0.2
Cervix uteri	71.4	69.6	1.8	58.8	62.9	–4.1
Lung and bronchus	16.4	16.7	–0.3	14.0	15.4	–1.4
Corpus uteri	85.4	87.6	–2.2	56.1	59.1	–3.0

Source: National Center for Health Statistics, Health, United States, 2000; *calculations by New Strategist*

AIDS Cases by Sex and Age, through June 1999

(cumulative number and percent distribution of AIDS cases diagnosed by sex and age at diagnosis; through June 1999)

	number	percent
Total cases	**687,863**	**100.0%**
Under age 1	3,224	0.5
Aged 1 to 12	4,969	0.7
Aged 13 to 19	3,404	0.5
Aged 20 to 29	116,390	16.9
Aged 30 to 39	309,456	45.0
Aged 40 to 49	177,641	25.8
Aged 50 to 59	53,076	7.7
Aged 60 or older	19,703	2.9
Males		
Aged 13 or older	570,211	82.9
Aged 13 to 19	2,036	0.3
Aged 20 to 29	92,540	13.5
Aged 30 to 39	259,917	37.8
Aged 40 to 49	153,154	22.3
Aged 50 to 59	46,314	6.7
Aged 60 or older	16,250	2.4
Females		
Aged 13 or older	109,459	15.9
Aged 13 to 19	1,368	0.2
Aged 20 to 29	23,850	3.5
Aged 30 to 39	49,539	7.2
Aged 40 to 49	24,487	3.6
Aged 50 to 59	6,762	1.0
Aged 60 or older	3,453	0.5

Source: National Center for Health Statistics, Health, United States, 2000*; calculations by New Strategist*

Chronic Circulatory Conditions, 1990–92

(average annual number of chronic circulatory conditions, rate per 1,000 persons by age, and percent of conditions causing activity limitation, hospitalization, and physician visits, 1990–92)

	total conditions (number in 000s)	rate by age						percent of conditions causing		
		total	< age 18	18 to 44	45 to 64	65 to 74	75+	limitation of activity	1 or more hospitalizations	1 or more physician visits
Heart disease	20,480	82.4	18.9	37.4	129.4	262.0	364.9	24.7%	45.1%	98.2%
Ischemic heart disease	7,732	31.1	0.1	4.1	60.3	131.8	168.9	31.5	72.4	99.5
Heart rhythm disorders	7,868	31.6	14.1	25.8	40.7	65.1	91.7	6.4	14.8	96.4
Tachycardia or rapid heart	1,911	7.7	0.8	4.3	13.7	22.7	28.0	7.0	25.1	94.2
Heart murmurs	4,276	17.2	12.6	18.3	18.5	18.9	24.6	2.2	7.3	97.4
Other and unspecified heart rhythm disorders	1,681	6.8	0.7	3.1	8.5	23.5	39.1	16.3	22.4	96.3
Congenital heart disease	741	3.0	2.6	2.4	2.9	5.6	6.5	17.9	49.3	99.1
Other selected diseases of heart (excl. hypertension)	4,148	16.7	2.1	5.2	25.4	59.5	97.8	47.8	50.9	99.2
Rheumatic fever, with or without heart disease	2,029	8.2	0.7	7.9	16.1	13.6	11.8	15.1	31.3	99.6
High blood pressure (hypertension)	27,600	111.0	1.6	52.1	229.7	364.3	369.8	10.6	7.8	99.1
Cerebrovascular disease	3,002	12.1	0.5	1.4	16.7	57.9	80.8	35.9	70.3	99.6
Hardening of arteries	2,074	8.3	–	0.5	11.5	40.0	61.8	9.6	38.1	96.2
Aneurysm	226	0.9	0.1	0.1	1.8	3.4	5.4	15.5	61.9	100.0

(continued)

(continued from previous page)

	total conditions (number in 000s)	rate by age						percent of conditions causing		
		total	< age 18	18 to 44	45 to 64	65 to 74	75+	limitation of activity	1 or more hospital-izations	1 or more physician visits
Phlebitis, thrombophlebitis	727	2.9	–	1.7	4.6	9.4	13.0	17.2%	47.6%	98.1%
Varicose veins of lower extremities	7,403	29.8	0.3	24.8	52.8	73.3	77.2	2.2	8.9	60.1
Hemorrhoids	9,441	38.0	0.5	39.8	70.2	65.8	56.7	0.4	6.0	67.3
Poor circulation	980	3.9	–	1.4	5.9	14.3	24.8	27.7	19.9	92.8

Note: (–) means sample is too small to make a reliable estimate.
Source: National Center for Health Statistics, Prevalence of Selected Chronic Conditions: United States, 1990–92, Vital and Health Statistics, Series 10, No. 194, 1997

Chronic Digestive Conditions, 1990–92

(average annual number of chronic digestive conditions, rate per 1,000 persons by age, and percent of conditions causing activity limitation, hospitalization, and physician visits, 1990–92)

	total conditions (number in 000s)	rate by age						percent of conditions causing		
		total	< age 18	18 to 44	45 to 64	65 to 74	75+	limitation of activity	1 or more hospital- izations	1 or more physician visits
Gallbladder stones	1,068	4.3	0.2	3.4	7.8	12.2	8.8	11.0%	54.9%	99.1%
Liver diseases incl. cirrhosis	766	3.1	0.9	2.7	5.7	4.7	5.2	17.0	26.9	97.4
Ulcer, gastric, duodenal, and/or peptic	4,201	16.9	1.0	18.1	27.1	31.3	30.9	7.8	26.5	97.3
Gastric ulcer	3,121	12.5	0.9	14.1	20.2	19.9	20.9	7.7	25.1	96.8
Duodenal ulcer	613	2.5	0.1	2.0	4.0	7.3	6.2	10.4	29.5	100.0
Peptic ulcer	468	1.9	0.1	2.0	2.9	4.1	3.8	5.3	32.1	97.2
Hernia of abdominal cavity	4,768	19.2	3.4	10.1	35.5	55.0	66.3	9.8	21.5	96.8
Disease of the esophagus	834	3.4	0.6	2.7	6.1	5.7	9.7	5.4	27.7	97.6
Gastritis and duodenitis	3,003	12.1	2.4	12.0	19.3	23.1	20.8	1.0	12.8	88.4
Indigestion and other functional disorders of the stomach and digestive system	6,437	25.9	2.9	28.3	38.3	48.2	47.6	1.1	5.8	64.1
Enteritis and colitis	2,333	9.4	2.7	9.4	12.8	17.4	20.1	6.9	20.6	85.6
Spastic colon	1,686	6.8	0.4	7.5	11.3	11.5	10.2	2.7	13.3	94.7
Diverticula of intestines	1,999	8.0	0.0	1.8	12.3	42.2	37.9	4.3	27.9	97.7
Constipation	4302	17.3	6.5	13.1	18.1	36.4	80.7	0.7	3.8	69.4
Other stomach and intestinal disorders	2060	8.3	2.6	7.2	11.9	17.6	20.5	8.9	16.1	85.4
Malignant neoplasms of stomach, intestines, colon, and rectum	322	1.3	–	0.2	2.2	6.5	6.2	62.1	67.7	100.0

Note: (–) means sample is too small to make a reliable estimate.
Source: National Center for Health Statistics, Prevalence of Selected Chronic Conditions: United States, 1990–92, Vital and Health Statistics, Series 10, No. 194, 1997

Chronic Endocrine, Nutritional, Metabolic, Immune, Blood, and Genitourinary Conditions, 1990–92

(average annual number of chronic endocrine, nutritional, and metabolic diseases; immunity disorders; diseases of the blood and blood-forming organs; and genitourinary conditions; rate per 1,000 persons by age; and percent of conditions causing activity limitation, hospitalization, and physician visits, 1990–92)

	total conditions (number in 000s)	rate by age						percent of conditions causing		
		total	< age 18	18 to 44	45 to 64	65 to 74	75+	limitation of activity	1 or more hospital-izations	1 or more physician visits
Endocrine, nutritional, and metabolic diseases and immunity disorders										
Gout	2,167	8.7	–	3.8	18.0	31.1	29.2	9.6%	5.8%	93.8%
Goiter	478	1.9	0.3	1.6	3.4	5.6	1.6	5.6	15.5	100.0
Other diseases of the thyroid	3,303	13.3	1.0	9.3	26.6	34.9	30.3	6.5	13.0	99.3
Diabetes	6,962	28.0	1.0	11.7	54.7	106.7	92.8	34.7	26.5	100.0
Diseases of the blood and blood-forming organs										
Anemias	3,739	15.0	9.2	17.7	12.9	19.2	25.9	4.2	9.3	97.9
Genitourinary conditions										
Kidney stones	1,009	4.1	0.1	4.1	7.7	8.5	4.5	3.4	50.0	96.8
Kidney infections	1,325	5.3	1.5	6.1	6.6	8.5	9.7	3.5	24.0	96.2
Other kidney trouble, not elsewhere classified	862	3.5	1.8	2.5	3.8	8.5	11.4	27.5	35.8	95.0
Bladder infections	1,616	6.5	1.7	7.8	7.4	8.9	14.2	2.5	11.1	97.3
Other disorders of bladder	1,822	7.3	2.3	5.0	8.6	17.3	34.9	4.9	20.1	90.0

(continued)

(continued from previous page)

	total conditions (number in 000s)	rate by age						percent of conditions causing		
		total	< age 18	18 to 44	45 to 64	65 to 74	75+	limitation of activity	1 or more hospital-izations	1 or more physician visits
Diseases of prostate	1,513	6.1	–	1.9	11.0	27.2	24.2	5.2%	28.3%	97.2%
Inflammatory diseases of female genital organs	184	0.7	0.3	1.3	0.4	0.2	–	2.2	21.7	100.0
Noninflammatory diseases of female genital organs	1,219	4.9	0.8	9.1	3.4	1.6	1.3	3.0	37.7	99.7
Menstrual disorders	1,964	8.0	3.3	14.3	5.4	0.2	0.3	0.9	10.5	89.5
Other diseases of female genital organs	2,382	9.6	2.5	15.4	9.8	4.2	4.5	7.7	21.0	92.0
Female trouble, not otherwise specified	144	0.6	–	0.8	1.1	0.3	–	4.9	29.9	93.1
Malignant neoplasm of breast	802	3.2	–	0.7	5.4	14.3	17.3	23.7	85.3	100.0
Malignant neoplasm of female genital organs	221	0.9	–	1.1	1.0	2.0	1.4	16.3	57.5	100.0
Malignant neoplasm of prostate	344	1.4	–	0.1	1.3	8.8	9.4	22.1	70.6	100.0
Benign neoplasm of breast	73	0.3	–	0.4	0.3	0.5	0.8	2.7	30.1	100.0
Benign neoplasm of female genital organs	746	3.0	–	4.1	5.4	2.3	1.1	5.0	49.6	100.0

Note: (–) means sample is too small to make a reliable estimate.
Source: National Center for Health Statistics, Prevalence of Selected Chronic Conditions: United States, 1990–92, Vital and Health Statistics, Series 10, No. 194, 1997

Chronic Conditions and Impairments of the Nervous System and Sense Organs, 1990–92

(average annual number of impairments and chronic conditions of the nervous system and sense organs, rate per 1,000 persons by age, and percent of conditions causing activity limitations, hospitalization, and physician visits, 1990–92)

	total conditions (number in 000s)	rate by age						percent of conditions causing		
		total	< age 18	18 to 44	45 to 64	65 to 74	75+	limitation of activity	1 or more hospital-izations	1 or more physician visits
Blindness and other visual impairments	8,169	32.8	8.2	29.2	45.0	59.8	110.6	15.8%	14.9%	82.7%
Blind, both eyes	551	2.2	0.5	1.5	2.3	3.3	16.1	60.3	22.3	98.2
Other visual impairments	7,618	30.6	7.7	27.7	42.8	56.5	94.4	12.6	14.3	81.6
Deafness and other hearing impairments	23,266	93.5	17.3	50.7	148.6	262.6	410.3	5.5	6.1	74.8
Deaf, both ears	1,465	5.9	0.9	1.8	7.4	17.7	45.0	14.5	8.2	90.9
Other hearing impairments	21,801	87.6	16.4	48.9	141.3	244.9	365.3	4.9	6.0	73.7
Speech impairments	2,725	11.0	17.3	7.9	7.9	10.4	15.9	20.4	5.4	69.4
Impairment of sensation	1,142	4.6	0.1	2.7	7.7	12.2	21.3	5.8	9.6	64.4
Mental retardation	1,562	6.3	11.5	6.0	3.0	0.6	1.5	87.5	8.4	85.9
Absence of extremities	1,479	5.9	1.0	4.2	9.9	17.0	16.3	19.7	59.2	100.0
Absence of upper extremities or parts of upper extremities	946	3.8	0.7	3.0	6.0	9.7	9.8	12.4	52.3	100.0
Absence of lower extremities or parts of lower extremities	533	2.1	0.3	1.2	3.8	7.3	6.5	32.8	71.5	100.0

(continued)

(continued from previous page)

	total conditions (number in 000s)	rate by age						percent of conditions causing		
		total	< age 18	18 to 44	45 to 64	65 to 74	75+	limitation of activity	1 or more hospitalizations	1 or more physician visits
Absence of lung	236	0.9	–	0.3	2.1	3.9	2.6	22.5%	80.9%	100.0%
Absence of kidney	556	2.2	0.7	1.3	3.6	6.6	6.9	11.5	75.9	99.1
Absence of breast	1,153	4.6	–	0.7	8.2	18.8	28.5	4.7	91.8	100.0
Absence of bone, joint, or muscle of extremity	876	3.5	0.2	2.0	4.4	11.4	19.8	32.0	66.1	99.1
Absence of tips of fingers or toes	366	1.5	0.2	1.4	2.3	4.1	1.8	5.7	29.5	100.0
Paralysis of extremities, complete or partial	1,464	5.9	2.7	3.1	8.0	16.0	24.3	60.7	42.5	99.5
Paralysis of extremities, complete	626	2.5	0.6	1.2	4.6	6.5	10.8	54.5	53.8	100.0
Paralysis of extremities, partial	838	3.4	2.2	1.9	3.4	9.5	13.4	65.5	34.0	99.2
Cerebral palsy	258	1.0	2.0	1.0	0.4	–	0.3	74.4	43.8	100.0
Paralysis of other site, complete or partial	371	1.5	0.6	0.8	2.5	2.6	6.6	48.0	37.5	98.7
Deformities or orthopedic impairments, total	34,964	140.6	30.7	161.7	195.4	203.5	242.2	25.2	18.6	90.4
Deformities or orthopedic impairments of back	18,144	72.9	10.3	90.8	103.7	92.6	106.5	22.4	15.6	92.2
Curvature or other deformity of back or spine	5,078	20.4	7.9	25.1	21.8	23.3	37.8	12.2	8.9	93.4
Deformities or orthopedic impairments of upper extremities	3,846	15.5	2.1	16.2	23.5	29.3	29.0	30.0	26.1	94.2

(continued)

(continued from previous page)

	total conditions (number in 000s)	rate by age						percent of conditions causing		
		total	< age 18	18 to 44	45 to 64	65 to 74	75+	limitation of activity	1 or more hospital- izations	1 or more physician visits
Orthopedic impairment, shoulder	2,919	11.7	1.2	13.1	18.6	18.8	19.2	36.4%	24.6%	94.6%
Deformities or orthopedic impairments of lower extremities	12,518	50.3	18.0	52.8	66.1	79.2	98.6	26.8	20.8	86.4
Flat feet	3,698	14.9	10.0	15.7	18.6	17.9	15.0	1.2	2.6	69.5
Other deformities or orthopedic impairment	456	1.8	0.4	1.8	2.1	2.4	8.1	54.4	13.4	96.3
Cleft palate	217	0.9	1.0	0.8	1.2	0.7	0.3	3.2	63.1	95.4
Glaucoma	2,433	9.8	0.4	2.1	12.2	43.3	67.7	13.4	10.5	99.8
Cataracts	6,416	25.8	1.1	2.7	22.7	122.1	229.0	6.1	9.9	98.4
Color blindness	2,697	10.8	4.0	12.7	15.0	13.7	11.8	0.2	–	58.0
Diseases of retina	1,293	5.2	0.4	2.0	4.8	18.7	40.9	28.9	20.7	99.8
Tinnitus	7,144	28.7	1.8	16.8	54.6	91.6	82.5	0.8	1.5	69.2
Epilepsy	1,243	5.0	4.4	5.6	5.0	3.9	4.6	44.4	47.8	98.9
Migraine headache	9,992	40.2	13.2	57.2	51.6	22.9	19.1	3.4	7.7	81.8
Other headache (excluding tension headache)	10,279	41.3	12.7	57.6	50.3	34.7	29.1	1.8	2.8	63.6
Multiple sclerosis	180	0.7	–	0.9	1.4	0.9	0.2	69.4	43.9	100.0

Note: (–) means sample is too small to make a reliable estimate.
Source: National Center for Health Statistics, Prevalence of Selected Chronic Conditions: United States, 1990–92, Vital and Health Statistics, Series 10, No. 194, 1997

Chronic Respiratory Conditions, 1990–92

(average annual number of chronic respiratory conditions, rate per 1,000 persons by age, and percent of conditions causing activity limitation, hospitalization, and physician visits, by age, 1990–92)

	total conditions (number in 000s)	rate by age							percent of conditions causing		
		total	< age 18	18 to 44	45 to 64	65 to 74	75+		limitation of activity	1 or more hospital-izations	1 or more physician visits
Chronic bronchitis	12,884	51.8	53.4	45.1	56.6	70.4	54.8		2.0%	9.8%	94.9%
Emphysema	1,861	7.5	–	0.8	13.5	35.8	39.9		44.1	27.4	97.8
Asthma	11,482	46.2	61.2	41.2	41.5	38.2	37.3		21.8	21.9	96.8
Hay fever or allergic rhinitis without asthma	24,060	96.7	64.3	121.1	101.4	79.8	66.7		1.4	1.7	71.2
Nasal polyps	805	3.2	1.4	3.0	5.3	5.2	4.5		0.4	16.5	88.9
Chronic sinusitis	33,736	135.6	62.0	157.1	180.3	156.2	140.8		0.5	2.5	70.9
Deviated nasal septum	1,646	6.6	0.9	8.4	9.5	8.7	7.0		0.2	11.7	95.2
Chronic disease of tonsils and adenoids	2,836	11.4	24.9	9.7	2.9	2.2	0.6		0.4	12.1	94.2
Chronic laryngitis	1,508	6.1	2.2	7.1	7.2	10.3	6.5		–	3.4	68.2
Pleurisy	690	2.8	0.2	2.9	4.7	5.2	4.4		1.6	10.7	86.7
Pneumoconiosis/asbestosis	324	1.3	0.1	0.8	2.2	4.9	3.7		26.2	12.3	84.0
Malignant neoplasms of lung, bronchus, and other respiratory sites	218	0.9	–	0.1	1.9	4.0	3.6		60.6	71.6	100.0
Other diseases of the lung	1,141	4.6	3.7	2.8	5.9	8.8	13.5		16.2	31.2	99.6

Note: (–) means sample is too small to make a reliable estimate.
Source: National Center for Health Statistics, Prevalence of Selected Chronic Conditions: United States, 1990–92, Vital and Health Statistics, Series 10, No. 194, 1997

Chronic Conditions of the Skin, Musculoskeletal System, and Connective Tissue, 1990–92

(average annual number of chronic conditions of the skin and subcutaneous tissue and of the musculoskeletal system and connective tissue, rate per 1,000 persons by age, and percent of conditions causing activity limitation, hospitalization, and physician visits, 1990–92)

	total conditions (number in 000s)	rate by age						percent of conditions causing		
		total	< age 18	18 to 44	45 to 64	65 to 74	75+	limitation of activity	1 or more hospital-izations	1 or more physician visits
Condition of skin and subcutaneous tissue										
Sebaceous skin cyst	1,249	5.0	1.6	6.2	6.4	7.4	4.6	0.2%	6.0%	93.3%
Acne	4,904	19.7	25.7	28.4	4.3	1.2	3.0	–	0.4	67.6
Psoriasis	2,378	9.6	2.6	9.3	16.2	14.4	16.1	2.1	2.9	88.4
Dermatitis	9,273	37.3	34.5	39.5	38.5	36.7	29.2	1.5	1.6	85.2
Dry (itching) skin, not elsewhere classified	5,123	20.6	10.0	21.1	23.9	31.3	44.8	0.1	0.5	54.0
Chronic ulcer of skin	332	1.3	0.1	0.9	1.8	4.4	5.9	24.1	20.8	93.4
Ingrown nails	6,078	24.4	8.2	24.5	30.6	45.1	56.5	0.3	1.0	54.1
Corns and calluses	4,731	19.0	1.0	16.3	33.1	40.4	52.9	0.5	1.5	46.7
Benign neoplasms of the skin	862	3.5	1.1	3.0	5.4	7.4	7.3	2.1	3.4	97.2
Malignant neoplasms of the skin	2,269	9.1	0.1	2.0	16.9	34.4	51.8	3.9	3.4	97.1
Condition of musculoskeletal system and connective tissue										
Arthritis	31,788	127.8	2.3	49.8	250.2	433.0	550.0	21.2	7.4	82.6
Rheumatism, unspecified	454	1.8	0.1	1.2	3.0	5.6	6.8	17.0	8.6	78.9
Sciatica (including lumbago)	2,058	8.3	–	6.5	17.5	19.6	15.3	6.5	6.9	88.1

(continued)

(continued from previous page)

| | total conditions (number in 000s) | rate by age | | | | | | percent of conditions causing | | |
		total	< age 18	18 to 44	45 to 64	65 to 74	75+	limitation of activity	1 or more hospital-izations	1 or more physician visits
Intervertebral disc disorders	4,976	20.0	0.3	19.3	43.1	33.6	21.5	45.2%	38.4%	96.7%
Bone spur or tendinitis, not otherwise specified	2,633	10.6	0.9	9.2	21.1	23.1	15.6	9.6	9.6	92.1
Disorders of bone or cartilage	1,568	6.3	1.5	3.7	9.3	19.7	23.5	37.9	18.0	97.2
Bunions	2,907	11.7	0.9	7.9	22.3	28.0	37.2	0.9	5.0	58.0
Bursitis, not elsewhere classified	4,674	18.8	0.8	14.1	40.6	42.3	36.7	5.3	3.9	88.8
Neuritis or neuralgia, unspecified	518	2.1	0.0	0.9	4.2	6.8	7.9	4.6	8.7	77.8

Note: (−) means sample is too small to make a reliable estimate.
Source: National Center for Health Statistics, Prevalence of Selected Chronic Conditions: United States, 1990–92, Vital and Health Statistics, Series 10, No. 194, 1997

9

Living with Disability

Disability is a term much bandied about these days. Yet a precise definition of disability does not exist, making it difficult to examine the link between disability and health. Not only are there many different kinds of physical disabilities, but identifying the disabled depends on a society's definition of normal. In American society, technological and attitudinal change challenge the definitions of disabled and normal every day.

New technologies are removing people once considered disabled from the category. Take corrective lenses, for example. Before they became available, the nearsighted were visually impaired. Today, they are considered normal. The definition of disability is an equation that balances the state of adaptive technology with the cultural expectations of what a person should be able to do.

In the United States, attitudes towards disability have changed during the past century. Not long ago, the disabled were the main attraction at freak shows. Those spared this horror were often institutionalized to set them apart from normal society. There were some

Disability rises with age

(percent of people with a disability by age, 1994–95)

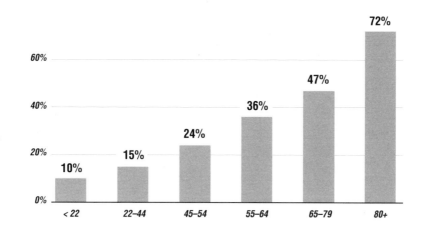

exceptions, of course—disabled people who set out to change society or at least not be limited by it. The textbook example is Helen Keller, the blind and deaf pioneer. But whether a freak, a heroine, or hidden in an institution, one fact was clear: to be disabled meant to be excluded.

Thanks to the efforts of many, this attitude first became unacceptable and then illegal with the passage of the Americans with Disabilities Act in 1990. The ADA extended civil rights protection to disabled people. Just as it was illegal to discriminate based on race or religion, it became illegal to discriminate on the basis of disability.

The ADA ushered in a new way of thinking about disability. Suddenly, there were powerful financial and legal incentives to understand the needs of the disabled and to accommodate those needs. The legislation was intended to bring disabled people out of the shadows and into society with as few limits as possible.

The ADA has brought to the public forefront the question of what disability means. It vaguely defines disability as any physical or mental impairment that substantially limits a major life activity. As the courts attempt to interpret the definition, it's clear that nothing is clear. Drug addiction, for example, is not considered a disability under ADA, although it is an impairment that substantially limits life activities. The New York State Court of Appeals has ruled that obesity is not a disability either. Yet, diabetes is a disability, as is dyslexia, according to other court rulings. A Chicago policewoman successfully claimed that infertility was a disability under the ADA, requiring her employer to cover the cost of treatment. The Supreme Court recently ruled that HIV is a disability under the ADA.

The debate over the definition of disability has created a backlash against the ADA. Critics see it as an expensive intrusion by the government, allowing some with so-called boutique disabilities—a term generally used to describe disabilities that seem to be designed or acquired specifically to trigger ADA protection—to benefit from the law. Studies show, however, that the law is abused far less often than media coverage may indicate. Of the 24,000 cases that came before the Equal Employment Opportunities Commission in 1997 (the Commission adjudicates ADA cases), 60 percent were thrown out, according to *The Economist*.[1] Only 12 percent had outcomes favorable to the complainant.

In the Supreme Court's 1998-99 session, three important cases set new precedent for the definition of disability: Sutton v. United Airlines, Albertsons Inc. v. Kirkingburg, and Murphy v. United Parcel. In these cases, the Supreme Court decided that the ADA does not cover people with a correctable impairment. If a person, after using a mitigating measure (such as medication, glasses, or other corrective device) does not continue to have a substantial limitation in a major life activity then he or she is not considered disabled under the law, explained the National Council on Disabilities in its 1998-1999 Progress Report.[2]

The three cases cited above involved people with poor uncorrected vision, monocular vision, and hypertension. All three were challenging disciplinary actions by their employers. "In deciding that these people fall outside the civil rights protections of ADA because their conditions are correctable, our highest court has left many people with treatable conditions such as epilepsy, diabetes and bipolar disorder outside the law's protection. . . . Anyone who is functioning well with their disability is now at risk of losing civil rights protections as a result of the Supreme Court's 'miserly' construction, to use Justice Steven's characterization in his eloquent report," the NCD states.

The fact that correctable problems are not considered disabilities under the law has enormous implications as the population ages and as medical technology marches on. The controversy is far from resolved.

Defining disability

While the definition of disability may be under debate, this hasn't stopped the adoption of definitions for the purposes of collecting data about the disabled.

According to the Census Bureau, 21 percent of Americans—54 million people— had some level of disability in 1994–95. To be considered disabled by the Bureau, a person had to meet at least one of the following criteria:

- Uses a wheelchair, cane, crutches, or walker.
- Has difficulty performing one or more functional activities, which include seeing, hearing, speaking, lifting, carrying, using stairs, or walking.
- Has difficulty with at least one activity of daily living (ADL). These include getting around inside the home, getting in and out of a bed or chair, bathing, dressing, eating, and toileting.
- Has difficulty with at least one instrumental activity of daily living (IADL). These include going outside, keeping track of money and bills, preparing meals, doing light housework, taking prescription medicine correctly, and using the telephone.
- Has a specified condition such as a learning disability, mental retardation, or Alzheimer's disease.
- Is limited in his or her ability to do housework.

- Is of working age (16 to 67) and unable to work.

- Receives federal benefits based on inability to work.

One in 10 Americans—or 26 million people—had a severe disability in 1994-95. To be classified as severely disabled, the person must need assistance with one or more activities of daily living or instrumental activities of daily living, or have a long-term need for a wheelchair, cane, crutches, or walker.

The incidence of disability increases with age. Only 9 percent of children under age 15 are disabled, but the proportion rises to 12 percent among young adults aged 15 to 21 and to 15 percent among people aged 22 to 44. Disability climbs sharply beginning in middle age. Twenty-four percent of 45-to-54-year-olds are disabled, as are 36 percent of 55-to-64-year-olds, and 47 percent of 65-to-79-year-olds. An enormous 72 percent of people aged 80 or older have some disability, according to the Census Bureau's definition.

The likelihood of having a severe disability also increases with age, from 2 percent of school-aged children to 54 percent of the oldest Americans. More than half the Americans who require the help of others to manage their daily lives are aged 65 or older.

Many of the disabled use what are called assistive technology devices to get around or communicate with others. Assistive technologies include a range of low- and high-tech devices from canes to hearing aids to computer equipment. The cane is the most common assistive technology device, used by 4.8 million Americans.

The most commonly used assistive technology devices

(number of people using the five most common assistive technology devices, 1994–95; in millions)

cane	4.8
hearing aid	4.2
walker	1.8
back brace	1.7
wheelchair	1.6

People aged 65 or older account for most of the users of assistive technologies, with the exception of anatomical devices such as back or neck braces. Younger people account for the majority or near-majority of users of more high-tech assistive technology devices such as TDD/TTY (telephone communication for the deaf), closed-caption television, Braille, and computer equipment for the sight impaired.

The use of assistive technology has soared over the past few years as the disabled integrate with society and as the new health care consumer resists the limitations of disability. The number of people using walkers, wheelchairs, and braces other than for neck or leg more than doubled between 1980 and 1994, according to the National Center for Health Statistics. Expect continued rapid growth in the use of assistive technology devices as boomers age and confront more disability.

Another of the Census Bureau classifications is "work disability." A work disability is a condition that limits the kind or amount of work that a person can do, and a severe work disability is a condition that prevents someone from working. By that definition, 17 million people—or 10 percent of the working-age population (aged 16 to 64)—had a work disability in 1999. The Census Bureau estimates that 11.5 million people have a severe work disability—or 68 percent of the total work-disabled population.

The probability of having a work disability increases with age. Only 4 percent of people aged 16 to 24 have a work disability compared with 22 percent of those aged 55 to 64. There

Rapid growth in the use of assistive technology

(percent change in number of people using assistive technology devices, by type of device, 1980–94)

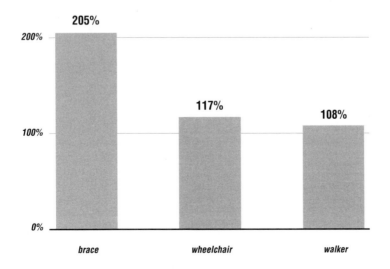

is little difference in the percentage of working-age men and women with a work disability. As education increases, the likelihood of having a work disability falls. Just 5 percent of people with 16 or more years of education have a work disability versus 24 percent of people with fewer than eight years of education.

Only 30 percent of people with a work disability are in the labor force compared with 82 percent of people without a work disability. Among the work disabled, the unemployment rate was 11 percent in 1999 compared with 4 percent among the population without a work disability. Younger people with work disabilities are more likely to participate in the labor force than their older counterparts.

Children and disability

According to the Census Bureau's definition of disability, 5 million children under age 15 (or 9 percent) were disabled in 1994–95. By another definition, the National Center for Health Statistics reports that 12 percent of noninstitutionalized children aged 5 to 17 have difficulty performing one or more daily activities.[3] The most common difficulty is with learning. In 1994, 11 percent of children aged 5 to 17 had a learning disability, while 6 percent had a communication disorder. Only about 1 percent had mobility limitations, and fewer than 1 percent had self-care limitations.

Boys are more likely than girls to have a limitation. Sixteen percent of boys have difficulty in at least one area compared with 9 percent of girls.

Children from families with low incomes and low educational levels are more likely to be limited in their daily activities, reports NCHS. Eighteen percent of children in single-parent households were limited versus 10 percent of children in two-parent households.

More than 12 million children have special health care needs, according to the Family Partners Project—a collaboration of Family Voices, an advocacy group, and Brandeis University.[4] Between March 1998 and April 1999, the Family Partners Project Surveyed 2,220 families with a disabled child, asking them about their health care experiences. The survey revealed a needy market of unique health care consumers.

The average annual income of the families with disabled children was $34,327, according to the survey's results. More than half the disabled children were boys, and more than one-quarter were minorities. Most of the disabled children had more than one health condition or disability. The most common conditions were orthopedic, such as cerebral palsy. Behavioral problems, mental retardation, seizure disorders, and asthma were also common conditions. Seventeen percent of the disabled children were technology assisted or dependent, requiring a feeding tube, ventilator, or some other device.

Fully 97 percent of the children had some kind of health insurance at the time of the survey, although 6 percent had been without health insurance within the past year. Half the families experienced financial hardship, nearly half spending more than $1,000 out-of-pocket on medical care for their child. Ten percent reported spending more than $5,000.

Nine out of 10 children with disabilities used prescription medications, 82 percent used specialty doctors, 40 percent received physical therapy. Almost half used durable medical equipment, more than one-third used disposable medical supplies, and 30 percent received respite services.

Many parents had problems accessing specialty services for their children, the report revealed. Among parents of children receiving home health care, nearly half reported difficulty finding skilled home health care providers. Among those receiving mental health services, 43 percent had trouble finding skilled providers. Of children using prescription medications, 21 percent had problems getting prescriptions.

Parents of children with disabilities are an important market for caregiver services. Nearly two-thirds of parents reported that they had reduced their hours of employment or stopped working altogether because of their child's condition. One-fifth of parents provide 20 or more hours a week of health care services to their child at home.

Disability culture

Two years ago, at the New School for Social Research in New York City, students could enroll in a course entitled, "Celebrating Differences—Disability Culture," taught by Professor Nadina LaSpina. According to the catalog description, the course was an exploration of the creative expression of disabled people through fiction, poetry, theater, and film. Rather than viewing disability as a medical problem, the course defined disability as an important part of what makes each person unique. Although the course is no longer offered, that sentiment is strong and growing in the U.S. today, says Joseph P. Shapiro in his landmark book, *No Pity: People with Disabilites Forging a New Civil Rights Movement*. Shapiro says there is "no pity or tragedy in disability. . . it is society's myths, fears and sterotypes that most make being disabled difficult."[5]

The emergence of disability culture is a new factor in the disability debate, reframing the discussion of physical and mental disabilities from limitations to celebrations. "Perhaps most surprising. . .is that many say they would reject being cured even if it was possible, explaining that they have a condition, not an illness," writes Douglas Martin in *The New York Times*.[6] His article quotes LaSpina: "We will not change to fit the mold. We will destroy the mold and change the world to make sure there is room for everyone." In his article, Martin quotes a women with cerebral palsy who expresses pity for newly disabled actor Christopher Reeve because he wants to be cured.

Twenty-five years ago, Susan Webb, President of Webb Transitions, Inc. of Phoenix, Arizona, fell off a motorcycle and sustained a spinal cord injury. Webb is in a wheelchair and exemplifies the new attitude of the disabled. Her company helps people with disabilities make the transition into the workplace. "We have to separate what is medical and what is disability," Webb says. "There's a point where disability is a lifestyle. It is no longer a medical condition. When someone has a disability, because we're compassionate, caring people, we think, 'Oh poor you. Isn't this a tragedy.' But while you're trying to provide support, you're creating a victim. Helping people get beyond it is truly much more compassionate than the pity party."[7]

While not every disabled person shares this point of view, it is clear the movement is growing. Years of isolation and seclusion from society, paired with new, legally mandated access and education, are producing an explosion of disability culture, art, and community. On the Internet, sites like Disability Cool (www.geocities.com/CapeCanaveral/Lab/1383/discool.html) skip the pity and focus on the positive.

This attitude has broad implications outside the disabled community. The rejection of the medical definition of disability in favor of the self-definition of health and ability is the ultimate consumer-directed health trend. As the baby-boom generation ages and encounters more disability, defining health as how you feel rather than how you are will become even more prevalent. An upbeat attitude may have significant health benefits itself. A study in the *Journal of Physical Education, Recreation and Dance* found that successful adjustment to a changed lifestyle such as that caused by a chronic health condition may be more important to long-term health than the actual prognosis.[8] People who are physically healthy but unhappy cannot be considered as healthy as those with physical problems and a positive outlook on life, the researchers concluded.

The rejection of the medical model does not mean rejection of medical treatment, however. The emergence of disability culture is possible in part only because medicine has advanced sufficiently to allow people with many types of impairments to live independently. But treatments are often expensive and long-term, two factors that hurt the bottom line of health insurance companies. This may be why working-age people with disabilities are more likely to be without health insurance (23 percent of 22-to-64-year-olds) than their able-bodied counterparts (17 percent), according to the Census Bureau.

Like Americans without disabilities, most of the disabled receive health insurance through an employer. Seventy-one percent of 22-to-64-year-olds with a disability receive health insurance through an employer compared with 79 percent of their nondisabled counterparts. Only 6 percent of the disabled rely on government-provided health insurance.

The picture is somewhat different for people with severe disabilities. Although 44 percent have private insurance, 40 percent have government-provided health insurance because the severely disabled are less likely to be employed. While the rate of severe disability is high for people who receive government assistance, the 63 percent majority of the severely disabled do not receive government help, according to the Census Bureau.

The introduction of managed care has created problems for the disabled, especially since most are privately insured. Media catering to the disabled focus much attention on how to manage HMOs. In *Accent on Living*, author Patti Makosky complains about the one-wheelchair-per-lifetime restriction, the disruption of long-term relationships between patient and doctor, and the unwillingness of insurers to cover experimental treatments.[9] The battle between insurers and people with disabilities is likely to be a long one, since insurers understandably regard people with disabilities as high risk for expensive medical costs. Insurers are slowly starting to cover experimental treatments—usually only after government prodding. New Jersey, for example, has begun to require coverage of experimental cancer treatments.[10]

Because most private health insurance comes through employers, the lack of insurance for the disabled who cannot work or who are between jobs is a serious problem. The disabled community is leading the way in finding alternatives to employer-provided health insurance. In *Inside MS*, for example, disability rights lawyer Laura Cooper suggests that the disabled join various organizations to share in their health benefits. "After a weekend of web browsing, I'm thinking about becoming a 'friend' of the University of Alabama," writes Cooper. "I've never been to that fine institution, but the alumni association seems to have a great major medical plan. . .if the required donation is reasonable enough, I'd be happy to join up."[11]

Internet use and people with disabilities

The Internet has become an important communication tool for people with disabilities. But according to a recent analysis of 1998 CPS data by the Disability Statistics Center, computer and Internet access among people with work disabilities is far less prevalent than it is for people without work disabilities.[12] While 51 percent of the nondisabled aged 15 or older have a computer in the household, and three in ten have Internet access, just 24 percent of people with a work disability have a computer at home and only 11 percent have Internet access. Among people aged 15 to 64 with a work disability, the numbers are better. Nearly one-third have a computer and 16 percent access the Internet at home.

As computer technology evolves to allow a wider range of the disabled to take advantage of its potential, the Internet could transform the lives of many disabled Americans in the decades ahead.

The future of disability culture

Just as racial and ethnic minority cultures are becoming part of mainstream America, so is disability culture. As businesses accommodate the disabled and more Americans face disability, the distinction between the abled and the disabled will blur. Several trends will shape that future.

TREND 1: UNIVERSAL DESIGN

When a product or service is universally designed, it is accessible to people of varying abilities. In the years ahead, health itself will take on a universal design. The definition of good health will no longer be the equation: perfection minus health problems equals current health status. Instead, health will be measured by how well a person adapts to his or her particular health challenges. Disabled people are at the vanguard of this movement, but the concept is certain to expand.

The adoption of universal design will be aided by the increasing number of disabled as the population ages. Indeed, everyone will experience a disability at some point during his or her life. (Some of the disabled, in fact, refer to the nondisabled as TABs—temporarily able-bodied persons.) The growing number of disabled, combined with their greater education and access to society, guarantees their position as powerful consumer group. Their lobbying will speed the adoption of universal design in products, services, and attitudes.

TREND 2: BECOMING NORMAL

Technological advances as well as the deinstitutionalization of medical care will shift the focus away from curing the disabled towards helping them improve the quality of their life. Community care of the disabled will become an even more powerful movement in the future. Consequently, the disabled who live a normal—even successful—life will no longer be remarkable as they are today. Typically, the disabled who live normally are considered so unusual that they merit special profiles by the media. In the future, more of the disabled will make the transition from tragic hero to average citizen.

TREND 3: MORE COMMUNITY CARE

Another watershed case recently before the Supreme Court, Olmstead v. L.C., changed the way disabled people will receive care. The Court ruled that placing disabled people in institutions when they would benefit more from care in a community or home setting was discrimination under the ADA. "Institutional placement of persons who can handle and benefit from community settings perpetuates unwarranted assumptions that persons so isolated or incapable are unworthy in participating in community life and cultural enrichment," the Court noted in its opinion.[13] This decision will put legal pressure on communities to provide noninstitutional care for more of the disabled.

TREND 4: THE DISABLED AS A MARKET

The marketing community is slowly discovering that the disabled are an important opportunity. The Internet is helping to make this happen. One company exploring the market is We Media, which publishes a successful magazine for the disabled. It has launched a portal site called WeMedia.com, allowing advertisers to tap into a market that, they claim, is worth $1 trillion in purchasing power.[14]

The disabled are not sitting back and waiting for the rest of the world to discover them, however. In recent years there has been an explosion of health care products and services designed by and for the disabled. Expect to see many more such efforts in the coming years.

TREND 5: PUBLIC BACKLASH

The transition to universally designed health will not be entirely smooth. Some business owners, for example, view the Americans with Disabilities Act as heavy-handed legislation that leaves them vulnerable to business-destroying lawsuits. Beyond the financial and legal concerns of businesses, discrimination by the public still exists and is not likely to disappear entirely. The able-bodied backlash against expanded access is similar to the backlash against Civil Rights legislation after its passage in the 1960s, says author Jan Little, writing in *Accent on Living*.[15] Many of the able-bodied will never accept the full integration of the disabled into society, just as some people have never accepted racial integration. But their numbers will diminish as the disabled demand more involvement in everyday life.

Notes

1. "The Halt, the Blind and the Dyslexic: Has the Americans with Disabilities Act Gone Too Far, or Not Far Enough?" *The Economist* (April 18, 1998): 25–27.

2. National Council on Disability, *National Disability Policy: A Progress Report, November 1, 1998–November 19, 1999* (Washington, D.C., 2000).

3. Federal Interagency Forum on Child and Family Statistics, *America's Children: Key National Indicators of Well-Being, 1999* (1999). <http://childstats.gov>.

4. Family Voices and Brandeis University, *What Do Families Say about Health Care for Children with Special Health Care Needs? The Family Partners Project Report to Families* (1998). <www.familyvoices.org>.

5. Joseph P. Shapiro, *No Pity: People with Disabilities Forging a New Civil Rights Movement* (New York: Times Books, 1994): 5.

6. Douglas Martin, "Eager to Bite the Hands That Would Feed Them," *The New York Times* (June 1, 1997): D1.

7. Interview with Susan Webb.

8. Lee Youngkhill and Thomas K. Skalko, "Redefining Health for People with Chronic Disabilities," *The Journal of Physical Education, Recreation and Dance* 67, no. 9 (November–December 1996): 64–66.

9. Patti Makosky, "HMOs," *Accent on Living* (Fall 1996): 34–38.

10. Harris Fleming Jr., "New Jersey Insurers to Cover Experimental Cancer Treatments," *Drug Topics* 144, no. 3 (February 7, 2000): 115.

11. Laura Cooper, "Finding Non-Employment Based Health Insurance," *Inside MS* (Spring 1998): 42–44.

12. H. Stephen Kaye, "Computer and Internet Use among People with Disabilities," *Disability Statistics Report* 13, U.S. Department of Education, National Institute on Disability and Rehabilitation Research (Washington, D.C., 2000).

13. National Council on Disability.

14. WeMedia.com, "People with Disabilities Are the Next Consumer Niche" (December 15, 1999). <www.wemedia.com>.

15. Jan Little," The Changing Images of Disability," *Accent on Living* (Winter 1995): 116–120.

People with Disabilities by Sex and Age, 1994–95

(total number of people, percent with a disability, and percent severely disabled, by sex and age, 1994–95; numbers in thousands)

	total	disabled	
		total	*severely*
Total people	**261,748**	**20.6%**	**9.9%**
Under age 22	84,527	10.0	1.7
Aged 22 to 44	95,002	14.8	6.4
Aged 45 to 54	30,316	24.4	11.5
Aged 55 to 64	20,647	36.3	21.9
Aged 65 to 79	24,470	47.3	27.8
Aged 80 or older	6,786	71.5	53.5
Total males	**127,908**	**19.8**	**8.3**
Under age 22	43,131	12.0	2.1
Aged 22 to 44	47,090	14.1	5.6
Aged 45 to 54	14,825	24.0	10.3
Aged 55 to 64	9,798	35.3	19.2
Aged 65 to 79	10,693	46.2	24.8
Aged 80 or older	2,371	66.3	44.9
Total females	**133,840**	**21.3**	**11.5**
Under age 22	41,369	8.0	1.4
Aged 22 to 44	47,912	15.6	7.2
Aged 45 to 54	15,491	24.9	12.5
Aged 55 to 64	10,849	37.2	24.4
Aged 65 to 79	13,777	48.1	30.1
Aged 80 or older	4,415	74.3	58.1

Note: People were considered to have a disability if they used a wheelchair; used a cane, crutches, or walker for at least six months; had difficulty with a functional activity or activity of daily living such as doing light housework or dressing; or had a learning disability, or developmental, mental, or emotional condition. In addition, people aged 16 to 67 were considered to have a disability if they had a condition that limited the kind or amount of work they could do at a job. People were classified as having a severe disability if they used a wheelchair or another mobility aid for at least six months; were unable to perform one or more functional activities or needed assistance with an activity of daily living; were prevented from working or doing housework; or had a selected condition such as autism or Alzheimer's disease. Persons under age 65 who received Medicare or SSI were considered to have a severe disability.

Source: Bureau of the Census, Internet web site <http://www.census.gov/hhes/www/disable/sipp/disable9495.html>

Children with Disabilities, 1994–95

(total number of children, and number and percent with a disability, by age, sex, and type of disability, 1994–95; numbers in thousands)

	number	percent
Total children under age 15	**59,380**	**100.0%**
With any disability	5,417	9.1
Children aged 0 to 2	**11,942**	**100.0**
With a developmental condition	303	2.6
Children aged 3 to 5	**12,427**	**100.0**
With any disability	652	5.2
With a developmental condition	510	4.1
Difficulty walking or running	235	1.9
Boys aged 3 to 5	6,419	100.0
With any disability	442	6.9
Girls aged 3 to 5	6,009	100.0
With any disability	210	3.5
Children aged 6 to 14	**35,011**	**100.0**
With any disability	4,462	12.7
With a severe disability	659	1.9
Difficulty doing regular schoolwork	2,170	6.2
With a learning disability	1,559	4.5
With a developmental disability	451	1.3
Difficulty with one or more ADLs	381	1.1
Needs personal assistance	272	0.8
Boys aged 6 to 14	17,896	100.0
With any disability	2,824	15.8
Girls aged 6 to 14	17,115	100.0
With any disability	1,638	9.6

Source: Bureau of the Census, Americans with Disabilities: 1994–95, *Current Population Reports, P70–61, 1997*

Adults with Disabilities by Type of Disability and Age, 1994–95

(total number of people aged 15 or older and percent with a disability, by type of disability and age, 1994–95)

	15 or older	15 to 21	22 to 44	45 to 54	55 to 64	65 to 79	80+
Total people (in thousands)	**202,367**	**25,146**	**95,002**	**30,316**	**20,647**	**24,471**	**6,785**
With any disability	24.0%	12.1%	14.9%	24.5%	36.3%	47.3%	71.5%
Severe	12.5	3.2	6.4	11.5	21.9	27.8	53.5
Not severe	11.5	8.9	8.5	13.0	14.4	19.5	18.1
With a mental disability	4.8	4.9	3.8	4.4	4.5	5.7	18.8
Uses wheelchair	0.9	0.3	0.3	0.4	1.3	2.1	6.9
Used cane/crutch/walker for 6+ mos.	2.6	0.2	0.5	1.4	3.3	7.8	24.3
Difficulty with or unable to perform one or more functional activities	**16.4**	**3.7**	**7.8**	**16.1**	**26.2**	**41.2**	**67.8**
Seeing words and letters	5.8	0.7	1.6	4.2	6.0	10.0	25.2
Hearing normal conversation	6.2	1.0	2.0	4.1	6.5	12.5	28.2
Having speech understood	1.0	1.0	0.6	0.7	1.3	2.0	4.5
Lifting, carrying 10 pounds	7.9	1.1	3.2	7.4	12.9	20.9	39.6
Climbing stairs without resting	8.9	1.2	3.1	7.8	15.3	25.2	45.3
Walking three city blocks	9.1	1.3	3.3	7.7	15.5	25.2	48.5
Difficulty with or unable to perform one or more ADLs	**4.0**	**0.6**	**1.5**	**3.1**	**6.0**	**10.5**	**27.5**
Getting around inside the home	1.7	0.3	0.5	1.0	2.3	4.6	14.7
Getting in and out of bed or chair	2.7	0.4	1.0	2.2	4.1	6.9	18.0
Bathing	2.2	0.3	0.7	1.3	3.0	5.8	19.4
Dressing	1.6	0.3	0.6	1.0	2.4	3.8	12.2
Eating	0.5	0.2	0.2	0.3	0.8	1.4	3.4
Getting to/using toilet	0.9	0.3	0.3	0.5	1.3	2.5	8.9
Difficulty with or unable to perform one or more IADLs	**6.1**	**1.5**	**2.5**	**4.5**	**8.1**	**15.3**	**40.4**
Going outside alone	4.0	0.7	1.2	2.6	5.5	10.8	31.4
Keeping track of money and bills	1.9	0.9	0.9	1.3	1.7	3.8	15.8
Preparing meals	2.1	0.6	0.8	1.1	2.2	5.0	17.8
Doing light housework	3.4	0.6	1.3	2.3	4.7	8.6	23.7
Taking prescribed medicines	1.5	0.8	0.6	1.0	1.3	3.4	12.8
Using the telephone	1.3	0.5	0.4	0.6	1.3	3.6	13.3
Needs personal assistance with an ADL or an IADL	4.7	1.3	1.9	3.3	6.1	11.5	34.1

Note: An ADL is an activity of daily living; an IADL is an instrumental activity of daily living.
Source: Bureau of the Census, Internet web sit < http://www.census.gov/hhes/www/disable/sipp/disable9495.html>

People Using Assistive Technology Devices by Age, 1994

(number of people using assistive technology devices, by type of device and age, 1994; numbers in thousands)

	total	under age 45	aged 45 to 64	aged 65 or older
Any anatomical device	**4,565**	**2,491**	**1,325**	**748**
Back brace	1,688	795	614	279
Neck brace	168	76	78	13
Hand brace	332	171	119	42
Arm brace	320	209	86	25
Leg brace	596	266	138	192
Foot brace	282	191	59	31
Knee brace	989	694	199	96
Other brace	399	239	104	56
Any artificial limb	199	69	59	70
Artificial leg or foot	173	58	50	65
Artificial arm or hand	21	9	6	6
Any mobility device	**7,394**	**1,151**	**1,699**	**4,544**
Crutch	575	227	188	160
Cane	4,762	434	1,116	3,212
Walker	1,799	109	295	1,395
Medical shoes	677	248	226	203
Wheelchair	1,564	335	365	863
Scooter	140	12	53	75
Any hearing device	**4,484**	**439**	**969**	**3,076**
Hearing aid	4,156	370	849	2,938
Amplified telephone	675	73	175	427
TDD/TTY	104	58	25	21
Closed-caption television	141	66	32	43
Listening device	106	26	22	58
Signaling device	95	37	23	35
Interpreter	57	27	21	9
Other hearing technology	93	28	24	41
Any vision device	**527**	**123**	**135**	**268**
Telescopic lenses	158	40	49	70
Braille	59	28	23	8
Readers	68	15	14	39
White cane	130	35	48	47
Computer equipment	34	19	8	7
Other vision technology	277	51	76	151

Note: Numbers will not add to total because people may use more than one device within a category.
Source: National Center for Health Statistics, Trends and Differential Use of Assistive Technology Devices: United States, 1994, *Advance Data, No. 292, 1997*

Percent Distribution of People Using Assistive Technology Devices by Age, 1994

(percent distribution of people using assistive technology devices by age, and type of device, 1994)

	total	under age 45	aged 45 to 64	aged 65 or older
Any anatomical device	**100.0%**	**54.6%**	**29.0%**	**16.4%**
Back brace	100.0	47.1	36.4	16.5
Neck brace	100.0	45.3	46.7	8.0
Hand brace	100.0	51.5	35.9	12.7
Arm brace	100.0	65.4	26.7	7.9
Leg brace	100.0	44.6	23.2	32.2
Foot brace	100.0	67.8	21.0	11.2
Knee brace	100.0	70.2	20.1	9.7
Other brace	100.0	59.9	26.1	14.0
Any artificial limb	100.0	35.0	29.6	35.4
Artificial leg or foot	100.0	33.5	29.1	37.6
Artificial arm or hand	100.0	42.7	30.9	26.4
Any mobility device	**100.0**	**15.6**	**23.0**	**61.5**
Crutch	100.0	39.4	32.7	27.8
Cane	100.0	9.1	23.4	67.5
Walker	100.0	6.1	16.4	77.5
Medical shoes	100.0	36.6	33.4	30.0
Wheelchair	100.0	21.4	23.4	55.2
Scooter	100.0	8.4	38.2	53.4
Any hearing device	**100.0**	**9.8**	**21.6**	**63.2**
Hearing aid	100.0	8.9	20.4	70.7
Amplified telephone	100.0	10.8	26.0	63.2
TDD/TTY	100.0	56.2	24.0	19.8
Closed-caption television	100.0	47.0	22.7	30.3
Listening device	100.0	24.1	21.1	54.8
Signaling device	100.0	38.8	23.9	37.3
Interpreter	100.0	46.4	37.5	16.2
Other hearing technology	100.0	30.1	26.0	44.1
Any vision device	**100.0**	**23.4**	**25.7**	**51.0**
Telescopic lenses	100.0	25.0	31.1	43.9
Braille	100.0	47.6	39.3	13.1
Readers	100.0	22.1	20.2	57.7
White cane	100.0	26.8	37.0	36.2
Computer equipment	100.0	57.2	22.3	20.5
Other vision technology	100.0	18.4	27.3	54.3

Source: National Center for Health Statistics, Trends and Differential Use of Assistive Technology Devices: United States, 1994, *Advance Data, No. 292, 1997*

Percent Distribution of People Using Assistive Technology by Type of Device, 1994

(percent distribution of assistive technology devices used by persons by age, 1994)

	total	under age 45	aged 45 to 64	aged 65 or older
Any anatomical device	100.0%	100.0%	100.0%	100.0%
Back brace	37.0	31.9	46.3	37.3
Neck brace	3.7	3.1	5.9	1.7
Hand brace	7.3	6.9	9.0	5.6
Arm brace	7.0	8.4	6.5	3.3
Leg brace	13.1	10.7	10.4	25.7
Foot brace	6.2	7.7	4.5	4.1
Knee brace	21.7	27.9	15.0	12.8
Other brace	8.7	9.6	7.8	7.5
Any artificial limb	4.4	2.8	4.5	9.4
Artificial leg or foot	3.8	2.3	3.8	8.7
Artificial arm or hand	0.5	0.4	0.5	0.8
Any mobility device	100.0	100.0	100.0	100.0
Crutch	7.8	19.7	11.1	3.5
Cane	64.4	37.7	65.7	70.7
Walker	24.3	9.5	17.4	30.7
Medical shoes	9.2	21.5	13.3	4.5
Wheelchair	21.2	29.1	21.5	19.0
Scooter	1.9	1.0	3.1	1.7
Any hearing device	100.0	100.0	100.0	100.0
Hearing aid	92.7	84.3	87.6	95.5
Amplified telephone	15.1	16.6	18.1	13.9
TDD/TTY	2.3	13.2	2.6	0.7
Closed-caption television	3.1	15.0	3.3	1.4
Listening device	2.4	5.9	2.3	1.9
Signaling device	2.1	8.4	2.4	1.1
Interpreter	1.3	6.2	2.2	0.3
Other hearing technology	2.1	6.4	2.5	1.3
Any vision device	100.0	100.0	100.0	100.0
Telescopic lenses	30.0	32.5	36.3	26.1
Braille	11.2	22.8	17.0	3.0
Readers	12.9	12.2	10.4	14.6
White cane	24.7	28.5	35.6	17.5
Computer equipment	6.5	15.4	5.9	2.6
Other vision technology	52.6	41.5	56.3	56.3

Note: Numbers will not add to total because people may use more than one device within a category.
Source: National Center for Health Statistics, Trends and Differential Use of Assistive Technology Devices: United States, 1994, *Advance Data, No. 292, 1997*

Trends in Use of Assistive Technology Devices, 1980 to 1994

(total number of people and number using selected assistive technology devices, by type of device, 1980 and 1994; percent change in number, 1980–94; numbers in thousands)

	1994	1980	percent change 1980–94
Total people	**259,626**	**217,923**	**19.1%**
Leg or foot brace	834	472	76.7
Brace other than leg or foot	3,651	1,000	265.1
Artificial limb	199	177	12.4
Crutch	575	588	−2.2
Cane	4,762	2,878	65.5
Walker	1,799	866	107.7
Wheelchair	1,564	720	117.2

Source: National Center for Health Statistics, Trends and Differential Use of Assistive Technology Devices: United States, 1994, *Advance Data, No. 292, 1997*

People with a Work Disability, 1999

(number and percent of people aged 16 to 64 with a work disability by sex, age, and disability status, 1999; numbers in thousands)

	total	with a work disability		with a severe work disability	
		number	percent	number	percent
Total people	**174,644**	**16,993**	**9.7%**	**11,549**	**6.6%**
Aged 16 to 24	33,891	1,292	3.8	849	2.5
Aged 25 to 34	38,205	2,132	5.6	1,428	3.7
Aged 35 to 44	44,453	3,928	8.8	2,611	5.9
Aged 45 to 54	35,194	4,532	12.9	3,022	8.6
Aged 55 to 64	22,901	5,108	22.3	3,640	15.9
Total men	**84,885**	**8,291**	**9.8**	**5,536**	**6.5**
Aged 16 to 24	16,626	675	4.1	477	2.9
Aged 25 to 34	19,230	987	5.1	652	3.4
Aged 35 to 44	21,810	2,029	9.3	1,450	6.6
Aged 45 to 54	16,552	2,123	12.8	1,317	8.0
Aged 55 to 64	10,667	2,477	23.2	1,639	15.4
Total women	**87,583**	**8,867**	**10.1**	**5,751**	**6.6**
Aged 16 to 24	16,375	693	4.2	408	2.5
Aged 25 to 34	19,785	1,144	5.8	710	3.6
Aged 35 to 44	22,389	2,006	9.0	1,255	5.6
Aged 45 to 54	17,454	2,365	13.5	1,590	9.1
Aged 55 to 64	11,580	2,659	23.0	1,786	15.4

Source: Bureau of the Census, Internet web site <http://www.census.gov/hhes/www/disable/cps/cps199.html>

Computer Ownership and Internet Use by Disability Status, 1998

(number and percent of people aged 15 or older with a computer in the household and with Internet access, by age and work disability status, 1998; numbers in thousands)

	work disability		no disability	
	number	*percent*	*number*	*percent*
Aged 15 or older	**20,877**	**100.0%**	**189,954**	**100.0%**
Computer in household	4,983	23.9	98,267	51.7
Internet access at home	2,379	11.4	59,132	31.1
Uses Internet	2,076	9.9	72,300	38.1
Aged 15 to 64	**12,579**	**100.0**	**164,928**	**100.0**
Computer in household	4,106	32.6	91,618	55.6
Internet access at home	1,991	15.8	55,903	33.9
Uses Internet	1,896	15.1	69,702	42.3
Aged 65 or older	**8,289**	**100.0**	**23,973**	**100.0**
Computer in household	877	10.6	6,056	25.3
Internet access at home	388	4.7	2,944	12.3
Uses Internet	180	2.2	2,134	8.9

Source: National Institute on Disability and Rehabilitation Research, "Computer and Internet Use among People with Disabilities," H. Stephen Kaye, Disability Statistics Report 13, *2000*

10

Mental Health Care Needs

Mental health has a new, powerful cheerleader: Tipper Gore, wife of Al Gore. During the Clinton administration, she was the mental health advisor, organizing the first White House Conference on Mental Health in June 1999. She also made public her own struggle with clinical depression, which has opened the door for media coverage and public discussion about mental health and its consequences.

At the 1999 White House Conference, several initiatives were announced that will shape the field of mental health for years to come. Health insurance plans for federal government employees, for example, must now offer the same level of coverage for mental health and substance abuse problems as for medical illnesses—and they must not charge a higher co-payment for doing so. This measure is meant to serve as an example for the private sector.[1] At the conference, the National Institute of Mental Health launched a five-year study of mental illness, which will help researchers better understand the number of Americans with mental illness and the treatments most commonly used.

Each year, 1 in 10 Americans experiences some degree of disability from a diagnosable mental illness, according to NIMH. Five million adults suffer from the most severe mental illnesses, at a cost of $150 billion annually including social services, disability payments, lost productivity, and premature mortality.

The definition of mental illness is inexact and changeable. Unfortunately for the people who suffer from mental illness, the quality of care and treatment is also inexact and changeable, depending in large part on the national mood. Today, public opinion about mental illness differs by disorder. Americans have sympathy for Alzheimer's patients, for example, but not much for substance abusers. Concern for the victims of mental illness also varies over time. When mental illness strikes the young and beautiful, the public responds with fascination—which explains the success of the movie "Girl, Interrupted," starring Winona Ryder and Angelina Jolie. On the other hand, when 29-year-old schizophrenic Andrew Goldstein pushed Kendra Webdale to her death in front of an oncoming subway in 1999, the public responded with horror. The tragedy might have been prevented had

Goldstein been admitted to the proper health care facility when he complained to doctors that he was hearing voices. The incident prompted new legislation, known as Kendra's Law, beefing up safeguards surrounding outpatient care—including court-ordered outpatient treatment and increased funding for intensive case management.[2]

Health insurance coverage for mental problems differs from that for other types of illnesses. It is more common and acceptable for a health insurance company to refuse to pay for the mental health care of a disturbed teenager than to refuse to pay for the same teenager's leukemia treatment, for example. The problem of unequal coverage is one of the issues the Clinton administration hoped to solve by creating the parity requirement for government employees. Proposed legislation in Congress to force insurers to pony up equal benefits has not met with much success. Yet Americans overwhelmingly support treatment for people with mental illness. According to a 1999 Time/CNN poll, 67 percent of Americans believe the government should spend more to treat mentally ill people who can't afford to pay. Only 4 percent think the government should pay less, while fewer than one-quarter think the amount should stay the same. When asked whether employers should be required to offer insurance for mental illness at the same level as insurance for physical illness, 77 percent of Americans say yes.[3]

Not only do the mentally ill suffer from a changeable definition of mental illness, but also from the significant social stigma that surrounds these diseases—including skepticism about mental illness itself. Some Americans see certain disorders that fall under the NIMH's definition of mental illness, such as extreme shyness or phobias, as nothing more than an unfortunate personality trait, a moral failing, or a lack of self-control. Pop psychology coverage in the media, which often creates more disdain for rather than understanding of mental illness, reinforces this perception.

The fact is, mental illness can be just as debilitating as physical illness. The belief that it is not has serious consequences. One arena in which this becomes patently clear is health care legislation and policy. The debate boils down to this: How much mental stress is normal? At what point do we classify people as mentally ill and worthy of assistance? The answers to these questions open hospital doors or set up roadblocks to treatment. Substance abusers, for example, have run into political and attitudinal obstacles. People who are addicted to drugs are specifically excluded from legislation designed to protect the rights of the mentally ill.

The most severe mental illnesses are schizophrenia, affective disorders, and anxiety disorders, according to the NIMH report, *Mental Illness in America*.[4] More than 2 million

Americans suffer from schizophrenia in any given year, and only one in five sufferers ever recovers completely from the disease. Symptoms include hallucinations, delusions, bizarre thought patterns, social isolation and withdrawal, blunting of emotional expressiveness, poor communication skills, and decreased motivation and self-care. Even with treatment, most victims continue to suffer chronically or episodically from the illness for the rest of their lives. An estimated 1 in 10 schizophrenics dies by suicide.

Nearly 18 million Americans aged 18 or older suffer from affective (or mood) disorders. The two most severe forms are major depression and manic-depressive, or bipolar, illness. Major depression is marked by persistent depressive thoughts and mood, accompanied by physiological disturbances in sleep, appetite, and energy level. Both depression and bipolar illness are recurrent disorders.

Anxiety disorders share a central, primary symptom of intense anxiety. Four of the most serious anxiety disorders are obsessive-compulsive disorder, phobias, panic disorder, and posttraumatic stress disorder. Obsessive-compulsive disorder is characterized by recurrent, unwanted thoughts and conscious, ritualized, seemingly purposeless acts. Phobias are persistent, irrational fears of an object or situation and the compelling desire to avoid the object of fear. Panic disorder is attacks of terror and irrational fear, with an overwhelming

Most Americans feel "blue" sometimes

(percent of people who couldn't shake the blues on at least one of the past seven days, by education, 1996)

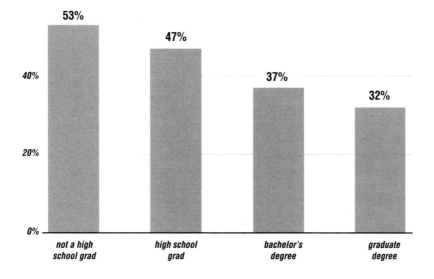

sense of impending doom and bodily symptoms such as racing heartbeat, gasping for air, sweating, weakness, dizziness, and feelings of unreality. Posttraumatic stress disorder, although most closely associated with wartime experience, can follow any traumatic event, such as rape or other violent acts, natural disasters, or accidents. Recollections of the event, sometimes occurring years later, intrude on everyday life and appear in disturbing dreams. Disabling symptoms commonly develop, such as avoiding important activities, feeling emotionally numb, experiencing sleep difficulties, hypervigilance, or other symptoms of physiological arousal.

Millions of Americans experience milder versions of mental health problems. Forty-five percent of adults could not shake the blues on at least one day during the past week, and 11 percent felt blue most of the past seven days, according to the 1996 General Social Survey of the University of Chicago's National Opinion Research Center. Those most likely to feel this way are women, blacks, young adults, and those without a high school diploma.

Most Americans (58 percent) know someone who has received mental health counseling. Those most likely to know someone who is seeing a mental health professional are people aged 50 to 59 (69 percent) and the college educated (72 to 75 percent). One-half of Americans also know someone who has been hospitalized because of mental illness, including 60 percent of people aged 40 to 49 and 74 percent of those with graduate degrees.

The well-educated are most likely to seek professional help

(percent of people who would seek professional help for a personal problem, by education, 1996)

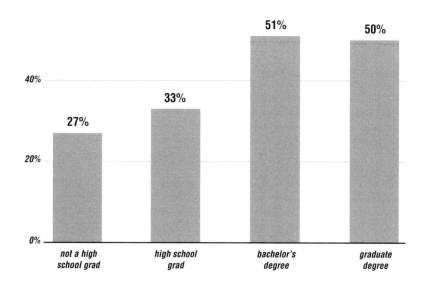

The best-educated Americans are most likely to know someone who has received professional help for mental problems because the higher the educational level, the more likely people are to seek professional help for problems. When asked how they would resolve a long-standing and troubling personal problem, half of those with college degrees said they would talk to a doctor, clergyman, psychologist, or counselor. Only 33 percent of high school graduates and 27 percent of those who did not graduate from high school would do likewise, according to the General Social Survey.

Paying for mental health care

The treatment of mental illness is often lengthy and, therefore, can be expensive. The high cost of treatment accounts in part for the spotty health insurance coverage for the mentally ill. Traditional fee-for-service health insurance plans typically do not cover mental health care. But because physical problems often have an underlying mental health component, the cost of not providing mental health coverage may outweigh savings in the long run. From 11 to 35 percent of patients who visit primary care physicians have an underlying mental health problem, according to an article in *Patient Care*.[5]

Managed care insurance is more likely to provide mental health benefits than traditional plans. But mental health benefits suffer from the same difficulties under managed care as physical health benefits do: limits on the number of treatment sessions, a disincentive to

Most Americans want government to take responsibility for providing mental health care

(percent agreeing it is and it is not government's responsibility to provide mental health care for people with mental illness, 1996)

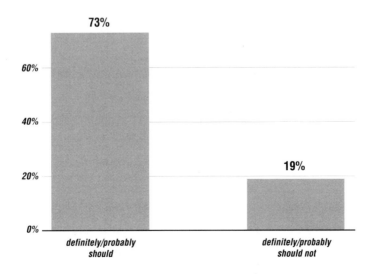

refer patients to specialists, and little time spent with primary care providers. These limits allow illnesses to go undiagnosed. On top of these problems, there is a lack of consensus about which mental problems deserve medical treatment. Schizophrenia clearly does, but what about people suffering from bereavement or marital difficulties?

Medicine by legislation is the American way of resolving these issues. Many states have introduced or passed legislation mandating mental health coverage parity. The Mental Health Parity Act took effect January 1, 1998. Although the act doesn't completely equalize mental and physical health benefits, it does require plans that provide mental health benefits to offer the same annual and lifetime payments for mental and physical health care. The law does not require health plans to cover mental health care, however.

The Mental Health Parity Act is further weakened by significant exemptions. The law does not apply to group plans sold to small businesses or individuals, for example. It doesn't apply to substance abuse. And if compliance with the act increases a company's costs more than 1 percent, a plan can be exempted from the requirements.

The public appears to be less uncertain about paying for mental health care than are the politicians are. When asked whether the government should provide care for the mentally ill, 73 percent of Americans agree thought it should, according to the General Social Survey. Those most likely to think it is government's responsibility are blacks (80 percent), young adults (80 percent), and those without a high school diploma (84 percent). Despite public support for government action on mental health care, only 46 percent of Americans would spend more on mental health care if it meant the possibility of higher taxes. Nevertheless, this figure is higher than the 36 percent who want to leave spending on mental health care unchanged and the 10 percent who want to spend less.

Children and mental health

School shootings—particularly the 1999 massacre at Columbine High School in Littleton Colorado—has focused attention on children's mental disorders. The NIMH considers children's mental health to be an important long-term focus, according to its director, Steven E. Hyman, in his testimony to Congress during fiscal year 2000 budget hearings. NIMH is funding several research studies that focus on the special problem of mental illness in children.[6]

Research indicates that acts of violence and other antisocial behavior by children or teenagers are not caused by a single factor or situation. Four decades of research has shown that many factors contribute to antisocial behavior. Although some are internal to the child, others are linked to the social environment—family, friends, school, and community. All play a role in the development of antisocial behavior, substance abuse, and conduct disorder. Expect to see more "holistic" attention to children's mental health as researchers take a broader look at the factors causing children to become violent.[7]

A far more common problem in children, although less dramatic, is attention deficit hyperactivity disorder. According to NIMH, ADHD is the most common of the psychiatric disorders that appear in childhood. It affects 3 to 5 percent of school-aged children, and it can have serious consequences. "Children with ADHD are unable to stay focused on a task, cannot sit still, act without thinking, and rarely finish anything. If untreated, the disorder can have long-term effects on a child's ability to make friends or do well at school or in other activities. Over time, children with ADHD may develop depression, lack of self-esteem, and other emotional problems," the NIMH fact sheet explains.[8]

To learn more about the disease, NIMH funded The Multimodal Treatment Study of Children with ADHD, taking place at six different university medical centers and hospitals and including nearly 600 elementary school children. NIMH is investigating four types of treatment: medication alone, psychosocial/behavioral treatment alone, a combination of both, or routine community care. In December 1999, NIMH released the first findings, reporting that medication is the key element in better outcomes for children with the ADHD. Long-term combination treatment, as well as medication-management alone, had significantly better results in reducing ADHD symptoms than intensive behavioral or routine community treatment. The findings were applicable across sociodemographic groups. Do these results mean behavioral therapy will be discredited as a treatment for ADHD? Not necessarily, because families and teachers report higher levels of consumer satisfaction when treatment includes behavioral therapy. The trick is to find the right mix of medication and therapy to help afflicted children.[9]

The future of mental health care

Mental health care is likely to receive much more attention in the years ahead. Behind the increase are advances in drug therapy, the growing population of teenagers and young adults prone to mental health problems, and a public more willing to talk about mental health needs.

Trend 1: Less talk, more drugs

The brain's mysteries are slowly yielding to the investigations of modern researchers. There are two aspects to this research, the physical and the behavioral. Consequently, there are two methods for treating mental illness—drugs and behavioral therapy. Because of cost-cutting pressure, drug therapy is increasingly the treatment of choice. The antipsychotic medication clozapine (Clozaril), used for schizophrenia, saves an average of $23,000 in treatment costs per patient per year, for example, primarily by reducing the need for hospitalization, according to the NIMH.

Behavioral therapy is lengthy and expensive, requires trained professionals, office overhead, and other related expenses. Because of the cost, the talking cure will be used less in the future while drugs will be used more. Consumers have already shown their preference for popping pills to solve medical problems. As more is understood about the neurochemistry of the brain, new generations of effective drugs will emerge to treat mental problems. One family of drug compounds, serotonin-selective re-uptake inhibitors, has become mainstream thanks to fluoxetine, better known as Prozac. This family of drugs has been shown to be effective in treating depression, panic disorder, obsessive-compulsive disorder, and bulimia. It may also be useful in treating alcoholism and obesity. Expect more wonder drugs in the future.

Ultimately, behavioral therapy will be reserved for serious cases or for those who pay the bills themselves. Managed care companies are already controlling costs by placing caps on the number of therapy sessions they will cover. Consumers who want a cheaper alternative to talk therapy increasingly will turn to the Internet. Today, mental health professionals discourage the use of cybertherapy as a substitute for in-person treatment, but recommend it as a supplementary treatment. Yet in the future, consumers may not want or be able to afford the time or resources to seek in-person counseling. For better or worse, telemedicine will fill their needs.

TREND 2: MENTAL ILLNESS PREVENTION

Mental illnesses are to a certain extent preventable, according to the NIMH. The pressure to cut costs is likely to turn more attention to prevention strategies, especially in the workplace, where businesses bear a large financial burden from mental illness whether they provide mental health coverage or not. Untreated behavioral problems breed declining job performance, poor morale, increased turnover, frequent absenteeism, work site accidents, and compensation claims, writes S. Alan Savitz in *Best's Insurance Review*.[10] He points to a Massachusetts Institute of Technology report showing that a worker with untreated depression can cost a company more than $3,000 a year. The costs of employee substance abuse are also high. As the main consumers of managed care policies, businesses will likely insist on the implementation of less costly preventative measures to lessen their expenses.

The best way to prevent mental illness may be to target children with prevention programs. Depression and other severe psychiatric problems affect about 3 percent of children and adolescents, and millions more suffer other psychiatric and behavioral conditions. According to the NIMH, preliminary findings indicate that early mental health intervention in children can reduce problems in adolescence. Early intervention strategies can include child abuse prevention and other home outreach programs. A recent University of Michigan study found that children who witness domestic violence show symptoms similar to combat war veterans, including a tendency toward violent behavior.[11]

TREND 3: ON THE FRONT LINES: PRIMARY CARE PROVIDERS

Because most Americans see medical practitioners routinely, primary care doctors, nurses, and physician assistants are often the first to spot signs of mental illness. Primary care providers are likely to become more responsible for their patients' mental health in the future, playing an advocacy role in securing them appropriate mental health care.

Surgeon General David Satcher thinks that primary care physicians should play a more important role in the delivery of mental health services. "We are concerned that the primary care sector has not been playing that role as well as we think it could—but really no sector has," he said in an interview with *Patient Care*. Satcher would like to see primary care physicians get out of their offices and work in their communities with civic and athletic groups, schools, and religious organizations.[12]

TREND 4: ALTERNATIVE TREATMENTS

The NIMH is funding a three-year study of the efficacy of St. John's Wort—an herb thought to be beneficial in soothing mental distress, which is widely prescribed in Europe today. An overview of 23 clinical studies in Europe, published in the *British Medical Journal* in August 1996, found the herb potentially useful in cases of mild to moderate depression. The studies, which included 1,757 outpatients, concluded that St. John's Wort was superior to a placebo and appeared to produce fewer side effects than standard antidepressants. The NIMH is concerned, however, because a separate National Institutes of Health study found St. John's Wort to interact negatively with a drug used to treat HIV as well as a drug used to prevent organ transplant rejection. The NIMH hopes to provide definitive word on whether the botanical supplement is useful in the treatment of mental illness. Expect to hear more about the herb as the study progresses.[13]

TREND 5: MORE MENTAL ILLNESS AMONG THE ELDERLY

Mental illness among the elderly will rise dramatically over the next 30 years, according to a study by psychiatrist Dilip V. Jeste reported in *Science News*. The reasons: improved physical health among mentally ill young adults is allowing many more to reach old age; the rising number of older Americans means more older people will be at risk of mental illness; and aging baby boomers may be more susceptible to depression, anxiety disorders, and substance abuse than the current generation of older people, according to researchers. The study foresees a crisis in geriatric mental health care because of the shortage of professionals equipped to deal with it. Expect to see and hear more about geriatric mental health care over the next few years.[14]

Notes

1. Beverly D. Lucas, "White House Focuses on America's Mental Health Needs," *Patient Care* 33, no. 13 (August 15, 1999): 20.

2. Laura Newman, "U.S. Panel Examines Mental-Health Policies in New York," *The Lancet* 355, no. 9201 (January 29, 2000): 386.

3. "What It Would Really Take: Tipper Gore Has Brought a Welcome Focus on the Problem. But Millions of Mentally Ill Americans Aren't Getting the Treatment They Need. And There's No Easy Fix," *Time* 153, no. 22 (June 7, 1999): 54.

4. National Institute of Mental Health, *Mental Illness in America* (June 4, 1998). <www.nihm.nih.gov>.

5. Joi Barret, Thomas Detre, Harold Alan Pincus, et al., "Mental Health Benefits in the Era of Managed Care," *Patient Care* 31, no. 14 (September 15, 1997): 76–83.

6. Statement of Dr. Steven E. Hyman, Director of the National Institute of Mental Health, to the Subcommittee on Labor-DHHS, Education and Related Agencies, Committee on Appropriations, U.S. House of Representatives, March 4, 1999. <www.nimh.nih.gov>.

7. National Institute of Mental Health, NIH Expert Panel on Youth Violence Intervention Research, February 29, 2000. <www.nimh.nih.gov>.

8. National Institute of Mental Health, *NIMH Research on Treatment for Attention Deficit Hyperactivity Disorder (ADHD): The Multimodal Treatment Study—Questions and Answers* (March 2000). <www.nimh.nih.gov>.

9. Ibid.

10. S. Alan Savitz, "Mental Health Plans Help Employees, Reduce Costs," *Best's Insurance Review, Life-Health Insurance Edition* 96, no. 3 (July 1995): 60–63.

11. Marilyn Elias, "Violent Home Is a War Zone for Kids," *USA Today* (February 4, 1998): 8B.

12. Carol S. Saunders, "The Surgeon General Advocates for Mental Health," *Patient Care* 34, no. 115 (March 15, 2000): 11.

13. National Institute of Mental Health, "Questions and Answers about St. John's Wort" (March 10, 2000). <www.nimh.nih.gov>.

14. "Warning on Elderly Mental Health," *Science News* 156, no. 12 (September 18, 1999): 189.

Feeling Blue, 1996

"On how many days in the past seven days have you felt
that you couldn't shake the blues?"

(percent of people aged 18 or older responding by sex, race, age, and education, 1996)

	no days	*one to three days*	*four or more days*
Total persons	**54%**	**34%**	**11%**
Sex			
Male	60	29	10
Female	50	38	12
Race			
Black	45	36	16
White	56	33	9
Age			
Aged 18 to 29	46	40	12
Aged 30 to 39	51	36	11
Aged 40 to 49	54	34	12
Aged 50 to 59	61	33	5
Aged 60 to 69	66	21	10
Aged 70 or older	57	30	13
Education			
Not a high school graduate	46	32	21
High school graduate	52	36	11
Bachelor's degree	62	29	8
Graduate degree	68	29	3

Note: Numbers may not add to 100 because "don't know" and no answer are not included.
Source: 1996 General Social Survey, National Opinion Research Center, University of Chicago; calculations by New Strategist

Knowing Someone Receiving Mental Health Counseling, 1996

"Have you ever known anyone who was seeing a psychologist, mental health professional, social worker, or other counselor?"

(percent of people aged 18 or older responding by sex, race, age, and education, 1996)

	yes	no
Total persons	**58%**	**40%**
Sex		
Male	57	41
Female	59	40
Race		
Black	35	63
White	63	35
Age		
Aged 18 to 29	56	44
Aged 30 to 39	62	38
Aged 40 to 49	66	33
Aged 50 to 59	69	29
Aged 60 to 69	48	48
Aged 70 or older	30	66
Education		
Not a high school graduate	34	63
High school graduate	58	40
Bachelor's degree	72	28
Graduate degree	75	25

Note: Does not include persons hospitalized because of mental illness. Numbers may not add to 100 because "don't know" is not included.
Source: 1996 General Social Survey, National Opinion Research Center, University of Chicago; calculations by New Strategist

Knowing Someone in a Mental Hospital, 1996

"Did you ever know anyone who was in a
hospital because of a mental illness?"

(percent of people aged 18 or older responding by sex, race, age, and education, 1996)

	yes	no
Total persons	**50%**	**48%**
Sex		
Male	48	50
Female	52	46
Race		
Black	41	56
White	52	46
Age		
Aged 18 to 29	42	57
Aged 30 to 39	47	52
Aged 40 to 49	60	37
Aged 50 to 59	54	44
Aged 60 to 69	46	51
Aged 70 or older	46	49
Education		
Not a high school graduate	35	63
High school graduate	48	49
Bachelor's degree	58	42
Graduate degree	74	26

Note: Numbers may not add to 100 because "don't know" and no answer are not included.
Source: 1996 General Social Survey, National Opinion Research Center, University of Chicago; calculations by New Strategist

How Would You Resolve a Personal Problem? 1996

"Let's suppose you had a lot of personal problems and you're very unhappy
all the time. You've been that way for a long time and it isn't
getting any better. What do you think you would do about it?"

(percent of people aged 18 or older responding by sex, race, age, and education, 1996)

	deny/ignore problem*	try to figure it out myself**	talk with uninvolved friends, family	talk to doctor clergyman, psychologist, counselor, etc.
Total persons	14%	21%	19%	36%
Sex				
Male	11	24	21	32
Female	16	18	17	39
Race				
Black	23	22	23	22
White	13	20	18	38
Age				
Aged 18 to 29	9	32	28	24
Aged 30 to 39	14	18	17	41
Aged 40 to 49	14	17	20	39
Aged 50 to 59	13	16	19	42
Aged 60 to 69	15	20	15	34
Aged 70 or older	22	14	13	30
Education				
Not a high school graduate	18	26	14	27
High school graduate	17	22	17	33
Bachelor's degree	8	13	25	51
Graduate degree	8	15	19	50

Responses include "try to forget about it," "not think about it," "engage in distracting activity," "do nothing," "just let things take their course," "hope for the best," "just give up," "pray," "trust in the Lord."
**Responses include "try to figure out what's wrong," "see what the problem is," "who is at fault," "would do something," "just keep trying," "talk it over with person involved," "get another job," "move to another city," "eliminate or change relationship."*
Note: Numbers may not add to 100 because "don't know" and no answer are not included.
Source: 1996 General Social Survey, National Opinion Research Center, University of Chicago; calculations by New Strategist

Is Mental Health Care Government's Responsibility? 1996

"On the whole, do you think it should or should not be the government's responsibility to provide mental health care for persons with mental illnesses?"

(percent of people aged 18 or older responding by sex, race, age, and education, 1996)

	definitely should be	probably should be	probably should not be	definitely should not be	can't choose	definitely/ probably should be	definitely/ probably should not be
Total persons	34%	39%	12%	7%	6%	73%	19%
Sex							
Male	34	38	14	10	4	72	24
Female	34	39	11	5	7	73	16
Race							
Black	53	27	4	6	7	80	10
White	31	40	13	8	6	71	21
Age							
Aged 18 to 29	36	44	11	3	3	80	14
Aged 30 to 39	29	43	13	6	6	72	19
Aged 40 to 49	39	31	16	8	4	70	24
Aged 50 to 59	31	38	12	12	5	69	24
Aged 60 to 69	40	33	11	9	5	73	20
Aged 70 or older	34	37	5	12	12	71	17
Education							
Not a high school graduate	47	37	7	6	3	84	13
High school graduate	33	40	12	7	6	73	19
Bachelor's degree	33	40	14	10	2	73	24
Graduate degree	25	37	18	8	7	62	26

Note: Numbers may not add to 100 because no answer is not included.
Source: General Social Survey, National Opinion Research Center, University of Chicago; calculations by New Strategist

Government Spending on Mental Health Care, 1996

"Please indicate whether you would like to see more or less government spending in the area of mental health care. Remember that if you say 'much more,' it might require a tax increase to pay for it."

(percent of people aged 18 or older responding by sex, race, age, and education, 1996)

	spend much more	spend more	spend the same as now	spend less	spend much less	can't choose	spend more, total	spend less, total
Total persons	12%	34%	36%	8%	2%	7%	46%	10%
Sex								
Male	11	31	37	11	2	6	42	13
Female	12	36	36	6	2	7	48	8
Race								
Black	21	36	32	2	1	7	57	3
White	11	33	37	9	2	7	44	11
Age								
Aged 18 to 29	13	33	39	4	3	6	46	7
Aged 30 to 39	11	39	35	10	1	3	50	11
Aged 40 to 49	12	32	38	8	2	7	44	10
Aged 50 to 59	11	34	34	13	2	4	45	15
Aged 60 to 69	12	24	39	10	3	12	36	13
Aged 70 or older	8	35	31	5	2	14	43	7
Education								
Not a high school graduate	12	33	30	7	3	15	45	10
High school graduate	12	33	37	9	1	5	45	10
Bachelor's degree	8	32	39	9	4	7	41	13
Graduate degree	17	35	31	9	2	6	52	11

Note: Numbers may not add to 100 because no answer is not included.
Source: 1996 General Social Survey, National Opinion Research Center, University of Chicago; calculations by New Strategist

Additions to Mental Health Organizations, 1983 and 1994

(total number of additions to mental health organizations and number per 100,000 civilian population, by type of service and organization, 1983 and 1994; percent change in additions and rate, 1983–94; numbers in thousands)

	number			number per 100,000		
	1994	1983	percent change 1983–94	1994	1983	percent change 1983–94
INPATIENT AND RESIDENTIAL TREATMENT						
Total additions	**2,197**	**1,633**	**34.5%**	**840.3**	**701.4**	**19.8%**
State and county mental hospitals	236	339	−30.4	91.2	146.0	−37.5
Private psychiatric hospitals	480	165	190.9	185.5	70.9	161.6
Nonfederal general hospital psychiatric services	1,067	786	35.8	411.9	336.8	22.3
Department of Veterans Affairs psychiatric services	172	149	15.4	61.5	64.3	−4.4
Residential treatment centers for emotionally disturbed children	39	17	129.4	15.0	7.1	111.3
All other	203	177	14.7	75.2	76.3	−1.4
OUTPATIENT TREATMENT						
Total additions	**3,242**	**2,665**	**21.7**	**1,252.8**	**1,147.5**	**9.2**
State and county mental hospitals	38	84	−54.8	14.8	36.3	−59.2
Private psychiatric hospitals	145	78	85.9	56.1	33.4	68.0
Nonfederal general hospital psychiatric services	443	469	−5.5	171.0	202.1	−15.4
Department of Veterans Affairs psychiatric services	120	103	16.5	46.5	44.5	4.5
Residential treatment centers for emotionally disturbed children	156	33	372.7	60.3	14.1	327.7
Freestanding psychiatric outpatient clinics	567	538	5.4	218.9	231.7	−5.5
All other	1,773	1,360	30.4	685.2	585.4	17.0

(continued)

(continued from previous page)

	number			number per 100,000		
	1994	*1983*	*percent change 1983–94*	*1994*	*1983*	*percent change 1983–94*
PARTIAL CARE TREATMENT						
Total additions	**273**	**177**	**54.2%**	**105.3**	**76.3**	**38.0%**
State and county mental hospitals	3	4	–25.0	1.3	1.6	–18.8
Private psychiatric hospitals	68	6	1,033.3	26.4	2.4	1,000.0
Nonfederal general hospital psychiatric services	55	46	19.6	21.1	19.8	6.6
Department of Veterans Affairs psychiatric services	12	10	20.0	4.6	4.4	4.5
Residential treatment centers for emotionally disturbed children	12	3	300.0	4.3	1.5	186.7
Freestanding psychiatric outpatient clinics	–	5	–	–	2.3	–
All other	123	103	19.4	47.6	44.3	7.4

Note: (–) means data not available.
Source: National Center for Health Statistics, Health, United States, 2000; *calculations by New Strategist*

11

Treating Addictions

There are many kinds of addictions in our society, from alcohol to tobacco to drugs. Even the Internet has become an addiction for some. Addiction equals compulsive use in spite of harmful effects and the inability to stop for any significant period of time, according to *The Columbia University College of Physicians and Surgeons Complete Home Medical Guide.*[1]

Most often, talk about addiction is talk about drugs. According to the *Medical Guide*, drug addiction occurs when reliance on drug use becomes the central focus of behavior despite harmful consequences. An estimated 14 million Americans aged 12 or older—6 percent of the population—used an illicit drug at least once in the past month, according to the 1998 National Household Survey on Drug Abuse by the U.S. Substance Abuse and Mental Health Services Administrations.[2] While this number is significant, it is far smaller than the 25 million (or 14.1 percent) who used illegal drugs in 1979. An estimated 4.1 million Americans met the criteria for drug addiction in 1998, including 1.1 million teenagers aged 12 to 17.

When politicians talk about the war on drugs or the goal of a drug-free America, their target is only five classes of drugs: amphetamines, cannabis, cocaine, hallucinogens, and opiates. Two other addictive substances, nicotine and alcohol, are legal, although age limits are placed on their use. Caffeine is unregulated.

The caffeine exception reveals what bothers Americans about the use of other addictive drugs. It also explains why we wage war on drugs instead of helping users recover from what is increasingly considered a mental illness. Unlike most other addictive drugs, caffeine does not interfere with the ability to work. Rather, it enhances productivity by helping users stay alert. The leniency toward caffeine shows that what really bothers us about a drug is not its addictive nature, but its interference with social obligations.

This attitude is nothing new. Alcohol addiction, for example, once was more acceptable than it is today. The temperance movement, which eventually resulted in prohibition, closely followed the industrialization of the United States for good reason. "Although a plowhorse could be driven by a drunk, the machines of industry—and the men who owned them—were less forgiving," writes Andrew A. Skolnick in the *Journal of the American Medical Association*.[3] The consequences of addiction—lowered productivity and potential harm to others—are the real enemies in the war on drugs.

Another issue surrounding addictive drugs is whether they harm innocent bystanders, either intentionally or unintentionally. Because drug and alcohol abuse is linked to crime and violence, especially against family members, we closely control the use of these substances. Even the live-and-let-live attitude toward tobacco smokers changed upon the discovery of the dangers of secondhand smoke.

Tobacco: The hot issue

Tobacco use is one of the most important determinants of human health trends worldwide, reports the Centers for Disease Control.[4] To recover the health care expenses of smokers, 46 states sued the tobacco industry in 1997. The industry recently negotiated settlements with the states, agreeing to pay billions of dollars over the next 25 years. Florida, for example, is slated to receive $11.3 billion.[5] But the tobacco industry will not write checks of equal size to the other states. In April 2000, for example, New York State received its first payment of $441 million—12 percent less than originally negotiated because the amount is tied to cigarette consumption. Since consumption dropped, so did the payment.[6]

Cigarette smoking is still common, especially among young adults

(percent of people aged 12 or older who have smoked cigarettes in the past month, by age, 1998)

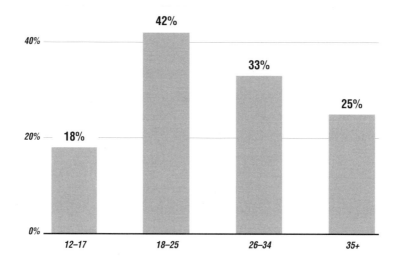

Legal settlements with the states do not mean the tobacco industry is finished with lawsuits. Individuals can still sue tobacco companies, as happened in a high-profile case in Florida. Three Floridian smokers were recently awarded $6.9 million in compensatory damages and punitive damages in the billions.[7]

Sometimes politicians are more zealous than the courts. When smoking was banned in most California bars beginning January 1, 1998, the new law raised the ire of smokers and, by most accounts, was largely ignored. Two years later, the anger is still fresh. Al Tolbert, a bar owner in San Carlos, California, hung a sign in his tavern in the style of Nazi-regime postings, complete with a swastika. "We had a guy who was opposed to hunting, to private gun ownership. He was a vegetarian and a rabid anti-smoker. That was Adolph Hitler," Tolbert is quoted as saying by Knight-Ridder/Tribune Business News. "It appears that a bunch of his adherents are running Sacramento."[8] Needless to say, his statements have raised the ire of the area's Jewish community.

The attention paid to the dangers of cigarette smoking over the past few decades seems to have had the desired effect—at least on adults. Only 28 percent of Americans aged 12 or older had smoked a cigarette during the past month, according to the 1998 National Household Survey on Drug Abuse. This figure was down significantly from 39 percent in 1985. In 1965, an even larger 42 percent of adults aged 18 or older smoked cigarettes, including fully 61 percent of men aged 25 to 34. Clearly, tobacco use has declined sharply over the past few decades as the public has become aware of its associated health problems.

In 1985, 29 percent of teens aged 12 to 17 had smoked a cigarette in the past month. This figure fell to 18 percent in 1992 and has remained at about that level ever since. The trend is more worrisome among young adults, those aged 18 to 25. While 47 percent of 18-to-25-year-olds smoked cigarettes in 1985, the figure fell to a low of 35 percent in 1994. Since then, however, the proportion of those who smoke has grown to 42 percent.

Men are more likely to smoke than women (30 versus 26 percent), and blacks are slightly more likely to smoke than non-Hispanic whites and Hispanics (29 percent of blacks versus 28 percent of non-Hispanic whites and 26 percent of Hispanics). Smoking is much more prevalent among those with less education. Thirty-seven percent of people aged 18 or older who did not complete high school are smokers versus only 15 percent of college graduates, according to the 1998 survey.

While the cigarette industry faced increased regulation during the past few years, the largely unregulated cigar industry experienced a rebound in popularity—perhaps because many smokers were under the mistaken impression that cigars are somehow safer than cigarettes. After a 20-year decline, cigar sales began to grow rapidly. This popularity caught the attention of federal regulators and brought an end to the relaxed oversight the industry had enjoyed. The percentage of people aged 12 or older who smoked a cigar in the past month grew from 6 to 7 percent between 1997 and 1998. Since then, cigar sales have declined.

Most Americans drink

The dangers of drinking seem to have faded a bit from the public mind, replaced first by concerns about harder substances such as crack cocaine and then by the media circus surrounding tobacco. Nevertheless, alcohol abuse continues to be an important problem. Alcohol is a factor in about 40 percent of all violent crimes, according to the Justice Department.[9]

Fifty-two percent of Americans aged 12 or older have had an alcoholic drink at least once in the past month, according to the 1998 National Household Survey of Drug Abuse. Sixteen percent of the population are binge drinkers, meaning they have had five or more drinks on one occasion in the past month. Six percent are heavy drinkers, meaning they have binged on five or more days of the past month. (Heavy drinkers are, by definition, binge drinkers.) In 1985, a slightly larger share of Americans had an alcohol problem—20 percent were binge drinkers and 8 percent were heavy drinkers.

Men are more likely to drink than women

(percent of people aged 11 or older who have drunk an alcoholic beverage in the past month, by sex, 1998)

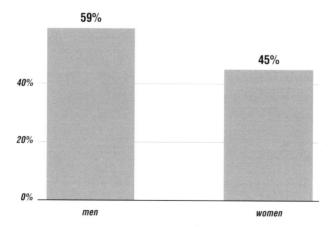

The public has gotten mixed messages about alcohol use in recent years. Researchers have touted the cardiovascular benefits of drinking wine, but alcohol consumption has also been linked to an increased risk of breast cancer. These contradictory reports mean Americans can use health reasons to justify just about any position they take on drinking. There is no waffling about drinking and driving, however. Between 1988 and 1998, the proportion of traffic deaths that were alcohol-related fell 33 percent, thanks to the focus on the dangers of drinking and driving as well as the increase in the drinking age from 18 to 21 across the country.[10]

Men are much more likely to drink than women—59 percent of men have had a drink in the past month versus 45 percent of women. Those most likely to drink are 21-to-25-year-olds, of whom 65 percent did so in the past month. Non-Hispanic whites are more likely to drink (55 percent) than blacks (40 percent) and Hispanics (45 percent).

Binge drinking peaks in the 21-to-25 age group, with 33 percent binge drinking in the past month. Among 18-to-20-year-olds, the proportion who binge drink is nearly as high, at 30 percent. Heavy drinking is most common among 18-to-20-year-olds, with 15 percent reporting heavy drinking in the past month. Among 21-to-25-year-olds, 13 percent are heavy drinkers.

In contrast to the pattern for smoking, the percentage of people who drink rises with educational attainment, according to the 1998 National Household Survey of Drug Abuse. Fully 65 percent of people aged 18 or older with a college degree are drinkers compared with only 40 percent of those without a high school diploma. This pattern does not hold for binge or heavy drinking. People with some college experience but no degree are most likely to binge drink, while those without a high school diploma are most likely to be heavy drinkers.

Many have used drugs

While only 6 percent of Americans aged 12 or older have used illegal drugs in the past month, the proportion is much higher among young adults—peaking at 20 percent among 18-to-20-year-olds. Sixteen percent of teenagers aged 16 and 17 have used illicit drugs in the past month, as have 13 percent of 21-to-25-year-olds. Drug use declines with age—just 3 percent of people aged 35 or older are drug users.

People in their forties and fifties are becoming increasingly likely to use drugs—not because they are discovering drugs in middle age, but because of the aging of the baby-boom generation. The shift in the age composition of drug users is also reflected in data from the Drug Abuse Warning Network, which shows an increasing number of drug-related deaths among people aged 45 to 54.[11] Between 1997 and 1998, the number of drug deaths in the age group increased 15 percent. Drug-related deaths among people aged 55 or older rose 13 percent during the same time period.

Men are more likely than women to have used illicit drugs in the past month—8 versus 4 percent. The rate of illicit drug use is somewhat higher among blacks (8 percent) than among non-Hispanic whites and Hispanics (6 percent). Less educated people are more likely to use illicit drugs than those with more education (6 percent of those without a high school diploma versus 4 percent of those with a college degree), according to the 1998 National Household Survey of Drug Abuse.

Five percent of people aged 12 or older currently use marijuana, the most popular illegal drug. Those most likely to be current marijuana smokers are people aged 18 to 20, of whom 18 percent have used marijuana during the past month, as have 15 percent of 16- and 17-year-olds. Just 0.8 percent of people aged 12 or older have used cocaine in the past month, including 2 percent of 18-to-25-year-olds.

While only a tiny fraction of Americans are current users of illicit drugs, 36 percent have used illegal drugs at some point in their lives. In some age groups (typically those encompassing the baby-boom generation), the majority have used illegal drugs. Fifty-five

Most baby boomers have smoked marijuana

(percent of people aged 12 or older who have ever used marijuana, by age, 1998)

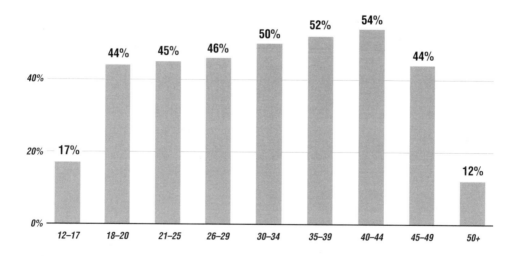

percent of people aged 40 to 44 in 1998 had ever used an illegal drug, as have 54 percent of 35-to-39-year-olds and 52 percent of 30-to-34-year-olds. Only 6 to 8 percent of 30-to-44-year-olds currently use illegal drugs.

Interestingly, baby boomers' experience with marijuana has not turned them into supporters of its legalization. Only 28 percent of Americans support legalizing marijuana, a figure that varies little by age and peaks at 34 percent among people aged 18 to 29, according to the General Social Survey of the University of Chicago's National Opinion Research Center. More than 60 percent of Americans in every age group are against legalizing the drug.

The government estimates that a tiny 0.1 percent of the population has used heroin in the past month, according to the National Household Survey of Drug Abuse. This estimate is admittedly conservative due to the probable undercoverage of the population of heroin users. Just 0.7 percent has used hallucinogens, and 0.3 percent, inhalants.

Protecting children

Much of the effort in the war on drugs has been directed at preventing drug, tobacco, and alcohol use among children. Typically, the teen years are a time of experimentation. Studies of teen risk behavior show many teens test the limits.

Most 12th graders, for example, have drunk alcohol in the past month, according to the National Institute on Drug Abuse.[12] Twenty-three percent have used marijuana, while 35 percent have smoked cigarettes.

Many teens experiment with drugs, alcohol, and cigarettes

(percent of 12-to-17-year-olds engaging in selected behaviors, 1998)

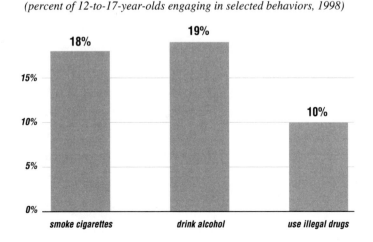

Since smoking is legal for adults, tobacco litigation has focused on the industry's efforts to recruit young smokers. Tobacco companies have long denied marketing to children, but documents uncovered during the investigations show the opposite to be the case. One tobacco company even had considered manufacturing honey- and cola-flavored cigarettes.

The CDC identifies cigarette advertising and marketing as just one of the influences that promote teen smoking.[13] Others include smoking by parents or older siblings, cigarette product placements in movies, easy access to cigarettes, and peer pressure. These influences have a powerful effect on teens. Fully 70 percent of 9th through 12th graders have tried cigarettes, according to the CDC. Among those who have experimented with cigarettes, one-third became regular smokers. Among regular smokers, 73 percent tried to quit but only 14 percent have been successful.

In the past few years, the public has gone to great lengths to control drinking by young adults. The greatest success has been in raising the legal drinking age from 18 to 21. Today, the focus is on binge drinking at college. A few well-publicized deaths due to alcohol poisoning have raised consciousness about the dangers of too much drink. In November 1999, 12 students at Texas A&M University were killed when a bonfire collapsed.[14] Although the college attributed the collapse to poor construction and design, alcohol may have played a role in the shoddy construction. Two of the dead were legally intoxicated, and empty beer cans were found in the construction area. But attempts to crack down on college drinking are sometimes met with resistance. In May 1998, police fired tear gas into a crowd of 3,000 students at Michigan State University who were protesting a ban on drinking at Munn Field, a popular drinking spot.

The Harvard School of Public Health has been monitoring college binge drinking throughout the 1990s, surveying students from more than 100 colleges in 39 states and the District of Columbia.[15] Its surveys have shown a polarization of students by drinking status. Some college students do not drink at all, while others are binge drinkers. The 1999 survey found that 23 percent of college students were frequent binge drinkers, and that another 19 percent of students had abstained from alcohol in the past year. The largest share of students—37 percent—were nonbinge drinkers, while 21 percent were occasional binge drinkers. The share of students who binge drink has not changed significantly since 1993, although binge drinking fell among students living in dormitories and increased among those living off campus.

The government closely monitors drug use by teens. Lately, the news has not been good. While drug use among teens is far less prevalent today than it was when the baby-boom generation filled the age group, it has been rising. Boomers now face the uncomfortable task of keeping their kids away from drugs, despite their own history of experimentation. So far, they don't seem to be doing a very good job. Illicit drug use by 12th graders during the past month grew from 16 percent in 1991 to 26 percent in 1999.[16] Drug use in the past month by 8th graders grew from 6 to 12 percent during those years. The only good news in the latest data is that drug use by 8th and 12th graders is down slightly from the levels of 1996 and 1997.

The future of substance abuse

Substance abuse is not about to disappear any time soon. In fact, it could worsen as the teen population grows. But the controlling hand of baby-boom parents and better drug treatment programs could help limit the destructive consequences of addiction.

TREND 1: TEEN SURVEILLANCE

In an affluent society such as ours, the search for a recreational high will be ever-present—especially among teens and young adults. This realization doesn't mean, however, that parents will just shrug their shoulders and wait for their children to grow up—and hopefully out of substance abuse. The hypervigilance of baby-boom parents insures a big market for products and services to monitor their children's behavior. Companies in the monitoring business have a friend in the Food and Drug Administration, which is considering loosening the regulation of home drug-testing kits. Kids going to market today must have received prior individual approval by the FDA. The new rules would remove the approval requirement as long as testing kits adhere to certain standards. American Bio Medica is marketing its drug-testing kits to schools who are using them to test their athletes, according to the Knight Ridder/Tribune News Service.[17]

In Japan, there's a healthy market for surveillance products and services, according to newspaper reports—including everything from wiretapping devices to private detectives.[18] Look for this trend to emerge in the United States in the years ahead.

TREND 2: NEW DIRECTIONS IN TREATMENT

High levels of alcohol, cigarette, and marijuana use among teens, coupled with the rapidly growing teen and young-adult population during the next decade, insure a renewed interest in addiction prevention and treatment. More research into addiction is likely to improve treatment programs as new ideas about substance abuse and therapy arise. There has been new attention to the problem of smoking among alcoholics, and whether alcoholics should quit smoking and drinking at the same time. Until recently, doctors believed that quitting smoking made it harder for alcoholics to stay with a recovery program. But now they think this may not be the case because smoking and drinking are linked for many alcoholics. By quitting smoking, an alcoholic may improve his chances of staying sober.[19]

Notes

1. Herbert Kleber, "Chapter Six: Abuse and Addiction," in *The Columbia University College of Physicians and Surgeons Complete Home Medical Guide*, 3rd ed. (Crown Publishers, 1995).

2. Department of Health and Human Services, Substance Abuse and Mental Health Services Administrations, Office of Applied Studies,*Summary of Findings from the 1998 National Household Survey on Drug Abuse* (Washington, D.C., 1999).

3. Andrew A. Skolnick, "Lessons from U.S. History of Drug Abuse," *The Journal of the American Medical Association 277*, no. 24 (June 25, 1996): 1919–1921.

4. Centers for Disease Control and *Prevention* Magazine, "World No-Tobacco Day, May 31, 1999," *Mortality and Morbidity Weekly Report 7*, no. 19 (May 22, 1998): 1.

5. Christopher McEntee, "Florida to Receive $11.3 Billion from Tobacco Industry in Settlement," *The Bond Buyer 321*, no. 30217 (August 26, 1997): 2.

6. Joel Stashenko, "New York State Gets First Tobacco Settlement Payment," *Marketing News* 34, no. 10 (May 8, 2000): 27.

7. "Why Big Tobacco Can't Be Killed," *Business Week* (April 24, 2000): 68.

8. Marilee Enge, "San Carlos, California, Bar Owner's Smoking-Ban Protest Draws Fire," Knight-Ridder/ Tribune News Service (January 4, 2000).

9. United States Department of Justice, "Statement by Attorney General Janet Reno on Impending Television Advertisements for Hard Liquor" (April 1, 1997).

10. U.S. Department of Transportation, National Center for Statistics and Analysis, *Traffic Safety Facts 1998* <www.nhtsa.dot.gov>.

11. Department of Health and Human Services, Substance Abuse and Mental Health Services Administrations, *Drug Abuse Warning Network, Annual Examiner Data 1998* (March 2000).

12. Lloyd D. Johnston, Patrick M. O'Malley, and Jerald G. Bachman, *Monitoring the Future National Results on Adolescent Drug Use, Overview of Key Findings, 1999* (National Institutes of Health, Public Health Service, National Institute on Drug Abuse, 2000).

13. Centers for Disease Control and Prevention, "Selected Cigarette Smoking Initiation and Quitting Behaviors Among High School Students—United States, 1997," *Mortality and Morbidity Weekly Report 47*, no. 19 (1998): 386–389.

14. United Press International, "Texas A&M Bonfire Suspended Two Years" (June 19, 2000).

15. Henry Wechsler, Jae Eun Lee, Meichun Kuo, and Hang Lee, "College Binge Drinking in the 1990s: A Continuing Problem—Results of the Harvard School of Public Health 1999 College Alcohol Study" <www.hsph.harvard.edu/cas/rpt2000/CAS2000rpt2.html> (2000).

16. Johnston, O'Malley, and Bachman.

17. Danielle Furfaro, "New York Based Maker of Drug Testing Kits Markets Products to Schools," Knight Ridder Tribune Business News (August 25, 1999).

18. "Japanese Fearful Parents Seek Ways to Track Kids," *The Democrat and Chronicle* (June 18, 1998): 14A.

19. "Smoking Cessation in Recovering Alcoholics: Fiction Versus Fact," *American Family Physician* 61, no. 6 (March 15, 2000): 1883.

Cigarette Smoking, 1998

(percent of people aged 12 or older who have smoked cigarettes in the past month, by sex, age, race, Hispanic origin, and education, 1998)

	percent
Total people	**27.7%**
Male	29.7
Female	25.7
Aged 12 to 17	18.2
Aged 12 to 13	8.0
Aged 14 to 15	18.2
Aged 16 to 17	29.3
Aged 18 to 25	41.6
Aged 18 to 20	43.1
Aged 21 to 25	40.6
Aged 26 to 34	32.5
Aged 26 to 29	33.1
Aged 30 to 34	32.0
Aged 35 or older	25.1
Aged 35 to 39	32.8
Aged 40 to 44	29.0
Aged 45 to 49	29.8
Aged 50 or older	20.2
Black, non-Hispanic	29.4
White, non-Hispanic	27.9
Other, non-Hispanic	23.8
Hispanic	25.8
Not a high school graduate	36.9
High school graduate	34.3
Some college	29.2
College graduate	15.2

Source: U.S. Substance Abuse and Mental Health Services Administrations, Summary of Findings from the 1998 National Household Survey on Drug Abuse, *1999*

Smoking during Pregnancy by Age and Education, 1989 and 1998

(percent of women giving birth who smoked during pregnancy, by age and education, 1989 and 1998; percentage point change, 1989–98)

	1998	1989	percentage point change 1989–98
Total women giving birth	**12.9%**	**19.5%**	**–6.6**
Age			
Under age 15	7.7	7.7	0.0
Aged 15 to 17	15.5	19.0	–3.5
Aged 18 to 19	19.2	23.9	–4.7
Aged 20 to 24	16.5	23.5	–7.0
Aged 25 to 29	11.4	19.0	–7.6
Aged 30 to 34	9.3	15.7	–6.4
Aged 35 to 39	10.6	13.6	–3.0
Aged 40 to 49	10.0	13.2	–3.2
Education			
Eight or fewer years	11.7	18.9	–7.2
Nine to eleven years	25.5	42.2	–16.7
High school graduate	16.8	22.8	–6.0
Some college	9.6	13.7	–4.1
College graduate	2.2	5.0	–2.8

Source: National Center for Health Statistics, Health, United States, 2000; *and* Births: Final Data for 1998, *National Vital Statistics Report, Vol. 48, No. 3, 2000; calculations by New Strategist*

Acohol Use, 1998

(percent of people aged 12 or older who have drunk an alcoholic beverage in the past month, by sex, age, race, Hispanic origin, and education, 1998)

	percent
Total people	**51.7%**
Male	58.7
Female	45.1
Aged 12 to 17	19.1
Aged 12 to 13	4.9
Aged 14 to 15	20.9
Aged 16 to 17	32.0
Aged 18 to 25	60.0
Aged 18 to 20	53.5
Aged 21 to 25	64.6
Aged 26 to 34	60.9
Aged 26 to 29	61.1
Aged 30 to 34	60.7
Aged 35 or older	53.1
Aged 35 to 39	63.5
Aged 40 to 44	61.9
Aged 45 to 49	54.8
Aged 50 or older	46.7
Black, non-Hispanic	39.8
White, non-Hispanic	55.3
Other, non-Hispanic	35.8
Hispanic	45.4
Not a high school graduate	40.4
High school graduate	52.3
Some college	60.1
College graduate	65.5

Source: U.S. Substance Abuse and Mental Health Services Administrations, Summary of Findings from the 1998 National Household Survey on Drug Abuse, *1999*

Binge and Heavy Drinking, 1998

(percent of people aged 12 or older who were binge or heavy drinkers of alcoholic beverages in the past month, by sex, age, race, Hispanic origin, and education, 1998)

	binge drinkers	heavy drinkers
Total people	**15.6%**	**5.9%**
Male	23.2	9.7
Female	8.6	2.4
Aged 12 to 17	7.7	2.9
Aged 12 to 13	1.4	0.5
Aged 14 to 15	7.6	2.5
Aged 16 to 17	14.8	6.0
Aged 18 to 25	31.7	13.8
Aged 18 to 20	30.1	14.9
Aged 21 to 25	32.8	13.1
Aged 26 to 34	22.0	7.2
Aged 26 to 29	24.6	8.0
Aged 30 to 34	19.9	6.6
Aged 35 or older	11.9	4.4
Aged 35 to 39	20.2	5.5
Aged 40 to 44	17.0	6.6
Aged 45 to 49	15.8	6.3
Aged 50 or older	6.8	2.9
Black, non-Hispanic	11.4	4.9
White, non-Hispanic	16.5	6.0
Other, non-Hispanic	11.1	4.7
Hispanic	15.7	6.5
Not a high school graduate	15.3	7.8
High school graduate	17.0	6.6
Some college	17.7	6.8
College graduate	15.8	4.1

Note: Binge drinking is defined as having drunk five or more drinks on the same occasion on at least one day in the past 30 days. Heavy alcohol use is defined as having drunk five or more drinks on the same occasion on each of five or more days in the past 30 days. Occasion means at the same time or within a couple of hours of each other. All heavy alcohol users are also binge drinkers.
Source: U.S. Substance Abuse and Mental Health Services Administrations, Summary of Findings from the 1998 National Household Survey on Drug Abuse, *1999* .

Illegal Drug Use, 1998

(percent of people aged 12 or older who have used illegal drugs in the past month, by sex, age, race, Hispanic origin, and education, 1998)

	percent
Total people	**6.2%**
Male	8.1
Female	4.5
Aged 12 to 17	9.9
Aged 12 to 13	2.9
Aged 14 to 15	10.8
Aged 16 to 17	16.4
Aged 18 to 25	16.1
Aged 18 to 20	19.9
Aged 21 to 25	13.5
Aged 26 to 34	7.0
Aged 26 to 29	7.4
Aged 30 to 34	6.8
Aged 35 or older	3.3
Aged 35 to 39	7.6
Aged 40 to 44	5.9
Aged 45 to 49	5.1
Aged 50 or older	0.7
Black, non-Hispanic	8.2
White, non-Hispanic	6.1
Other, non-Hispanic	3.8
Hispanic	6.1
Not a high school graduate	6.5
High school graduate	6.2
Some college	6.9
College graduate	3.7

Source: U.S. Substance Abuse and Mental Health Services Administrations, Summary of Findings from the 1998 National Household Survey on Drug Abuse, *1999*

Lifetime Use of Any Illegal Drug and Marijuana by Age, 1998

(percent of people aged 12 or older who have used any illegal drug and marijuana in their lifetime, by age, 1998)

	any illegal drug	marijuana
Total people	**35.8%**	**33.0%**
Aged 12 to 17	21.3	17.0
Aged 12 to 13	8.3	3.4
Aged 14 to 15	21.8	16.9
Aged 16 to 17	34.7	31.5
Aged 18 to 25	48.1	44.6
Aged 18 to 20	47.7	44.0
Aged 21 to 25	48.3	45.0
Aged 26 to 34	50.6	47.9
Aged 26 to 29	48.2	45.8
Aged 30 to 34	52.5	49.6
Aged 35 or older	31.8	29.4
Aged 35 to 39	54.4	51.2
Aged 40 to 44	55.5	53.8
Aged 45 to 49	46.1	44.4
Aged 50 or older	14.0	11.5

Source: U.S. Substance Abuse and Mental Health Services Administrations, Summary of Findings from the 1998 National Household Survey on Drug Abuse, *1999*

Should Marijuana Be Legal? 1998

"Do you think the use of marijuana should be made legal or not?"

(percent of people aged 18 or older responding by sex, race, age, and education, 1998)

	should	should not	don't know
Total	**28%**	**66%**	**6%**
Men	34	60	6
Women	22	71	6
Black	24	71	5
White	28	65	6
Other	26	67	7
Aged 18 to 29	34	60	6
Aged 30 to 39	29	63	8
Aged 40 to 49	32	64	4
Aged 50 to 59	29	66	6
Aged 60 to 69	16	77	6
Aged 70 or older	16	78	6
Not a high school graduate	21	72	7
High school graduate	26	68	6
Bachelor's degree	35	59	6
Graduate degree	31	61	7

Source: General Social Survey, National Opinion Research Center, University of Chicago; calculations by New Strategist

Cigarette Smoking Behavior of High School Students, 1997

(percent of 9th through 12th graders who report selected cigarette smoking initiation and quitting behaviors, by sex, race, Hispanic origin, and grade, 1997)

	lifetime smokers*	percent of lifetime smokers who have ever smoked daily**	percent of ever-daily smokers who have ever tried to quit	former smokers***
Total high school students	**70.2%**	**35.8%**	**72.9%**	**13.5%**
Male	70.9	34.7	68.7	13.0
Female	69.3	37.1	77.6	14.0
White, non-Hispanic	70.4	41.7	76.0	13.4
Black, non-Hispanic	68.4	14.9	64.8	16.9
Hispanic	75.0	24.5	61.9	14.3
Ninth grade	67.7	35.7	66.1	17.8
Tenth grade	70.0	34.9	77.3	14.6
Eleventh grade	68.8	37.1	73.2	10.0
Twelfth grade	73.7	35.5	74.4	12.4

* Ever tried cigarette smoking, even one or two puffs.
** Have ever smoked at least one cigarette every day for at least 30 days.
*** Did not smoke on any of the 30 days preceding the survey.
Source: Centers for Disease Control and Prevention, Selected Cigarette Smoking Initiation and Quitting Behaviors among High School Students—United States, 1997, Mortality and Morbidity Weekly Report, Vol. 47, No. 19, 1998

12

Birth, Aging, and Death

Each year, nearly 4 million babies are born in the United States. Thus begins the demand for health care that lasts—for most—a long lifetime. At each stage of life, health care consumers have different needs that must be met. Childbirth once routinely took place at home. Today, it is an often costly and highly medicalized experience. The aging process itself is increasingly treated as a medical problem to be cured, with cosmetic surgery on the rise as well as long-term treatment for once-fatal but now chronic conditions. The dying put extraordinary demands on the health care system—much of it unavoidable, but some of it could be better spent elsewhere.

In the next few decades, the greatest increase in demand on the health care system will be in the vast middle, where millions of baby boomers are attempting to stall the aging process. In contrast, demands at either end could lessen because a growing share of Americans favor a more natural approach to birth and death.

In the beginning: birth

In 1998, the number of births in the United States increased for the first time since 1990, rising to 3.9 million—1.6 percent more births than in 1997. The rise in the number of births is due to an upward bump in the birth rate of twenty- and thirtysomething women. The birth rate among women in their thirties is higher than it has been at any time in the past three decades as women who postponed childbearing have their long-awaited babies. Nevertheless, most births (52 percent) are to women in their twenties. Only 36 percent of births in 1998 were to women aged 30 or older.

The Census Bureau projects a rise in the number of births in the United States, with the figure topping 4 million in 2004 and continuing upward from there. Behind the rising number of births is population growth as well as the higher fertility of Hispanics—one of the most rapidly growing minority groups in the U.S. In 1998, 19 percent of all births were to Hispanic women. Another 15 percent were to black women. Just 60 percent of births were to non-Hispanic whites.

While the birth rate among women aged 20 or older is up, the rate among women under age 20 has fallen to an all-time low. In 1998, the birth rate for women aged 15 to 19 was 15 percent lower than in 1990 and 37 percent lower than in 1950. The teen birth rate is falling because more young women are seeking economic opportunity by going to college and entering the workforce, postponing childbearing until they are established in a career. The teen birth rate is also falling because of teens' increased use of contraceptives.

Out-of-wedlock births are much more common than teen births. Today, 33 percent of births are to unmarried women—more than 1 million babies were born to single women in 1998. Among blacks, the figure is an enormous 69 percent, while 42 percent of births to Hispanic women are out-of-wedlock. Children raised by single parents are much more likely to live in poverty and experience other social problems. Until out-of-wedlock births become much less common, the elimination of childhood poverty is unlikely.

Although there continues to be much hand-wringing about out-of-wedlock and teen births, many of the public health campaigns surrounding pregnancy and childbirth are proving to be successful. More women of all ages are using contraceptives, for example. The proportion rose from 56 percent in 1982 to 64 percent in 1995, according to the National Center for Health Statistics. Perhaps because of the greater use of contraception, the abortion

Most babies are born to women under age 30

(percent distribution of births by age of mother, 1998)

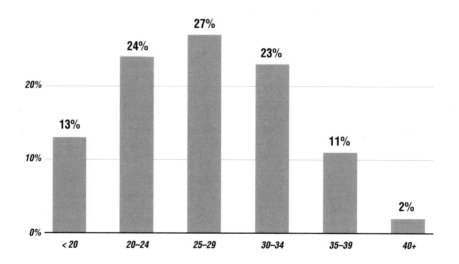

rate has declined from 29 abortions per 1,000 women aged 15 to 44 in 1980 to 23 abortions per 1,000 women aged 15 to 44 in 1996.

The percentage of women who smoke during pregnancy is also down, falling from 20 percent in 1989 to 13 percent in 1998. At the same time, the proportion of women receiving prenatal care during the first trimester rose to 83 percent in 1998, up from 76 percent in 1980. Breast-feeding also has become much more common—58 percent of babies were breast-fed in 1993–94 compared to 30 percent in 1972–74.

With a lower birth rate among teens, more contraceptive use, more prenatal care and breast feeding, the medical complications of childbirth appear to be increasingly under control. Yet the proportion of babies born with low birth weight rose slightly between 1980 and 1998. The heroic efforts of doctors and hospitals to save these infants have raised serious ethical questions—such as how to determine the proper distribution of medical resources, and at what point doctors and families should allow ailing infants to die. The debate surrounding these issues is likely to intensify as medical advances extend the possibility of life to smaller and frailer infants.

One of the greatest debates surrounding childbirth is the result of astounding advances in medical science. New fertility technologies are allowing more of the infertile to have children, including women well beyond their reproductive years. Among the nation's 60 million women aged 15 to 44 in 1995, 15 percent have sought fertility services at some point, according to the National Center for Health Statistics. These services range from simple advice from a doctor to assisted reproductive technologies such as artificial insemination, in vitro fertilization, or gamete intrafallopian transfer (egg donation). Two percent of women aged 35 to 44 in 1995 had tried assisted reproductive technologies, including 5 percent of childless women in the age group.

One consequence of fertility intervention is an increase in multiple births. Between 1980 and 1998, the number of twin births rose 62 percent, according to the National Center for Health Statistics. The number of triplet and "higher order" births increased 470 percent. The rate of triplet or higher order births per 100,000 live births has more than quadrupled. The debate over multiple births came to the forefront of national attention in 1997, when seven siblings, known as the McCaughey septuplets, were brought into the world. "The fertility business is a rapidly expanding $4 billion industry," writes John Leo in *US News and World Report*.[1] "The industry is by and large for profit and unregulated." This situation is likely to change given the controversy surrounding high-tech fertility techniques and their consequences.

Assisted reproductive technologies create complex legal and ethical issues. The courts are only slowly coming to terms with new, more precise definitions of what it means to be a mother or father. While many Americans disapprove of the extraordinary efforts of some to have children, those who can afford to do so will continue to stretch the boundaries of medical science in order to procreate.

In the middle: the aging process

Aging is a relatively new stage of life. In the past, most people did not survive to old age. Even 100 years ago, life expectancy was just 47 years—meaning about half the population died before age 47, most of them in infancy and childhood. Thanks to medical advances during the 20th century, millions of Americans are living to old age. Consequently, knowledge about the effects of aging on the body's physical and mental processes is growing by leaps and bounds. Worry about the consequences of aging is also growing.

The process of aging is in the midst of change, and stereotypes of what it means to be old are falling by the wayside. The current generation of older Americans is the most active and affluent in history. As baby boomers age, they promise to rewrite the rules of aging even more. The generation that changed society's conception of youth will also change its conception of age. No industry will be affected more strongly by this development than health care. Although boomers will not be able to halt the aging process, they will do their best to delay it.

The physical aspects of aging are many and complex. "Aging involves the steady decline of organ functioning and of the regulation of body systems," writes Mark E. Williams in *The American Geriatric Society's Complete Guide to Aging and Health*.[2] Translation: older people get sick and die more easily than younger people. The eyes become less sensitive, and the senses of smell and hearing weaken. In particular, the body's barriers to infection are compromised. Hormonal changes in both men and women can also lead to physical problems, such as the increased risk of osteoporosis in women and the loss of virility in men. One of the most infamous hormonal changes is menopause, when women's ovaries stop producing the hormone estrogen, which regulates or affects many critical body functions.

Aging also affects the mind. Older people require more time and effort to process information than younger people. Short-term memory also decreases. In the past few years, the specter of Alzheimer's disease has loomed large. This dreaded disease slowly impairs memory to the point where its victims can no longer remember who they are. Alzheimer's disease has gained more recognition, in part because of its celebrity victim—former president Ronald Reagan. It has also gained more recognition because, for our more educated society, the thought of losing the knowledge of a lifetime is particularly frightening. "People are very frightened of the possibilities because they know it represents a loss of one's self," says Steven T. DeKosky, M.D., director of the Alzheimer's Disease Research Center at the University of Pittsburgh, in *FDA Consumer*.[3] Nearly 23,000 people died of Alzheimer's disease in 1998, according to the National Center for Health Statistics. The Alzheimer's Association estimates that by 2050 as many as 14 million Americans could have the disease. Early diagnosis and treatment will become an important issue, particularly among boomers.

The multitude of potential health problems that accompany aging, coupled with a powerful desire to avoid them, creates a marketing opportunity of gigantic proportion. Each of the problems of aging will have a market of consumers eager for products and services that promise to solve or alleviate it. Examples range from the growing interest in antibacterial products and germ-filtration systems to the intensifying demand for methods to remove unwanted hair. The key to success with any aging-related product is to keep in mind that most people—particularly baby boomers—will shun products aimed at old people and their problems. An example of how a business can sidestep the "old" label is the positioning of Dr. Scholl's foot care products as an important part of a beauty regimen—such as the company's launch of a new line called Pedicure Essentials.[4] Toothpaste brands from Crest to Arm and Hammer have introduced teeth whitening pastes. And Oil of Olay, Proctor and Gamble's venerable old lady of skin care products, dropped the "Oil" from its name in an effort to shed years from its image.[5]

Women will account for the majority of the consumers of health care products and services designed to ease the problems of aging for two reasons. First, women live longer than men, on average, and increasingly outnumber them in old age. Second, women are more interested than men in prolonging their youth because society's notion of feminine beauty is a youthful one. Generally, as women approach the end of their reproductive years, they are considered to be at the end of their youth. With millions of baby boomers now entering menopause, the market for youth-enhancing products and services will grow enormously—from health and beauty products that promise to cover up the symptoms of aging to surgical procedures that promise to remove them altogether. Of the 4.6 million cosmetic surgery procedures performed in 1999, fully 89 percent were performed on women, according to The American Society for Aesthetic Plastic Surgery.

Baby-boom women are redefining aging, however. They are the first generation in which the majority of women have careers. The end of their reproductive potential will not have the impact it did on previous generations of women, who saw themselves primarily as mothers. As life expectancy has grown over the decades, women have gained an extra 20 years of life—the time between the end of their fertile years and old age, according to Martha Farnsworth Riche, former director of the Census Bureau. The glossy magazine, *More*, published by Meredith Corporation, uses the slogan "there's more in the middle" to advertise the new vitality and consumer power of women in middle age.

Men, too, are more active in middle age than they once were. Baby-boom men are more concerned with their looks and health than their fathers were. Aging in men is not as clearly marked as it is by menopause for women, although men do experience a version of menopause (or, as author Gail Sheehy calls it, "MANopause"). The symptoms of manopause include irritability, sluggishness, mild mood swings, impotence, and decreased muscle mass and strength.[6] But because hormonal changes in men are far more gradual than those occurring during menopause, men's change of life will never capture the same marketing attention as menopause. Nevertheless, the mania over the male impotence pill, Viagra, shows that alleviating the symptoms of aging in men can be extremely lucrative.

As science progresses, consumers catch glimpses of the tantalizing possibility of expanding life beyond its current limits. It remains to be seen whether consumers will be eager for technologies that extend life past the 100-year mark. The Pew Research Center for The People & The Press found in one of its surveys that just 41 percent of men and 31 percent of women were interested in adding an extra 100 years to their life.[7]

At the end: death

As life expectancy creeps upward and chronic diseases become more widespread in our aging population, the quest for learning more about the end of life will intensify. Attitudes toward death, which are already changing, are likely to be transformed by this greater knowledge and by the demands of the new health care consumer.

Until recently, death wasn't a subject for polite conversation. Today, although the topic still causes many to squirm, public debate is growing about the manner and meaning of death. Increasingly, death is being viewed as a personal growth experience. "The end of life is a potentially rich and rewarding period for human development. Our goal must be to maximize the opportunity for each dying individual to live well on their own terms, right up to the time of death," writes Dr. Joanne Lynn in *The Journal of the American Medical Association*.[8]

The notion of death as a personal growth experience is the result of medical advances which are prolonging fatal illnesses, giving the dying and their friends and relatives a chance to say good-bye and make their peace. This attitude does not extend to the deaths of young people, however. Generally, patients under age 80 are treated more aggressively than those aged 80 or older—who tend to be treated for pain and other symptoms rather than being cured.[9]

Hand in hand with changing attitudes towards aging is the rise of the hospice industry—agencies and facilities that make death more comfortable for those suffering from fatal illnesses. Only about 60,000 Americans are receiving hospice care at any one time—most of them aged 65 or older, according to the National Center for Health Statistics. During a year's time, however, the number of Americans cared for in a hospice program is much greater. Still, hospice programs care for only a small portion of the 2 million Americans who die each year.

Heart disease and cancer are the two greatest killers of Americans, accounting for 54 percent of all deaths. Heart disease is the cause of death for 31 percent of those who die each year, while cancer kills 23 percent. Among people under age 35, however, accidents are the leading cause of death. Most deaths (55 percent) occur to people aged 75 or older, including 65 percent of deaths due to heart disease.

Because of continuing advances in medical care, life expectancy rises each year. In 1998 it stood at 73.8 years for men and 79.5 years for women. Those figures are projected to climb to 79.5 for men and 84.9 for women by 2050, according to the Census Bureau.

Most deaths are to people aged 75 or older

(percent distribution of deaths by age, 1998)

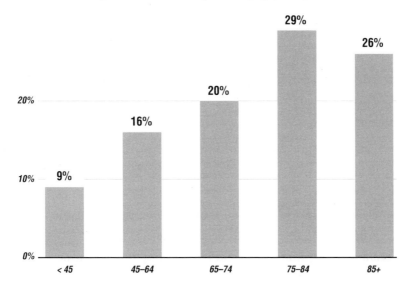

Despite increasing life expectancy, the annual number of deaths in the U.S. will grow enormously as the large baby-boom generation ages. The number is projected to rise 69 percent between 1998 and 2050, from 2.3 million to 4.0 million a year. This increase guarantees an intensifying debate over death and dying.

The most heated debate surrounding the issue of death today concerns physician-assisted suicide, with Dr. Jack Kevorkian at the center of the maelstrom. Physician-assisted suicide, or euthanasia, occurs when a terminally ill person takes his or her own life with the help of a physician. At the heart of the debate is one issue: Who controls the death decision? Some say God does, and that nature must be allowed to run its course. But an increasing proportion of Americans want to put the power in the hands of patients and family members. Sixty-eight percent of Americans think a doctor should be able to end a patient's life painlessly if a patient with a terminal illness wants it, according to the General Social Survey of the University of Chicago's National Opinion Research Center. This figure is up from 58 percent in 1978. Public support is likely to continue to grow since younger people are more supportive of physician-assisted suicide than older generations. But even older people have grown more supportive than they once were. In 1978, only 45 percent of people aged 70 or older supported euthanasia. By 1998, the figure had grown to the 59 percent majority.

As with abortion, it's likely that consensus on this issue will never be reached, making physician-assisted suicide difficult to legislate. The Supreme Court has held that there is no constitutional right to physician-assisted suicide, but it has also overturned laws prohibiting it.

The fuzzy legal status of euthanasia has more than a theoretical effect on patients. Eighteen percent of physicians reported patients asking for medication to end their life, but only 11 percent of physicians said there were circumstances in which they would be willing to hasten a patient's death by prescribing medication. Just 7 percent said they would be willing to provide a lethal injection. But if it were legal to do so, a larger 36 percent of doctors said they would prescribe death-inducing medication, and 24 percent said they would provide a lethal injection.[10]

Less extreme than euthanasia but also a topic of debate is palliative medicine, or therapy designed to relieve pain and discomfort but not to produce a cure. When dying is painful, it poses an ethical dilemma not only for physicians and family members, but for society as a whole. The main goal of palliative treatments is to relieve pain. The problem with this approach is that it sometimes speeds death. A balance is necessary, but as yet no clear guidelines exist that doctors, families, or individuals can follow to achieve that balance. As the dying grow in number, however, and as more of them are members of the vocal and demanding baby-boom generation, look for some resolution to these issues in the years to come.

The Future of birth, aging, and death

The baby-boom generation now being in middle age, the aging process will occupy the minds of these important health care consumers. The unique attitudes of boomers have already tranformed the birth process. Aging is next. Eventually, boomers will upset the status quo surrounding death itself.

TREND 1: DIFFERENT CAST OF CHARACTERS ATTENDING BIRTHS

Although doctors are the most common attendant at a birth, the percentage of physicians attended births has been falling over the past decade. In 1989, a physician was present at 96 percent of births, according to the National Center for Health Statistics. By 1997, a smaller 92 percent of births had a doctor present. At the same time, the percentage of births attended by a midwife grew from just under 4 percent in 1989 to 7 percent in 1997. Expect the proportion of births attended by doctors to continue to drop as managed care pushes more medical procedures into the hands of less-expensive practitioners.

TREND 2: LIVING YOUNG

As the baby-boom generation seeks to prolong its youth, the real concern will be to minimize the signs and symptoms of aging. The pharmaceutical industry is hot in pursuit of treatments that promise a more youthful lifestyle, the anti-impotence drug Viagra probably being the most celebrated of these lifestyle drugs. Others are on the way that will fight everything from memory loss to wrinkles. Such drugs, which are worth billions of dollars to pharmaceutical companies, offer a quick and easy alternative to living carefully. "Industry executives figure baby boomers would gladly pay to pop a pill rather than diet, exercise, watch their cholesterol—or do without sex," comments *Business Week*.[11]

If one of these magic pills turned out to have nasty side effects, however, the market could collapse. The promise of a fountain of youth is a centuries-old scam, and future generations of elderly will be more resistant to false claims because they will be highly educated, cynical, and suspicious. It will be increasingly important for businesses marketing new anti-aging products to promise only what they can deliver.

Trend 3: New ways of segmenting the old

Aging is different for everyone, determined not so much by chronology but by how a person responds to the aging process. Because of this variety, the older market will be increasingly segmented not by age but by physical condition. Physical health, and the resulting need for products and services, will be strongly influenced by nondemographic factors such as smoking status, economic status, social status, family support, and self-esteem.[12]

Another way the old will be segmented is across cultural lines. A diverse society necessarily includes diverse perspectives on aging. The symptoms of menopause, for example, may be a matter of cultural expectation, according to an article in *Menopause News*.[13] In Japan, the number one menopause-related complaint is shoulder stiffness, according to researcher Margaret Locke. Shoulder stiffness does not even make the list of complaints in North America, where hot flashes rank number one. In Japan, hot flashes rank a lowly ninth.

Trend 4: Alternative medicine to the rescue

Alternative medicine has found a lucrative niche in treating the symptoms of aging because of the lack of medical research in the area. For women, in particular, alternative products have become an important means of treating a variety of aging symptoms such as menopause.

Although menopause is a physiological event, there is debate over whether it is a condition that needs to be cured or a natural event that should be allowed to run its course without medical interference. For women who choose the latter option, alternative medicine is a perfect fit. These women object to what they call the "medicalization" of menopause, such as the recommendation that menopausal women start hormone replacement therapy to restore estrogen levels. Low estrogen levels are a risk factor for osteoporosis and cardiovascular disease. Unfortunately, estrogen is a risk factor for breast and uterine cancer.

The cancer concern is one reason why not many women have adopted hormone replacement therapy. According to *Drug Store News*, only 15 to 20 percent of postmenopausal women use hormone replacement therapy. The reasons women who are not taking hormone replacement therapy most commonly cite are fear of cancer and the inconvenience of vaginal bleeding.[14] The development of better estrogen replacements, which provide heart and bone benefits without the cancer risk, may erode part of the demand for alternative treatments.

Trend 5: Acceptance of aging

The resistance to the medicalization of menopause may spread to other symptoms of aging. After all, most older people believe they are in good health, and they are satisfied with their lives. "Except for extremely old people, life satisfaction does not seem to decrease with aging, despite age associated events such as poorer health, reduced financial resources, widow-hood, loss of friends and reduced activity," writes Williams in *The American Geriatric Society's Complete Guide to Aging and Health*.[15] A study by the North American Menopause Society backs up this notion, finding that the 52 percent majority of American women aged 45 to 60 view menopause as the beginning of a new and fulfilling stage of life.[16] As the American population ages, the aging process will be not only accepted but, increasingly, celebrated.

TREND 6: MORE CONTROL OVER DEATH

Just as aging will become more acceptable, so will death—including euthanasia. In the next few years, expect the debate over physician-assisted suicide to intensify as more people face painful deaths. Because this is a highly charged political issue, it is difficult to predict the outcome. But one thing is certain: Even if physician-assisted suicide were outlawed entirely, euthanasia would continue to be an option for some in old age. Just as the baby-boom generation demanded more choice in foods, cars, and shoes, it will also demand choice in death. For some, that choice will be euthanasia. At the very least, the heroic efforts to save the terminally ill and very old will become less common, to be replaced by a more naturalistic approach to death. Behind this shift will be society's attempt to reduce the enormous cost of treating people in the last stages of life and also the desires of the terminally ill to control the end.

Along with greater tolerance for euthanasia will come greater acceptance of palliative medicine to treat the pain of the dying. As research produces more effective pain control medication, its use will become widespread. According to the Quality of Life's End Missoula Demonstration Project (a long-term project to determine how Missoula, Montana, could best meet the needs of its residents at the end of life), pain assessment should be the fifth vital sign, along with pulse, blood pressure, body temperature, and respiratory rate.[17]

TREND 7: DEATH SERVICE PROVIDERS

Many professionals are involved in a death—from general practitioners to medical special-ists, from therapists to administrators and clergy. This complex situation calls for coordina-tion, giving rise to a new profession—the death service provider. This person would have special knowledge of a patient's cultural and religious practices. He or she would be familiar with a patient's attitude toward death, as well as the attitudes of family members. The death service provider would continually update, translate, and coordinate a patient's living will and advance directives. He or she would have a legal understanding of the choices available to a patient and would advocate for the patient's wishes.

Death service providers will have an additional duty as well. They will help care for family caregivers. Because physicians are not trained to deal with grieving relatives and friends, many caregivers are left in limbo after a loved one's death. Death service providers will provide counseling and referrals for this ample and underserved market.

Notes

1. John Leo, "A New Medical Skill: Counting," *US News and World Report* (December 8, 1997): 20.

2. Mark E. Williams, *The American Geriatric Society's Complete Guide to Aging and Health* (Harmony Books, 1995): 14.

3. Audrey T. Hingley, "Alzheimers: Few Clues on the Mystery of Memory," *FDA Consumer* 32, no. 2 (May-June 1998): 26.

4. Virna Sanabria, "Dr. Scholl's in Step," *Global Cosmetic Industry* 166, no. 5 (May 2000): 64.

5. "Body Wash and Logo Revamp Enliven Olay's Image," *Drug Store News* (March 6, 2000): 41.

6. Gail Sheehy, "Beyond Virility, A New Vision: Men and Their Doctors Need to Understand That Impotence Is Just One Part of a Complicated Midlife Passage: Call it MANopause," *Newsweek* (November 17, 1997): 69.

7. Mark Dolliver, "100," *Adweek* eastern edition 40, no. 150 (December 13, 1999): 74.

8. Joanne Lynn, "An 88-Year-Old Woman Facing the End of Life," *Journal of the American Medical Association* 277, no. 20 (May 28, 1997): 1633–1641.

9. Ibid.

10. Diane E. Meier, Carol-Ann Emmons, Sylvan Wallenstein, Timothy Quill, R. Sean Morrison, and Christine K. Cassel, "A National Survey of Physician-Assisted Suicide and Euthanasia in the United States," *The New England Journal of Medicine* 338, no. 17 (April 23, 1998): 1193–2000.

11. Joseph Weber and Amy Barrett, "The New Era of Lifestyle Drugs: Viagra and Other Blockbusters Are Transforming the $300 Billion Industry," *Business Week* (May 11, 1998): 98.

12. Williams, 38–40.

13. "Japanese Menopause Is Different," *Menopause News* (November-December 1996): 1–3.

14. Janet McCombs, "Hormone Replacement Therapy," *Drug Store News* (September 22, 1997): 31–35.

15. Williams, 38.

16. North American Menopause Society, "NAMS 1997 Menopause Survey," abstracted on <www.menopause.org>.

17. Larry Beresford, "The Good Death: The People of Missoula, Montana, Open a Dialogue on Better Ways to Die," *Hospitals and Health Networks* 71, no. 12 (June 20, 1997): 60–63.

Contraceptive Use by Age, 1982 and 1995

(percent of women aged 15 to 44 who use contraception by method and age, 1982 and 1995; percentage point change, 1982–95)

	1995	1982	percentage point change 1982–95
ANY METHOD			
Total, aged 15 to 44	**64.2%**	**55.7%**	**8.5**
Aged 15 to 19	29.8	24.2	5.6
Aged 20 to 24	63.5	55.8	7.7
Aged 25 to 34	71.1	66.7	4.4
Aged 35 to 44	72.3	61.6	10.7
BIRTH CONTROL PILL			
Total, aged 15 to 44	**26.9**	**28.0**	**−1.1**
Aged 15 to 19	43.8	63.9	−20.1
Aged 20 to 24	52.1	55.1	−3.0
Aged 25 to 34	33.3	25.7	7.6
Aged 35 to 44	8.7	3.7	5.0
CONDOM			
Total, aged 15 to 44	**20.4**	**12.0**	**8.4**
Aged 15 to 19	36.7	20.8	15.9
Aged 20 to 24	26.4	10.7	15.7
Aged 25 to 34	21.1	11.4	9.7
Aged 35 to 44	14.7	11.3	3.4
DIAPHRAGM			
Total, aged 15 to 44	**1.9**	**8.1**	**−6.2**
Aged 15 to 19	0.1	6.0	−5.9
Aged 20 to 24	0.6	10.2	−9.6
Aged 25 to 34	1.7	10.3	−8.6
Aged 35 to 44	2.8	4.0	−1.2
INTRAUTERINE DEVICE			
Total, aged 15 to 44	**0.8**	**7.1**	**−6.3**
Aged 15 to 19	0.0	1.3	−1.3
Aged 20 to 24	0.3	4.2	−3.9
Aged 25 to 34	0.8	9.7	−8.9
Aged 35 to 44	1.1	6.9	−5.8

(continued)

(continued from previous page)

	1995	1982	percentage point change 1982–95
STERILIZATION, FEMALE			
Total, aged 15 to 44	**27.7%**	**23.2%**	**4.5**
Aged 15 to 19	0.3	0.0	0.3
Aged 20 to 24	4.0	4.5	–0.5
Aged 25 to 34	23.8	22.1	1.7
Aged 35 to 44	45.0	43.5	1.5
STERILIZATION, MALE			
Total, aged 15 to 44	**10.9**	**10.9**	**0.0**
Aged 15 to 19	0.0	0.4	–0.4
Aged 20 to 24	1.1	3.6	–2.5
Aged 25 to 34	7.8	10.1	–2.3
Aged 35 to 44	19.4	19.9	–0.5

Note: Method of contraception used in the month of interview.
Source: National Center for Health Statistics, Health, United States, 1998; *calculations by New Strategist*

Pregnancy Outcomes, 1976 to 1996

(number of pregnancies, live births, induced abortions, and fetal losses, 1976 to 1996; percent change for selected years; numbers in thousands)

	total pregnancies	live births	induced abortions	fetal losses
1996	6,240	3,891	1,366	983
1995	6,245	3,900	1,364	982
1994	6,373	3,953	1,431	989
1993	6,494	4,000	1,500	993
1992	6,596	4,065	1,529	1,002
1991	6,674	4,111	1,557	1,007
1990	6,778	4,158	1,609	1,011
1980	5,912	3,612	1,554	746
1976	5,002	3,168	1,179	655
Percent change				
1990–1996	–7.9%	–6.4%	–15.1%	–2.8%
1976–1990	35.5	31.3	36.5	54.4

Source: National Center for Health Statistics, Highlights of Trends in Pregnancies and Pregnancy Rates by Outcome: Estimates for the United States, 1976–96, *National Vital Statistics Reports, Vol. 47, No. 29, 1999; calculations by New Strategist*

Legal Abortions by Age, 1976 to 1996

(total number of legal abortions and rate per 1,000 women in specified age group, 1976 to 1996; percent change for selected years; numbers in thousands)

	total number	rate	< 15	15–19	20–24	25–29	30–34	35–39	40+
1996	1,366	22.9	1.1	29.2	50.7	33.6	18.2	9.9	3.2
1995	1,364	22.9	1.2	30.0	50.3	32.6	17.9	9.8	3.2
1994	1,431	24.1	1.3	32.2	53.0	33.1	18.4	10.0	3.2
1993	1,500	25.4	1.4	34.3	55.8	33.9	18.9	10.2	3.2
1992	1,529	25.9	1.5	35.5	56.3	33.9	19.0	10.4	3.2
1991	1,557	26.3	1.4	37.6	56.6	33.7	19.1	10.4	3.0
1990	1,609	27.4	1.5	40.3	56.7	33.9	19.7	10.8	3.2
1980	1,554	29.4	1.7	42.7	51.6	31.0	17.2	9.4	3.5
1976	1,179	24.2	1.6	34.3	39.6	24.1	15.0	9.3	3.7

Percent change

1990–1996	−15.1%	−16.4%	−26.7%	−27.5%	−10.6%	−0.9%	−7.6%	−8.3%	0.0%
1976–1990	36.5	13.2	−6.3	17.5	43.2	40.7	31.3	16.1	−13.5

Note: The total abortion rate is the number of abortions per 1,000 women aged 15 to 44.
Source: National Center for Health Statistics, Highlights of Trends in Pregnancies and Pregnancy Rates by Outcome: Estimates for the United States, 1976–96, *National Vital Statistics Reports, Vol. 47, No. 29, 1999; calculations by New Strategist*

Women by Fecundity Status, 1995

(total number and percent distribution of women aged 15 to 44 by selected characteristics and fecundity status, 1995; numbers in thousands)

	total number	percent	surgically sterile contra-ceptive	surgically sterile noncontra-ceptive	impaired fecundity	fecund
TOTAL WOMEN	**60,201**	**100.0%**	**24.2%**	**3.1%**	**10.2%**	**62.5%**
Age						
Aged 15 to 24	18,002	100.0	1.6	0.1	6.1	92.2
Aged 25 to 34	20,758	100.0	22.0	1.2	11.2	65.6
Aged 35 to 44	21,440	100.0	45.3	7.4	12.8	34.6
Marital status						
Never married	22,679	100.0	4.5	0.9	6.7	87.9
Currently married	29,673	100.0	36.6	4.1	12.9	46.3
Formerly married	7,849	100.0	34.1	5.8	10.2	50.0
Education (aged 22 to 44)						
Not a high school graduate	5,424	100.0	44.1	5.1	12.9	37.9
High school graduate	18,169	100.0	38.0	5.0	12.3	44.8
Some college	12,399	100.0	26.3	3.5	10.7	59.5
Bachelor's degree or more	11,748	100.0	17.0	2.0	10.7	70.3
Race and Hispanic origin						
Hispanic	6,702	100.0	22.9	2.3	10.8	64.0
Non-Hispanic white	42,522	100.0	24.7	3.2	10.0	62.2
Non-Hispanic black	8,210	100.0	25.5	3.7	10.1	60.7
Non-Hispanic other	2,767	100.0	15.6	2.3	13.1	69.1
CHILDLESS WOMEN						
Total, aged 15 to 44	**25,242**	**100.0**	**2.8**	**1.5**	**11.0**	**84.7**
Aged 15 to 24	14,113	100.0	0.2	0.1	5.5	94.3
Aged 25 to 34	7,139	100.0	2.9	0.7	13.9	82.5
Aged 35 to 44	3,991	100.0	11.9	8.1	25.7	54.3
WOMEN WITH CHILDREN						
Total, aged 15 to 44	**39,458**	**100.0**	**39.7**	**4.2**	**9.6**	**46.5**
Aged 15 to 24	3,889	100.0	6.7	0.3	8.4	84.6
Aged 25 to 34	13,620	100.0	32.1	1.5	9.8	56.7
Aged 35 to 44	17,449	100.0	52.9	7.2	9.8	30.1

Source: National Center for Health Statistics, Fertility, Family Planning, and Women's Health: New Data from the 1995 National Survey of Family Growth, *Vital and Health Statistics, Series 23, No. 19, 1997*

Women Ever Receiving Fertility Services, 1995

(total number of women aged 15 to 44 and percent ever receiving fertility services, by type of service, 1995; numbers in thousands)

				percent receiving			
	total	any service	advice*	test on woman or man	ovulation drugs	surgery or treatment for blocked tubes	assisted reproductive technology**
TOTAL WOMEN	**60,201**	**15.4%**	**6.4%**	**4.2%**	**3.0%**	**1.5%**	**1.0%**
Age							
Aged 15 to 24	18,002	4.4	1.1	0.2	0.3	0.1	0.0
Aged 25 to 34	20,758	17.1	6.3	3.7	3.1	1.2	0.8
Aged 35 to 44	21,440	22.9	10.9	8.1	5.2	2.9	2.1
Education (aged 22 to 44)							
Not a high school graduate	5,424	14.9	3.3	2.0	1.2	0.7	0.2
High school graduate	18,169	20.0	7.8	4.9	3.9	2.0	1.1
Some college	12,399	19.4	7.8	5.6	3.3	2.0	1.2
Bachelor's degree or more	11,748	18.0	10.3	7.1	5.3	1.9	2.2
Race and Hispanic origin							
Hispanic	6,702	13.4	4.9	2.4	1.7	0.9	0.6
Non-Hispanic white	42,522	16.3	7.2	4.9	3.5	1.6	1.2
Non-Hispanic black	8,210	13.0	3.8	2.2	1.4	0.9	0.3
Non-Hispanic other	2,767	12.3	5.0	3.9	2.9	1.9	1.4
CHILDLESS WOMEN							
Total, aged 15 to 44	**25,242**	**6.4**	**4.6**	**3.7**	**2.2**	**1.1**	**1.2**
Aged 15 to 24	14,113	1.2	0.5	0.2	0.2	0.1	0.1
Aged 25 to 34	7,139	8.7	6.5	4.6	3.0	1.0	1.1
Aged 35 to 44	3,991	20.7	15.5	14.5	8.0	4.8	5.3
Married	5,685	20.9	16.0	13.6	8.3	4.1	4.7
Unmarried	19,558	2.2	1.2	0.8	0.4	0.2	0.1
WOMEN WITH CHILDREN							
Total, aged 15 to 44	**39,458**	**21.8**	**7.7**	**4.6**	**3.6**	**1.8**	**0.9**
Aged 15 to 24	3,889	16.1	3.3	0.3	0.6	0.5	0.0
Aged 25 to 34	13,620	21.5	6.2	3.1	3.1	1.3	0.6
Aged 35 to 44	17,449	23.4	9.8	6.7	4.6	2.4	1.4
Married	23,988	24.1	9.2	6.0	4.6	2.1	1.1
Unmarried	10,970	16.8	4.3	1.6	1.3	0.9	0.5

* Includes services to help get pregnant as well as to help prevent miscarriage.
** Includes artificial insemination, in vitro fertilization, gamete intrafallopian transfer, and other techniques not shown separately.
Source: National Center for Health Statistics, Fertility, Family Planning, and Women's Health: New Data from the 1995 National Survey of Family Growth, *Vital and Health Statistics, Series 23, No. 19, 1997*

Women Adopting Children, 1973 and 1995

(number of ever-married women aged 18 to 44 and percent who have ever adopted a child, by selected characteristics, 1973 and 1995; numbers in thousands)

	1995	1973
Total number of women	**37,448**	**30,701**
Number who have ever adopted	**487**	**645**
Percent who have adopted	**1.3%**	**2.1%**
Age		
Aged 18 to 24	0.2	0.4
Aged 25 to 34	0.4	1.8
Aged 35 to 39	1.9	3.1
Aged 40 to 44	2.5	4.0
Race and Hispanic origin		
Non-Hispanic white	1.4	2.3
Non-Hispanic black	1.9	1.6
Hispanic	0.6	1.2
Number of births		
None	3.6	5.9
One birth	0.8	2.7
Two births	0.9	1.1
Three or more births	0.5	0.8
Education		
Not a high school graduate	0.8	1.8
High school graduate	1.2	2.4
Some college	1.4	1.6
College graduate	1.7	4.6

Source: National Center for Health Statistics, Adoption, Adoption Seeking, and Relinquishment for Adoption in the United States, *Advance Data, Number 306, 1999*

Projections of Births, 2000 to 2050

(annual number of births, 2000 to 2050; numbers in thousands)

year	number	year	number
2000	3,914	2026	4,759
2001	3,932	2027	4,785
2002	3,953	2028	4,813
2003	3,978	2029	4,844
2004	4,009	2030	4,878
2005	4,045	2031	4,915
2006	4,086	2032	4,953
2007	4,133	2033	4,992
2008	4,183	2034	5,032
2009	4,234	2035	5,074
2010	4,283	2036	5,116
2011	4,328	2037	5,159
2012	4,370	2038	5,201
2013	4,408	2039	5,244
2014	4,443	2040	5,286
2015	4,476	2041	5,327
2016	4,507	2042	5,367
2017	4,536	2043	5,407
2018	4,563	2044	5,446
2019	4,589	2045	5,483
2020	4,613	2046	5,520
2021	4,636	2047	5,556
2022	4,660	2048	5,592
2023	4,684	2049	5,626
2024	4,709	2050	5,661
2025	4,736		

Source: Bureau of the Census, Projections of the Resident Population by Age, Sex, Race, and Hispanic Origin: 1999 to 2100, *Internet web site <http://www.census.gov/population/www/projections/natproj.html>*

Birth Rates by Age, 1950 to 1998

(number of births per 1,000 women aged 15 to 44, and per 1,000 women in specified age group, 1950 to 1998; percent change for selected years)

	total	15 to 19	20 to 24	25 to 29	30 to 34	35 to 39	40 to 44	45 to 49
1998	65.6	51.1	111.2	115.9	87.4	37.4	7.3	0.4
1997	65.0	52.3	110.4	113.8	85.3	36.1	7.1	0.4
1996	65.3	54.4	110.4	113.1	83.9	35.3	6.8	0.3
1995	65.6	56.8	109.8	112.2	82.5	34.3	6.6	0.3
1994	66.7	58.9	111.1	113.9	81.5	33.7	6.4	0.3
1993	67.6	59.6	112.6	115.5	80.8	32.9	6.1	0.3
1992	68.9	60.7	114.6	117.4	80.2	32.5	5.9	0.3
1991	69.6	62.1	115.7	118.2	79.5	32.0	5.5	0.2
1990	70.9	59.9	116.5	120.2	80.8	31.7	5.5	0.2
1980	68.4	53.0	115.1	112.9	61.9	19.8	3.9	0.2
1970	87.9	68.3	167.8	145.1	73.3	31.7	8.1	0.5
1960	118.0	89.1	258.1	197.4	112.7	56.2	15.5	0.9
1950	106.2	81.6	196.6	166.1	103.7	52.9	15.1	1.2

Percent change

	total	15 to 19	20 to 24	25 to 29	30 to 34	35 to 39	40 to 44	45 to 49
1990–1998	–7.5%	–14.7%	–4.5%	–3.6%	8.2%	18.0%	32.7%	100.0%
1950–1990	–33.2	–26.6	–40.7	–27.6	–22.1	–40.1	–63.6	–83.3

Source: Bureau of the Census, Historical Statistics of the United States: Colonial Times to 1970, Part 1, *1975; and National Center for Health Statistics,* Health, United States, 1999; *and* Births: Final Data for 1998, *National Vital Statistics Report, Vol. 48, No. 3, 2000; calculations by New Strategist*

Births by Age of Mother and Birth Order, 1998

(number and percent distribution of births by age of mother and birth order, 1998)

	total births	first birth	second birth	third birth	fourth birth or more
Total births	**3,941,553**	**1,576,478**	**1,280,805**	**646,539**	**411,540**
Under age 20	494,357	384,397	87,974	15,275	2,248
Aged 20 to 24	965,122	437,632	334,566	133,872	52,311
Aged 25 to 29	1,083,010	394,268	376,634	193,783	111,988
Aged 30 to 34	889,365	248,986	321,412	186,685	127,004
Aged 35 to 39	424,890	93,428	137,137	99,453	92,122
Aged 40 to 44	81,027	16,897	22,217	16,821	24,519
Aged 45 to 54	3,782	870	865	650	1,348

Percent distribution by birth order

	total births	first birth	second birth	third birth	fourth birth or more
Total births	**100.0%**	**40.0%**	**32.5%**	**16.4%**	**10.4%**
Under age 20	100.0	77.8	17.8	3.1	0.5
Aged 20 to 24	100.0	45.3	34.7	13.9	5.4
Aged 25 to 29	100.0	36.4	34.8	17.9	10.3
Aged 30 to 34	100.0	28.0	36.1	21.0	14.3
Aged 35 to 39	100.0	22.0	32.3	23.4	21.7
Aged 40 to 44	100.0	20.9	27.4	20.8	30.3
Aged 45 to 54	100.0	23.0	22.9	17.2	35.6

Percent distribution by age

	total births	first birth	second birth	third birth	fourth birth or more
Total births	**100.0%**	**100.0%**	**100.0%**	**100.0%**	**100.0%**
Under age 20	12.5	24.4	6.9	2.4	0.5
Aged 20 to 24	24.5	27.8	26.1	20.7	12.7
Aged 25 to 29	27.5	25.0	29.4	30.0	27.2
Aged 30 to 34	22.6	15.8	25.1	28.9	30.9
Aged 35 to 39	10.8	5.9	10.7	15.4	22.4
Aged 40 to 44	2.1	1.1	1.7	2.6	6.0
Aged 45 to 54	0.1	0.1	0.1	0.1	0.3

Note: Births by birth order will not add to total because "not stated" is not included.
Source: National Center for Health Statistics, Births: Final Data for 1998, *National Vital Statistics Report, Vol. 48, No. 3, 2000; calculations by New Strategist*

Births by Age, Race, and Hispanic Origin of Mother, 1998

(number and percent distribution of births by age, race, and Hispanic origin of mother, 1998)

		race				Hispanic origin	
	total births	white	black	Asian	Native American	non-Hispanic white	Hispanic
Total births	**3,941,553**	**3,118,727**	**609,902**	**172,652**	**40,272**	**2,361,462**	**734,661**
Under age 20	494,357	345,495	131,226	9,238	8,398	221,301	124,104
Aged 20 to 24	965,122	736,664	189,088	26,324	13,046	511,101	223,113
Aged 25 to 29	1,083,010	880,688	139,302	53,491	9,529	678,227	196,012
Aged 30 to 34	889,365	737,532	93,785	52,118	5,930	603,639	125,702
Aged 35 to 39	424,890	349,799	46,657	25,639	2,795	291,202	54,195
Aged 40 to 44	81,027	65,485	9,496	5,491	555	53,480	11,056
Aged 45 to 54	3,782	3,064	348	351	19	2,512	479
Percent distribution by race and Hispanic origin							
Total births	**100.0%**	**79.1%**	**15.5%**	**4.4%**	**1.0%**	**59.9%**	**18.6%**
Under age 20	100.0	69.9	26.5	1.9	1.7	44.8	25.1
Aged 20 to 24	100.0	76.3	19.6	2.7	1.4	53.0	23.1
Aged 25 to 29	100.0	81.3	12.9	4.9	0.9	62.6	18.1
Aged 30 to 34	100.0	82.9	10.5	5.9	0.7	67.9	14.1
Aged 35 to 39	100.0	82.3	11.0	6.0	0.7	68.5	12.8
Aged 40 to 44	100.0	80.8	11.7	6.8	0.7	66.0	13.6
Aged 45 to 54	100.0	81.0	9.2	9.3	0.5	66.4	12.7
Percent distribution by age							
Total births	**100.0%**	**100.0%**	**100.0%**	**100.0%**	**100.0%**	**100.0%**	**100.0%**
Under age 20	12.5	11.1	21.5	5.4	20.9	9.4	16.9
Aged 20 to 24	24.5	23.6	31.0	15.2	32.4	21.6	30.4
Aged 25 to 29	27.5	28.2	22.8	31.0	23.7	28.7	26.7
Aged 30 to 34	22.6	23.6	15.4	30.2	14.7	25.6	17.1
Aged 35 to 39	10.8	11.2	7.6	14.9	6.9	12.3	7.4
Aged 40 to 44	2.1	2.1	1.6	3.2	1.4	2.3	1.5
Aged 45 to 54	0.1	0.1	0.1	0.2	0.0	0.1	0.1

Note: Births by race and Hispanic origin will not add to total because Hispanics may be of any race and "not stated" is not included.
Source: National Center for Health Statistics, Births: Final Data for 1998, National Vital Statistics Report, Vol. 48, No. 3, 2000; calculations by New Strategist

Births by Marital Status of Mother, 1998

(total number of births and number and percent to unmarried women, by age, race, and Hispanic origin of mother, 1998)

	total	race white	race black	non-Hispanic white	Hispanic
Total births	**3,941,553**	**3,118,727**	**609,902**	**2,361,462**	**734,661**
Under age 20	494,357	345,495	131,226	221,301	124,104
Aged 20 to 24	965,122	736,664	189,088	511,101	223,113
Aged 25 to 29	1,083,010	880,688	139,302	678,227	196,012
Aged 30 to 34	889,365	737,532	93,785	603,639	125,702
Aged 35 to 39	424,890	349,799	46,657	291,202	54,195
Aged 40 or older	84,809	68,549	9,844	55,992	11,535
Births to unmarried women	**1,293,567**	**821,441**	**421,383**	**517,153**	**305,442**
Under age 20	390,005	250,346	125,728	159,561	91,045
Aged 20 to 24	460,367	291,677	151,903	185,985	106,020
Aged 25 to 29	243,280	153,310	79,344	92,542	61,079
Aged 30 to 34	124,624	77,883	40,927	47,449	30,725
Aged 35 to 39	61,087	38,905	19,367	25,491	13,403
Aged 40 or older	14,204	9,320	4,114	6,125	3,170
Percent of births to unmarried women	**32.8%**	**26.3%**	**69.1%**	**21.9%**	**41.6%**
Under age 20	78.9	72.5	95.8	72.1	73.4
Aged 20 to 24	47.7	39.6	80.3	36.4	47.5
Aged 25 to 29	22.5	17.4	57.0	13.6	31.2
Aged 30 to 34	14.0	10.6	43.6	7.9	24.4
Aged 35 to 39	14.4	11.1	41.5	8.8	24.7
Aged 40 or older	16.7	13.6	41.8	10.9	27.5

Note: Births by race and Hispanic origin will not add to total because Hispanics may be of any race and "not stated" is not included.
Source: National Center for Health Statistics, Births: Final Data for 1998, *National Vital Statistics Report, Vol. 48, No. 3, 2000; calculations by New Strategist*

Births by Age and Educational Attainment of Mother, 1998

(number and percent distribution of births by age and educational attainment of mother, 1998)

	total	not a high school graduate	high school graduate only	some college	college graduate
Total births	**3,941,553**	**848,156**	**1,266,102**	**859,688**	**907,220**
Under age 20	494,357	304,958	157,085	23,469	—
Aged 20 to 24	965,122	254,708	423,593	222,605	49,613
Aged 25 to 29	1,083,010	154,301	341,622	287,684	284,171
Aged 30 to 34	889,365	84,932	222,470	211,046	358,152
Aged 35 to 39	424,890	39,508	102,106	96,496	179,773
Aged 40 to 54	84,809	9,749	19,226	18,388	35,511

Percent distribution by educational attainment

Total births	**100.0%**	**21.5%**	**32.1%**	**21.8%**	**23.0%**
Under age 20	100.0	61.7	31.8	4.7	—
Aged 20 to 24	100.0	26.4	43.9	23.1	5.1
Aged 25 to 29	100.0	14.2	31.5	26.6	26.2
Aged 30 to 34	100.0	9.5	25.0	23.7	40.3
Aged 35 to 39	100.0	9.3	24.0	22.7	42.3
Aged 40 to 54	100.0	11.5	22.7	21.7	41.9

Percent distribution by age

Total births	**100.0%**	**100.0%**	**100.0%**	**100.0%**	**100.0%**
Under age 20	12.5	36.0	12.4	2.7	—
Aged 20 to 24	24.5	30.0	33.5	25.9	5.5
Aged 25 to 29	27.5	18.2	27.0	33.5	31.3
Aged 30 to 34	22.6	10.0	17.6	24.5	39.5
Aged 35 to 39	10.8	4.7	8.1	11.2	19.8
Aged 40 to 54	2.2	1.1	1.5	2.1	3.9

Note: Births by education will not add to total because "not stated" is not shown. (–) means not applicable.
Source: National Center for Health Statistics, Births: Final Data for 1998, *National Vital Statistics Report, Vol. 48, No. 3, 2000; calculations by New Strategist*

Twin and Triplet Births, 1980 to 1998

(number of twin and triplet/higher order births, 1980 to 1998; rate of twin births per 1,000 live births and rate of triplet/higher order births per 100,000 live births; percent change for selected years; numbers in thousands)

	number		rate	
	twin	triplet/ higher order	twin	triplet/ higher order
1998	110,670	7,625	28.1	193.5
1997	104,137	6,737	25.9	173.6
1996	100,750	5,939	24.8	152.6
1995	96,736	4,973	24.6	127.5
1994	97,064	4,594	24.1	116.2
1993	96,445	4,168	23.5	104.2
1992	95,372	3,883	23.1	95.5
1991	94,779	3,346	22.6	81.4
1990	93,865	3,028	22.3	72.8
1985	77,102	1,925	20.5	51.2
1980	68,339	1,337	18.9	37.0
Percent change				
1990–1998	17.9%	151.8%	26.0%	165.8%
1980–1990	37.4	126.5	18.0	96.8

Source: National Center for Health Statistics, Trends in Twin and Triplet Births: 1980–97, *National Vital Statistics Reports, Vol. 47, No. 24, 1999; and* Births: Final Data for 1998, *Vital Statistics Report, Vol. 48, No. 3, 2000; calculations by New Strategist*

Births by Delivery Method, 1998

(number and percent distribution of births by age of mother and method of delivery, 1998)

	total births	vaginal total	vaginal after previous Caesarean	Caesarean total	Caesarean first	Caesarean repeat
Total births	**3,941,553**	**3,078,537**	**108,903**	**825,870**	**519,975**	**305,895**
Under age 20	494,357	418,743	3,614	71,195	63,425	7,770
Aged 20 to 24	965,122	789,395	20,742	166,403	114,822	51,581
Aged 25 to 29	1,083,010	847,952	31,292	224,878	140,031	84,847
Aged 30 to 34	889,365	666,110	32,966	215,010	121,144	93,866
Aged 35 to 39	424,890	300,150	17,228	120,604	64,451	56,153
Aged 40 to 54	84,809	56,187	3,061	27,780	16,102	11,678
Total births	**100.0%**	**78.1%**	**2.8%**	**21.0%**	**13.2%**	**7.8%**
Under age 20	100.0	84.7	0.7	14.4	12.8	1.6
Aged 20 to 24	100.0	81.8	2.1	17.2	11.9	5.3
Aged 25 to 29	100.0	78.3	2.9	20.8	12.9	7.8
Aged 30 to 34	100.0	74.9	3.7	24.2	13.6	10.6
Aged 35 to 39	100.0	70.6	4.1	28.4	15.2	13.2
Aged 40 to 54	100.0	66.3	3.6	32.8	19.0	13.8

Source: National Center for Health Statistics, Births: Final Data for 1998, *National Vital Statistics Report, Vol. 48, No. 3, 2000; calculations by New Strategist*

Births by Place of Delivery and Attendant, 1998

(number and percent distribution of births by place of delivery and attendant, 1997)

| | total births | attendant | | |
		physician	midwife	other
Total births	**3,941,553**	**3,625,043**	**293,386**	**21,852**
In hospital	3,903,770	3,619,406	272,261	11,516
Not in hospital	37,049	5,517	20,897	10,101
Freestanding birthing center	10,693	1,767	8,714	206
Clinic or doctor's office	857	336	233	282
Residence	23,232	2,664	11,634	8,538
Other	2,267	750	316	1,075
Total births	**100.0%**	**92.0%**	**7.4%**	**0.6%**
In hospital	100.0	92.7	7.0	0.3
Not in hospital	100.0	14.9	56.4	27.3
Freestanding birthing center	100.0	16.5	81.5	1.9
Clinic or doctor's office	100.0	39.2	27.2	32.9
Residence	100.0	11.5	50.1	36.8
Other	100.0	33.1	13.9	47.4

Note: Numbers will not add to total because unspecified is not shown.
Source: National Center for Health Statistics, Births: Final Data for 1998, *National Vital Statistics Report, Vol. 48, No. 3, 2000; calculations by New Strategist*

Cosmetic Surgery by Sex, 1999

(total number of cosmetic surgery procedures and percent performed on women by type of procedure, 1999; ranked by total number of procedures)

	total	percent performed on women
Total procedures	**4,606,954**	**88.7%**
Chemical peel	841,777	90.2
Botox injection	498,204	91.3
Laser hair removal	481,978	80.7
Collagen injection	474,756	91.8
Sclerotherapy	414,797	97.5
Lipoplasty (liposuction)	287,150	81.5
Microdermabrasion	286,614	91.8
Breast augmentation	191,583	100.0
Blepharoplasty (cosmetic eyelid surgery)	183,580	85.3
Laser skin resurfacing	133,454	82.0
Rhinoplasty (nose reshaping)	102,943	67.9
Facelift	100,203	88.0
Laser treatment of leg veins	93,517	98.7
Breast reduction (women)	89,769	100.0
Cellulite treatment (mechanical roller massage therapy)	63,059	99.0
Abdominoplasty (tummy tuck)	59,665	95.9
Fat injection	52,289	91.3
Forehead lift	48,815	91.3
Breast lift	44,861	100.0
Hair transplantation	33,665	18.1
Dermabrasion	28,355	74.3
Otoplasty (cosmetic ear surgery)	22,368	53.3
Lip augmentation (other than injectable materials)	21,729	97.7
Gynecomastia, treatment of	16,413	0.0
Chin augmentation	15,979	75.6
Cheek implants	5,382	81.3
Thigh lift	5,133	98.1
Upper arm lift	4,641	98.5
Lower body lift	2,870	95.4
Buttock lift	1,408	96.4

Source: The American Society for Aesthetic Plastic Surgery, Internet web site <http://www.surgery.org>

Cosmetic Surgery by Age, 1999

(total number of cosmetic surgery procedures and percent distribution by age of patient and type of procedure, 1999; ranked by total number of procedures)

	total	< age 19	19–34	35–50	51–64	65+
Total procedures	**4,606,954**	**3.8%**	**26.4%**	**42.5%**	**21.6%**	**5.7%**
Chemical peel	841,777	10.2	26.1	36.7	19.2	7.8
Botox injection	498,204	0.2	18.9	50.3	24.8	5.9
Laser hair removal	481,978	7.5	36.9	37.6	15.5	2.5
Collagen injection	474,756	0.3	17.3	45.7	27.4	9.3
Sclerotherapy	414,797	0.6	24.2	49.4	22.0	3.7
Lipoplasty (liposuction)	287,150	0.9	34.3	45.8	16.2	2.8
Microdermabrasion	286,614	2.8	28.7	45.5	18.2	4.8
Breast augmentation	191,583	1.4	59.2	35.3	3.9	0.2
Blepharoplasty (cosmetic eyelid surgery	183,580	0.1	4.8	41.2	41.7	12.2
Laser skin resurfacing	133,454	0.8	14.0	36.6	37.9	10.8
Rhinoplasty (nose reshaping)	102,943	12.6	49.1	29.5	8.2	0.7
Facelift	100,203	0.0	1.1	31.1	53.3	14.5
Laser treatment of leg veins	93,517	0.5	27.5	47.3	19.3	5.3
Breast reduction (women)	89,769	3.8	38.4	41.9	13.6	2.2
Cellulite treatment (mechanical roller massage therapy)	63,059	0.5	29.0	54.3	16.1	0.2
Abdominoplasty (tummy tuck)	59,665	0.1	19.4	58.6	19.5	2.3
Fat injection	52,289	1.0	20.8	42.3	27.0	9.0
Forehead lift	48,815	0.1	4.3	40.7	43.6	11.2
Breast lift	44,861	0.5	27.0	56.2	15.4	1.0
Hair transplantation	33,665	0.1	24.3	57.0	15.6	3.1
Dermabrasion	28,355	3.7	26.6	37.4	24.8	7.3
Otoplasty (cosmetic ear surgery)	22,368	49.5	35.0	12.9	2.3	0.5
Lip augmentation (other than injectable materials)	21,729	1.3	38.9	38.4	17.8	3.5
Gynecomastia, treatment of	16,413	18.9	46.2	29.6	4.9	0.5
Chin augmentation	15,979	2.7	45.9	35.6	14.1	1.6
Cheek implants	5,382	1.0	42.7	48.0	8.1	0.7
Thigh lift	5,133	0.0	14.7	69.7	14.7	0.7
Upper arm lift	4,641	0.0	13.5	50.1	28.5	6.0
Lower body lift	2,870	0.0	19.0	65.2	15.1	0.8
Buttock lift	1,408	0.0	21.5	62.5	14.4	0.6

Source: The American Society for Aesthetic Plastic Surgery, Internet web site <http://www.surgery.org>

Caregiving by Sex, 1996

(selected characteristics of persons aged 15 or older providing regular unpaid care to a family member or friend with a long-term illness or disability, by sex, 1996; numbers in thousands)

	total	men	women
Number of caregivers	**9,323**	**3,208**	**6,116**
Caregivers as a percent of people aged 15+	**4.5%**	**3.3%**	**5.5%**
PROVIDED CARE TO ONE OR MORE PERSONS INSIDE THE HOUSEHOLD			
Number	4,472	1,667	2,805
Average hours of care per week	42	36	46
Average years care has been provided	8.1	7.8	8.3
Type of care provided			
Helped with activities of daily living			
Number providing care	2,518	939	1,579
Percent providing care	56.3%	56.4%	56.3%
Helped with medical needs			
Number providing care	3,131	1,061	2,070
Percent providing care	70.0%	63.7%	73.8%
Helped with money management			
Number providing care	3,044	1,065	1,980
Percent providing care	68.1%	63.9%	70.6%
Helped with trips outside the home			
Number providing care	3,910	1,476	2,434
Percent providing care	87.4%	88.5%	86.8%
PROVIDED CARE TO ONE OR MORE PERSONS OUTSIDE THE HOUSEHOLD			
Number	5,027	1,594	3,434
Average hours of care per week	16	12	18
Average years care has been provided	4.1	4.4	4.0
Type of care provided			
Helped with activities of daily living			
Number providing care	1,596	388	1,208
Percent providing care	31.7%	24.3%	35.2%
Helped with medical needs			
Number providing care	2,032	521	1,511
Percent providing care	40.4%	32.7%	44.0%

(continued)

(continued from previous page)

	total	men	women
Helped with money management			
Number providing care	2,523	784	1,739
Percent providing care	50.2%	49.2%	50.6%
Helped with household chores			
Number providing care	2,814	682	2,133
Percent providing care	56.0%	42.8%	62.1%
Helped with trips outside the home			
Number providing care	3,627	1,063	2,564
Percent providing care	72.2%	66.7%	74.7%

Note: If more than one person is cared for, data are for first person cared for.
Source: Bureau of the Census, Preliminary Estimates on Caregiving from Wave 7 of the 1996 Survey of Income and Program Participation, *by John M. McNeil, No. 231, The Survey of Income and Program Participation, 1999*

Hospice Care Patients, 1996

(number and percent distribution of current hospice care patients by age, sex, race, and marital status, 1996)

	number	percent distribution
Total patients	**59,400**	**100.0%**
Age		
Under age 45	4,300	7.3
Aged 45 to 54	2,700	4.5
Aged 55 to 64	6,100	10.3
Aged 65 or older	46,100	77.7
Aged 65 to 69	5,000	8.4
Aged 70 to 74	9,600	16.2
Aged 75 to 79	9,800	16.6
Aged 80 to 84	9,100	15.2
Aged 85 or older	12,700	21.3
Sex		
Female	32,700	55.1
Male	26,600	44.9
Race		
White	49,700	83.7
Black	4,900	8.3
Other	800	1.3
Unknown	4,000	6.7
Marital status		
Never married	5,000	8.5
Married	25,900	43.7
Divorced or separated	5,500	9.3
Widowed	19,100	32.2
Unknown	3,800	6.3

Source: National Center for Health Statistics, An Overview of Home Health and Hospice Care Patients: 1996 National Home and Hospice Care Survey, *Advance Data, No. 297, 1998*

Hospice Care Patients by Current Residence, Living Arrangement, and Caregiver, 1996

(number and percent distribution of patients currently receiving hospice care by residence, living arrangement, and relationship to primary caregiver, 1996)

	number	percent
Total patients	**59,400**	**100.0%**
Current residence		
Private or semiprivate residence	46,600	78.5
Board and care or residential care facility	5,800	9.8
Health facility (including mental health facility)	6,700	11.3
Living arrangement		
Noninstitutionalized patients	46,600	78.5
Lives with family members	36,700	61.8
Lives alone	6,400	10.8
Lives with only nonfamily members	3,100	5.2
Primary caregiver		
Has no primary caregiver	4,700	7.9
Has primary caregiver	54,600	91.9
Lives with primary caregiver	42,200	71.0
Relationship to primary caregiver		
Spouse	22,200	37.4
Child/child-in-law	17,800	30.0
Sister or brother*	2,400	4.0
Other relative	3,900	6.6
Friend or neighbor	2,000	3.4
Hired help or staff of residential facility	4,500	7.6
Other nonrelative or unknown	1,900	3.2

* Includes sister- or brother-in-law.
Source: National Center for Health Statistics, Characteristics of Hospice Care Users: Data from the 1996 National Home and Hospice Care Survey, Advance Data No. 299, 1998

Hospice Care Patients by Diagnosis, 1996

(number and percent distribution of current hospice care patients by first-listed and all listed diagnoses at admission, 1996)

	primary diagnosis		all listed diagnoses	
	number	percent	number	percent
Total patients	**59,400**	**100.0%**	**146,900**	**100.0%**
Infectious and parasitic diseases	2,100	3.5	4,500	3.1
Human immunodeficiency virus (HIV) disease	2,000	3.3	2,000	1.4
Neoplasms	35,400	59.6	56,500	38.4
Malignant neoplasms	34,600	58.3	55,300	37.6
Endocrine, nutritional, and metabolic diseases and immunity disorders	–	–	7,300	5.0
Diabetes mellitus	–	–	3,200	2.2
Diseases of the blood and blood-forming organs	–	–	1,900	1.3
Mental disorders	–	–	5,400	3.7
Diseases of the nervous system and sense organs	4,800	8.1	8,800	6.0
Diseases of the circulatory system	7,300	12.3	28,600	19.4
Essential hypertension	–	–	4,200	2.9
Heart disease	4,900	8.3	16,000	10.9
Diseases of the respiratory system	4,400	7.3	9,800	6.7
Diseases of the digestive system	1,500	2.5	4,500	3.1
Diseases of the genitourinary system	–	–	2,400	1.6
Diseases of the skin and subcutaneous tissue	–	–	–	–
Diseases of the musculoskeletal system and connective tissue	–	–	4,300	2.9
Symptoms, signs, and ill-defined conditions	1,300	2.2	5,900	4.0
Injury and poisoning	–	–	–	–

Note: (–) means sample too small to make a reliable estimate.
Source: National Center for Health Statistics, An Overview of Home Health and Hospice Care Patients: 1996 National Home and Hospice Care Survey, *Advance Data, No. 297, 1998*

Hospice Care Patients by Services Received and Type of Provider, 1996

(number and percent distribution of current hospice care patients by services received and type of provider seen during the last 30 days, 1996)

	number	percent
Total patients	**59,400**	**100.0%**
Services received		
Nursing services	55,400	93.3
Social services	46,700	78.6
Medications	33,400	56.2
Counseling	31,200	52.5
Volunteers	23,000	38.7
Homemaker-household services	17,000	28.6
Physician services	15,200	25.6
Mental health services	7,200	12.1
Nutritionist services	5,800	9.8
Continuous home care	3,700	6.2
Spiritual care	2,900	4.9
Transportation	2,300	3.9
All other services	6,900	11.6
Service provider		
Registered nurse	54,100	91.1
Social worker	46,100	77.6
Home health aide	32,400	54.5
Volunteer	18,400	31.0
Chaplain	18,100	30.5
Nursing aide or attendant	10,000	16.8
Physician	8,200	13.8
Licensed practical or vocational nurse	8,100	13.6
Homemaker/personal caretaker	6,800	11.4
Dietitian/nutritionist	4,000	6.7
All other providers	4,700	7.9

Source: National Center for Health Statistics, Characteristics of Hospice Care Users: Data from the 1996 National Home and Hospice Care Survey, *Advance Data No. 299, 1998*

Physician-Assisted Suicide, 1978 and 1998

"When a person has a disease that cannot be cured, do you think doctors should be allowed by law to end the patient's life by some painless means if the patient and his family request it?"

(percent of people aged 18 or older responding by sex, race, age, and education, 1978 and 1998)

	yes		no	
	1998	1978	1998	1978
Total	**68%**	**58%**	**27%**	**38%**
Men	73	62	23	35
Women	63	55	30	41
Black	51	44	44	54
White	70	59	24	36
Aged 18 to 29	73	69	22	28
Aged 30 to 39	69	62	25	35
Aged 40 to 49	67	51	28	47
Aged 50 to 59	72	46	22	46
Aged 60 to 69	58	59	36	37
Aged 70 or older	59	45	34	49
Not a high school graduate	60	50	34	45
High school graduate	67	59	26	37
Bachelor's degree	71	66	23	30
Graduate degree	71	71	25	26

Note: Numbers may not add to 100 because "don't know" and no answer are not shown.
Source: General Social Surveys, National Opinion Research Center, University of Chicago; calculations by New Strategist

Experience with Terminal Illness, 1998

"Have you or any close friend or family members been faced
with a terminal or life-threatening illness?"

(percent of people aged 18 or older responding by sex, race, age, and education, 1998)

	total	yes, self	yes, friend	yes, immediate relative	yes, other relative	more than one	no
Total	**100.0%**	**5.2%**	**7.3%**	**23.6%**	**27.0%**	**2.4%**	**33.5%**
Men	100.0	4.0	7.5	20.9	29.3	2.4	34.6
Women	100.0	6.0	7.1	25.6	25.3	2.4	32.7
Black	100.0	1.5	7.0	19.1	24.1	1.5	46.2
White	100.0	6.3	7.5	25.3	27.1	2.7	30.0
Other	100.0	0.0	5.7	12.6	32.2	1.1	48.3
Aged 18 to 24	100.0	2.5	7.4	12.3	32.8	0.8	44.3
Aged 25 to 34	100.0	2.6	6.9	14.4	32.5	2.0	41.0
Aged 35 to 44	100.0	2.9	8.8	20.5	31.7	1.2	33.4
Aged 45 to 54	100.0	7.5	7.9	28.6	27.8	2.6	24.7
Aged 55 to 64	100.0	9.0	6.9	38.6	15.9	3.4	25.5
Aged 65 or older	100.0	8.7	5.2	32.0	16.0	4.8	31.6
Not a high school graduate	100.0	6.7	5.2	31.1	11.9	1.6	42.5
High school graduate	100.0	4.9	6.5	23.2	28.7	2.0	33.5
Bachelor's degree	100.0	5.8	9.5	22.8	27.4	4.1	29.0
Graduate degree	100.0	3.2	10.5	18.9	43.2	3.2	21.1

Note: Numbers may not add to 100 because "don't know" is not shown.
*Source: 1998 General Social Survey, National Opinion Research Center, University of Chicago; calculations by
New Strategist*

Worry about Economic Burden of Terminal Illness, 1998

"I worry about the economic burden that a
terminal illness might cause my family."

(percent of people aged 18 or older responding by sex, race, age, and education, 1998)

	agree	neither agree nor disagree	disagree
Total	**60.9%**	**10.6%**	**27.2%**
Men	60.3	10.9	27.6
Women	61.2	10.4	27.0
Black	53.2	11.9	33.3
White	62.7	10.3	25.7
Other	54.7	11.6	32.6
Aged 18 to 24	53.3	18.3	28.3
Aged 25 to 34	64.1	11.1	22.5
Aged 35 to 44	64.1	10.4	24.3
Aged 45 to 54	63.9	7.8	26.5
Aged 55 to 64	64.6	8.8	25.9
Aged 65 or older	50.4	10.3	38.5
Not a high school graduate	58.2	10.3	27.3
High school graduate	63.2	10.5	25.2
Bachelor's degree	58.1	9.8	31.3
Graduate degree	60.8	13.4	25.8

Note: Numbers may not add to 100 because "don't know" is not shown.
Source: 1998 General Social Survey, National Opinion Research Center, University of Chicago; calculations by New Strategist

Emotional Burden of Terminal Illness, 1998

"I worry about the emotional burden that my family
might face making decisions for me at the end of life."

(percent of people aged 18 or older responding by sex, race, age, and education, 1998)

	agree	neither agree nor disagree	disagree
Total	**61.6%**	**8.6%**	**28.3%**
Men	58.3	8.5	31.6
Women	63.9	8.6	25.9
Black	57.8	9.0	30.2
White	62.2	8.6	27.9
Other	62.8	7.0	29.1
Aged 18 to 24	68.3	10.0	20.0
Aged 25 to 34	70.3	7.5	20.3
Aged 35 to 44	69.8	7.0	22.4
Aged 45 to 54	58.8	7.5	31.6
Aged 55 to 64	54.4	13.6	31.3
Aged 65 or older	41.9	9.4	46.6
Not a high school graduate	55.2	7.7	32.5
High school graduate	65.1	7.3	26.1
Bachelor's degree	58.5	11.8	29.3
Graduate degree	60.4	12.5	26.0

Note: Numbers may not add to 100 because "don't know" is not shown.
Source: 1998 General Social Survey, National Opinion Research Center, University of Chicago; calculations by New Strategist

Religious Community and Terminal Illness, 1998

"My religious community would be very helpful if I were terminally ill."

(percent of people aged 18 or older responding by sex, race, age, and education, 1998)

	agree	neither agree nor disagree	disagree
Total	**54.3%**	**14.5%**	**26.4%**
Men	48.5	15.4	30.5
Women	58.5	13.8	23.4
Black	60.1	11.1	22.7
White	53.5	14.7	27.2
Other	51.2	19.8	24.4
Aged 18 to 24	49.6	19.3	28.6
Aged 25 to 34	44.7	18.8	29.6
Aged 35 to 44	55.1	15.7	24.2
Aged 45 to 54	56.3	10.5	30.1
Aged 55 to 64	56.8	12.3	25.3
Aged 65 or older	64.7	9.9	21.1
Not a high school graduate	56.8	10.9	23.4
High school graduate	52.8	15.9	27.0
Bachelor's degree	54.5	14.8	27.5
Graduate degree	54.2	11.5	30.2

Note: Numbers may not add to 100 because "don't know" is not shown.
Source: 1998 General Social Survey, National Opinion Research Center, University of Chicago; calculations by New Strategist

Pain at End of Life, 1998

"At the end of my life, I believe that the doctors
will be able to control my pain."

(percent of people aged 18 or older responding by sex, race, age, and education, 1998)

	agree	neither agree nor disagree	disagree
Total	**60.3%**	**17.9%**	**17.1%**
Men	61.5	17.2	16.8
Women	59.4	18.5	17.4
Black	53.2	18.4	22.4
White	63.2	17.2	15.6
Other	38.8	25.9	24.7
Aged 18 to 24	50.0	24.2	21.7
Aged 25 to 34	51.5	22.0	21.6
Aged 35 to 44	57.7	20.0	18.3
Aged 45 to 54	61.9	15.6	17.3
Aged 55 to 64	73.5	12.2	10.9
Aged 65 or older	70.9	12.4	11.1
Not a high school graduate	64.9	15.5	13.4
High school graduate	59.0	16.9	20.0
Bachelor's degree	56.9	22.8	15.0
Graduate degree	63.9	18.6	13.4

Note: Numbers may not add to 100 because "don't know" is not shown.
Source: 1998 General Social Survey, National Opinion Research Center, University of Chicago; calculations by New Strategist

Second Class Care at End of Life, 1998

"At the end of my life, I worry that if I run out of money or health insurance I will get second class health care."

(percent of people aged 18 or older responding by sex, race, age, and education, 1998)

	agree	neither agree nor disagree	disagree
Total	**55.2%**	**12.8%**	**29.0%**
Men	54.7	11.8	30.9
Women	55.6	13.6	27.6
Black	58.5	13.0	25.5
White	54.4	12.9	29.9
Other	58.1	11.6	25.6
Aged 18 to 24	62.5	12.5	22.5
Aged 25 to 34	59.2	14.4	23.9
Aged 35 to 44	61.4	14.3	22.5
Aged 45 to 54	57.6	10.0	29.0
Aged 55 to 64	49.7	10.9	36.1
Aged 65 or older	38.5	12.8	44.0
Not a high school graduate	48.5	11.3	32.0
High school graduate	59.2	13.4	25.0
Bachelor's degree	50.0	14.6	33.7
Graduate degree	54.2	11.5	32.3

Note: Numbers may not add to 100 because "don't know" is not shown.
Source: 1998 General Social Survey, National Opinion Research Center, University of Chicago; calculations by New Strategist

Trust in Decision Makers at End of Life, 1998: Family

"People sometimes are incapable of making decisions about their care and medical treatment at the end of life. If you were incapable, how much trust would you put in your family to do what was best for you?"

(percent of people aged 18 or older responding by sex, race, age, and education, 1998)

	total	completely	a great deal	somewhat	only a little or not at all
Total	**100.0%**	**74.3%**	**17.5%**	**5.6%**	**2.5%**
Men	100.0	73.8	18.9	5.0	1.9
Women	100.0	74.6	16.6	6.0	2.9
Black	100.0	68.7	17.9	8.5	5.0
White	100.0	75.2	17.6	5.0	2.0
Other	100.0	75.6	16.3	5.8	2.3
Aged 18 to 24	100.0	72.5	20.8	3.3	3.3
Aged 25 to 34	100.0	72.5	18.6	6.9	2.0
Aged 35 to 44	100.0	71.9	21.7	5.5	0.9
Aged 45 to 54	100.0	73.0	15.7	7.0	3.5
Aged 55 to 64	100.0	76.2	15.0	6.1	2.7
Aged 65 or older	100.0	81.0	11.6	3.4	3.9
Not a high school graduate	100.0	72.7	13.4	8.8	4.6
High school graduate	100.0	77.0	15.6	5.1	2.2
Bachelor's degree	100.0	70.7	24.0	2.8	2.4
Graduate degree	100.0	66.0	25.8	7.2	1.0

Note: Numbers may not add to 100 because "don't know" is not shown.
Source: 1998 General Social Survey, National Opinion Research Center, University of Chicago; calculations by New Strategist

Trust in Decision Makers at End of Life, 1998: Doctor

"People sometimes are incapable of making decisions about their care and medical treatment at the end of life. If you were incapable, how much trust would you put in your doctor to do what was best for you?"

(percent of people aged 18 or older responding by sex, race, age, and education, 1998)

	total	completely	a great deal	somewhat	only a little or not at all
Total	**100.0%**	**27.5%**	**28.9%**	**31.9%**	**10.3%**
Men	100.0	24.4	27.4	34.5	12.1
Women	100.0	29.8	30.0	30.0	9.1
Black	100.0	25.9	25.4	34.3	13.4
White	100.0	28.7	29.4	31.0	9.4
Other	100.0	16.3	31.4	37.2	15.1
Aged 18 to 24	100.0	13.3	35.0	35.0	16.7
Aged 25 to 34	100.0	16.7	31.0	36.6	14.7
Aged 35 to 44	100.0	20.0	28.1	40.3	10.4
Aged 45 to 54	100.0	29.0	27.7	35.9	5.6
Aged 55 to 64	100.0	37.4	29.3	19.0	11.6
Aged 65 or older	100.0	52.6	25.2	15.8	5.1
Not a high school graduate	100.0	41.8	21.1	23.7	11.3
High school graduate	100.0	26.4	29.6	32.5	10.4
Bachelor's degree	100.0	21.5	31.7	34.1	10.6
Graduate degree	100.0	22.7	35.1	32.0	9.3

Note: Numbers may not add to 100 because "don't know" is not shown.
Source: 1998 General Social Survey, National Opinion Research Center, University of Chicago; calculations by New Strategist

Trust in Decision Makers at End of Life, 1998: The Courts

"People sometimes are incapable of making decisions about their care and medical treatment at the end of life. If you were incapable, how much trust would you put in the courts to do what was best for you?"

(percent of people aged 18 or older responding by sex, race, age, and education, 1998)

	total	completely	a great deal	somewhat	only a little or not at all
Total	**100.0%**	**3.7%**	**4.0%**	**26.9%**	**62.4%**
Men	100.0	3.6	3.6	26.5	63.8
Women	100.0	3.7	4.2	27.2	61.4
Black	100.0	5.0	5.0	28.4	57.7
White	100.0	3.5	3.8	26.2	63.5
Other	100.0	3.5	3.5	32.6	59.3
Aged 18 to 24	100.0	2.5	2.5	28.3	65.0
Aged 25 to 34	100.0	2.3	2.9	26.5	67.3
Aged 35 to 44	100.0	2.3	4.1	28.1	63.5
Aged 45 to 54	100.0	4.3	3.9	28.6	60.6
Aged 55 to 64	100.0	4.8	4.1	25.9	62.6
Aged 65 or older	100.0	6.8	6.0	23.9	54.7
Not a high school graduate	100.0	6.7	5.7	30.9	49.0
High school graduate	100.0	3.8	3.6	25.2	64.8
Bachelor's degree	100.0	2.8	5.3	28.0	62.2
Graduate degree	100.0	2.1	1.0	28.9	67.0

Note: Numbers may not add to 100 because "don't know" is not shown.
Source: 1998 General Social Survey, National Opinion Research Center, University of Chicago; calculations by New Strategist

Projections of Deaths, 2000 to 2050

(annual number of deaths, 2000 to 2050; numbers in thousands)

year	number	year	number
2000	2,393	2026	3,076
2001	2,410	2027	3,120
2002	2,427	2028	3,165
2003	2,444	2029	3,211
2004	2,462	2030	3,257
2005	2,480	2031	3,304
2006	2,499	2032	3,351
2007	2,518	2033	3,398
2008	2,537	2034	3,445
2009	2,558	2035	3,491
2010	2,578	2036	3,537
2011	2,600	2037	3,580
2012	2,622	2038	3,622
2013	2,645	2039	3,663
2014	2,670	2040	3,702
2015	2,695	2041	3,738
2016	2,721	2042	3,772
2017	2,749	2043	3,804
2018	2,778	2044	3,833
2019	2,808	2045	3,859
2020	2,840	2046	3,883
2021	2,876	2047	3,904
2022	2,913	2048	3,923
2023	2,952	2049	3,939
2024	2,992	2050	3,952
2025	3,033		

Source: Bureau of the Census, Projections of the Resident Population by Age, Sex, Race, and Hispanic Origin: 1999 to 2100, *Internet web site <http://www.census.gov/population/www/projections/natproj.html>*

Deaths from Selected Causes, 1998

(number of deaths by cause and age, 1998; ranked by total number of deaths)

	total	< age 1	1 to 4	5 to 14	15 to 24	25 to 34	35 to 44	45 to 54	55 to 64	65 to 74	75 to 84	85+
Total deaths	2,337,256	28,045	5,251	7,791	30,627	42,516	88,866	146,476	233,724	458,982	681,663	612,575
Heart disease	724,859	609	214	326	1,057	3,207	13,593	35,056	65,068	135,295	226,769	243,609
Cancer	541,532	78	365	1,013	1,699	4,385	17,022	45,747	87,024	154,753	158,517	70,916
Cerebrovascular disease	158,448	296	57	82	178	670	2,650	5,709	9,653	23,912	54,428	60,804
Chronic obstructive pulmonary disease	112,584	39	49	152	239	328	884	2,828	10,162	31,102	43,718	23,076
Accidents	97,835	754	1,935	3,254	13,349	12,045	15,127	10,946	7,340	8,892	12,711	11,372
Motor vehicle accidents	43,501	162	759	1,868	10,026	7,132	6,963	4,996	3,420	3,410	3,457	1,278
Pneumonia and influenza	91,871	441	146	121	215	531	1,400	2,167	3,856	11,005	28,857	43,127
Diabetes mellitus	64,751	2	6	20	137	636	1,885	4,386	8,705	16,490	20,529	11,955
Suicide	30,575	–	–	324	4,135	5,365	6,837	5,131	2,963	2,597	2,355	851
Nephritis, nephrotic syndrome, nephrosis	26,182	138	12	20	43	149	436	932	1,812	4,778	9,058	8,804
Chronic liver disease and cirrhosis	25,192	16	1	4	22	506	3,370	5,744	5,279	5,655	3,703	887
Septicemia	23,731	216	89	56	104	257	671	1,231	2,093	4,474	7,431	7,107
Alzheimer's disease	22,725	–	1	–	–	–	9	39	259	1,907	8,367	12,142
Homicide and legal intervention	18,272	322	399	460	5,506	4,565	3,567	1,744	766	468	318	101
Atherosclerosis	15,279	1	1	–	2	10	41	172	560	1,687	4,407	8,398
Hypertension with or without renal disease	14,308	12	–	4	7	55	238	593	1,126	2,495	4,575	5,203

Note: Numbers will not add to total because "age not stated" is not shown; (–) means zero or not applicable.
Source: National Center for Health Statistics, Deaths: Final Data for 1998, National Vital Statistics Reports, Vol. 48, No. 11, 2000

Percent Distribution of Deaths by Cause, 1998

(percent distribution of deaths by cause and age, 1998)

	total	< age 1	1 to 4	5 to 15	15 to 24	25 to 34	35 to 44	45 to 54	55 to 64	65 to 74	75 to 84	85+
Total deaths	100.0%	100.0%	100.0%	100.0%	100.0%	100.0%	100.0%	100.0%	100.0%	100.0%	100.0%	100.0%
Heart disease	31.0	2.2	4.1	4.2	3.5	7.5	15.3	23.9	27.8	29.5	33.3	39.8
Cancer	23.2	0.3	7.0	13.0	5.5	10.3	19.2	31.2	37.2	33.7	23.3	11.6
Cerebrovascular disease	6.8	1.1	1.1	1.1	0.6	1.6	3.0	3.9	4.1	5.2	8.0	9.9
Chronic obstructive pulmonary disease	4.8	0.1	0.9	2.0	0.8	0.8	1.0	1.9	4.3	6.8	6.4	3.8
Accidents	4.2	2.7	36.9	41.8	43.6	28.3	17.0	7.5	3.1	1.9	1.9	1.9
Motor vehicle accidents	1.9	0.6	14.5	24.0	32.7	16.8	7.8	3.4	1.5	0.7	0.5	0.2
Pneumonia and influenza	3.9	1.6	2.8	1.6	0.7	1.2	1.6	1.5	1.6	2.4	4.2	7.0
Diabetes mellitus	2.8	0.0	0.1	0.3	0.4	1.5	2.1	3.0	3.7	3.6	3.0	2.0
Suicide	1.3	–	–	4.2	13.5	12.6	7.7	3.5	1.3	0.6	0.3	0.1
Nephritis, nephrotic syndrome, nephrosis	1.1	0.5	0.2	0.3	0.1	0.4	0.5	0.6	0.8	1.0	1.3	1.4
Chronic liver disease and cirrhosis	1.1	0.1	0.0	0.1	0.1	1.2	3.8	3.9	2.3	1.2	0.5	0.1
Septicemia	1.0	0.8	1.7	0.7	0.3	0.6	0.8	0.8	0.9	1.0	1.1	1.2
Alzheimer's disease	1.0	–	0.0	–	–	–	0.0	0.0	0.1	0.4	1.2	2.0
Homicide and legal intervention	0.8	1.1	7.6	5.9	18.0	10.7	4.0	1.2	0.3	0.1	0.0	0.0
Atherosclerosis	0.7	0.0	0.0	–	0.0	0.0	0.0	0.1	0.2	0.4	0.6	1.4
Hypertension with or without renal disease	0.6	0.0	–	0.1	0.0	0.1	0.3	0.4	0.5	0.5	0.7	0.8

Note: Percents will not add to total because not all causes of death are shown; (–) means zero or not applicable.
Source: National Center for Health Statistics, Deaths: Final Data for 1998, National Vital Statistics Reports, Vol. 48,
No. 11, 2000; calculations by New Strategist

Percent Distribution of Deaths by Age, 1998

(percent distribution of deaths by age and cause, 1998)

	total	< age 1	1 to 4	5 to 15	15 to 24	25 to 34	35 to 44	45 to 54	55 to 64	65 to 74	75 to 84	85+
Total deaths	100.0%	1.2%	0.2%	0.3%	1.3%	1.8%	3.8%	6.3%	10.0%	19.6%	29.2%	26.2%
Heart disease	100.0	0.1	0.0	0.0	0.1	0.4	1.9	4.8	9.0	18.7	31.3	33.6
Cancer	100.0	0.0	0.1	0.2	0.3	0.8	3.1	8.4	16.1	28.6	29.3	13.1
Cerebrovascular disease	100.0	0.2	0.0	0.1	0.1	0.4	1.7	3.6	6.1	15.1	34.4	38.4
Chronic obstructive pulmonary disease	100.0	0.0	0.0	0.1	0.2	0.3	0.8	2.5	9.0	27.6	38.8	20.5
Accidents	100.0	0.8	2.0	3.3	13.6	12.3	15.5	11.2	7.5	9.1	13.0	11.6
Motor vehicle accidents	100.0	0.4	1.7	4.3	23.0	16.4	16.0	11.5	7.9	7.8	7.9	2.9
Pneumonia and influenza	100.0	0.5	0.2	0.1	0.2	0.6	1.5	2.4	4.2	12.0	31.4	46.9
Diabetes mellitus	100.0	0.0	0.0	0.0	0.2	1.0	2.9	6.8	13.4	25.5	31.7	18.5
Suicide	100.0	–	–	1.1	13.5	17.5	22.4	16.8	9.7	8.5	7.7	2.8
Nephritis, nephrotic syndrome, nephrosis	100.0	0.5	0.0	0.1	0.2	0.6	1.7	3.6	6.9	18.2	34.6	33.6
Chronic liver disease and cirrhosis	100.0	0.1	0.0	0.0	0.1	2.0	13.4	22.8	21.0	22.4	14.7	3.5
Septicemia	100.0	0.9	0.4	0.2	0.4	1.1	2.8	5.2	8.8	18.9	31.3	29.9
Alzheimer's disease	100.0	–	0.0	–	–	–	0.0	0.2	1.1	8.4	36.8	53.4
Homicide and legal intervention	100.0	1.8	2.2	2.5	30.1	25.0	19.5	9.5	4.2	2.6	1.7	0.6
Atherosclerosis	100.0	0.0	0.0	–	0.0	0.1	0.3	1.1	3.7	11.0	28.8	55.0
Hypertension with or without renal disease	100.0	0.1	–	0.0	0.0	0.4	1.7	4.1	7.9	17.4	32.0	36.4

Note: Percents will not add to total because "age not stated" is not shown; (–) means zero or not applicable.
Source: National Center for Health Statistics, Deaths: Final Data for 1998, National Vital Statistics Reports, Vol. 48,
No. 11, 2000; calculations by New Strategist

Leading Causes of Death, 1998

(number and percent distribution of deaths accounted for by the ten leading causes of death, 1998)

		number	percent distribution
	All causes	**2,337,256**	**100.0%**
1.	Diseases of the heart	724,859	31.0
2.	Malignant neoplasms	541,532	23.2
3.	Cerebrovascular diseases	158,448	6.8
4.	Chronic obstructive pulmonary diseases and allied conditions	112,584	4.8
5.	Accidents and adverse effects	97,835	4.2
6.	Pneumonia and influenza	91,871	3.9
7.	Diabetes mellitus	64,751	2.8
8.	Suicide	30,575	1.3
9.	Nephritis, nephrotic syndrome, nephrosis	26,182	1.1
10.	Chronic liver disease and cirrhosis	25,192	1.1
	All other causes	463,427	19.8

Source: National Center for Health Statistics, Deaths: Final Data for 1998, *National Vital Statistics Reports, Vol. 48, No. 11, 2000; calculations by New Strategist*

Leading Causes of Death among Males, 1998

(number and percent distribution of deaths to males accounted for by the ten leading causes of death, 1998)

		number	percent distribution
	All causes	**1,157,260**	**100.0%**
1.	Diseases of the heart	353,897	30.6
2.	Malignant neoplasms	282,065	24.4
3.	Accidents and adverse effects	63,042	5.4
4.	Cerebrovascular diseases	61,145	5.3
5.	Chronic obstructive pulmonary diseases and allied conditions	57,018	4.9
6.	Pneumonia and influenza	40,979	3.5
7.	Diabetes mellitus	29,584	2.6
8.	Suicide	24,538	2.1
9.	Chronic liver disease and cirrhosis	16,343	1.4
10.	Homicide and legal intervention	14,023	1.2
	All other causes	214,626	18.5

Source: National Center for Health Statistics, Deaths: Final Data for 1998, *National Vital Statistics Reports, Vol. 48, No. 11, 2000; calculations by New Strategist*

Leading Causes of Death among Females, 1998

(number and percent distribution of deaths to females accounted for by the ten leading causes of death, 1998)

		number	percent distribution
	All causes	**1,179,996**	**100.0%**
1.	Diseases of the heart	370,962	31.4
2.	Malignant neoplasms	259,467	22.0
3.	Cerebrovascular diseases	97,303	8.2
4.	Chronic obstructive pulmonary diseases and allied conditions	55,566	4.7
5.	Pneumonia and influenza	50,892	4.3
6.	Diabetes mellitus	35,167	3.0
7.	Accidents and adverse effects	34,793	2.9
8.	Alzheimer's disease	15,671	1.3
9.	Nephritis, nephrotic syndrome, nephrosis	13,621	1.2
10.	Septicemia	13,506	1.1
	All other causes	233,048	19.7

Source: National Center for Health Statistics, Deaths: Final Data for 1998, *National Vital Statistics Reports, Vol. 48, No. 11, 2000; calculations by New Strategist*

Leading Causes of Death for Infants, 1998

(number and percent distribution of deaths accounted for by the ten leading causes of death for children under age 1, 1998)

		number	percent distribution
	All causes	**28,371**	**100.0%**
1.	Congenital anomalies	6,212	21.9
2.	Disorders relating to short gestation and low birthweight	4,101	14.5
3.	Sudden infant death syndrome	2,822	9.9
4.	Newborn affected by maternal complications of pregnancy	1,343	4.7
5.	Respiratory distress syndrome	1,295	4.6
6.	Newborn affected by complications of placenta, cord, and membranes	961	3.4
7.	Infections specific to the perinatal period	815	2.9
8.	Accidents and adverse effects	754	2.7
9.	Intrauterine hypoxia and birth asphyxia	461	1.6
10.	Pneumonia and influenza	441	1.6
	All other causes	9,166	32.3

Source: National Center for Health Statistics, Deaths: Final Data for 1998, National Vital Statistics Reports, Vol. 48, No. 11, 2000; calculations by New Strategist

Leading Causes of Death for Children Aged 1 to 4, 1998

(number and percent distribution of deaths accounted for by the ten leading causes of death for children aged 1 to 4, 1998)

		number	percent distribution
	All causes	**5,251**	**100.0%**
1.	Accidents and adverse effects	1,935	36.9
2.	Congenital anomalies	564	10.7
3.	Homicide	399	7.6
4.	Malignant neoplasms	365	7.0
5.	Diseases of heart	214	4.1
6.	Pneumonia and influenza	146	2.8
7.	Septicemia	89	1.7
8.	Certain conditions originating in the perinatal period	75	1.4
9.	Cerebrovascular diseases	57	1.1
10.	Benign neoplasms	53	1.0
	All other causes	1,354	25.8

Source: National Center for Health Statistics, Deaths: Final Data for 1998, *National Vital Statistics Reports, Vol. 48, No. 11, 2000; calculations by New Strategist*

Leading Causes of Death for Children Aged 5 to 14, 1998

(number and percent distribution of deaths accounted for by the ten leading causes of death for children aged 5 to 14, 1998)

		number	percent distribution
All causes		**7,791**	**100.0%**
1.	Accidents and adverse effects	3,254	41.8
2.	Malignant neoplasms	1,013	13.0
3.	Homicide	460	5.9
4.	Congenital anomalies	371	4.8
5.	Diseases of heart	326	5.9
6.	Suicide	324	4.2
7.	Chronic obstructive pulmonary diseases	152	2.0
8.	Pneumonia and influenza	121	1.6
9.	Benign neoplasms	84	1.1
10.	Cerebrovascular diseases	82	1.1
	All other causes	1,604	20.6

Source: National Center for Health Statistics, Deaths: Final Data for 1998, *National Vital Statistics Reports, Vol. 48, No. 11, 2000; calculations by New Strategist*

Leading Causes of Death for People Aged 15 to 24, 1998

(number and percent distribution of deaths accounted for by the ten leading causes of death for people aged 15 to 24, 1998)

		number	percent distribution
	All causes	**30,627**	**100.0%**
1.	Accidents and adverse effects	13,349	43.6
2.	Homicide	5,506	18.0
3.	Suicide	4,135	13.5
4.	Malignant neoplasms	1,699	5.5
5.	Diseases of the heart	1,057	3.5
6.	Congenital anomalies	450	1.5
7.	Chronic obstructive pulmonary diseases and allied conditions	239	0.8
8.	Pneumonia and influenza	215	0.7
9.	Human immunodeficiency virus infection	194	0.6
10.	Cerebrovascular diseases	178	0.6
	All other causes	3,605	11.8

Source: National Center for Health Statistics, Deaths: Final Data for 1998, *National Vital Statistics Reports, Vol. 48, No. 11, 2000; calculations by New Strategist*

Leading Causes of Death for People Aged 25 to 44, 1998

(number and percent distribution of deaths accounted for by the ten leading causes of death for people aged 25 to 44, 1998)

		number	percent distribution
	All causes	**131,382**	**100.0%**
1.	Accidents and adverse effects	27,172	20.7
2.	Malignant neoplasms	21,407	16.3
3.	Diseases of the heart	16,800	12.8
4.	Suicide	12,202	9.3
5.	Human immunodeficiency virus infection	8,658	6.6
6.	Homicide	8,132	6.2
7.	Chronic liver disease and cirrhosis	3,876	3.0
8.	Cerebrovascular diseases	3,320	2.5
9.	Diabetes mellitus	2,521	1.9
10.	Pneumonia and influenza	1,931	1.5
	All other causes	25,363	19.3

Source: National Center for Health Statistics, Deaths: Final Data for 1998, *National Vital Statistics Reports, Vol. 48, No. 11, 2000; calculations by New Strategist*

Leading Causes of Death for People Aged 45 to 64, 1998

(number and percent distribution of deaths accounted for by the ten leading causes of death for people aged 45 to 64, 1998)

		number	percent distribution
	All causes	**380,203**	**100.0%**
1.	Malignant neoplasms	132,771	34.9
2.	Diseases of the heart	100,124	26.3
3.	Accidents and adverse effects	18,286	4.8
4.	Cerebrovascular diseases	15,362	4.0
5.	Diabetes mellitus	13,091	3.4
6.	Chronic obstructive pulmonary diseases and allied conditions	12,990	3.4
7.	Chronic liver disease and cirrhosis	11,023	2.9
8.	Suicide	8,094	2.1
9.	Pneumonia and influenza	6,023	1.6
10.	Human immunodeficiency virus infection	4,099	1.1
	All other causes	58,340	15.3

Source: National Center for Health Statistics, Deaths: Final Data for 1998, *National Vital Statistics Reports, Vol. 48, No. 11, 2000; calculations by New Strategist*

Leading Causes of Death for People Aged 65 or Older, 1998

(number and percent distribution of deaths accounted for by the ten leading causes of death for people aged 65 or older, 1998)

		number	percent distribution
	All causes	**1,753,220**	**100.0%**
1.	Diseases of the heart	605,673	34.5
2.	Malignant neoplasms	384,186	21.9
3.	Cerebrovascular diseases	139,144	7.9
4.	Chronic obstructive pulmonary diseases and allied conditions	97,896	5.6
5.	Pneumonia and influenza	82,989	4.7
6.	Diabetes mellitus	48,974	2.8
7.	Accidents and adverse effects	32,975	1.9
8.	Nephritis, nephrotic syndrome, nephrosis	22,640	1.3
9.	Alzheimer's disease	22,416	1.3
10.	Septicemia	19,012	1.1
	All other causes	297,315	17.0

Source: National Center for Health Statistics, Deaths: Final Data for 1998, *National Vital Statistics Reports, Vol. 48, No. 11, 2000; calculations by New Strategist*

Life Expectancy by Sex, 1950 to 2050

(years of life remaining at birth by sex, 1950 to 2050; change in years of life remaining for selected years)

	males	females
2050	79.5	84.9
2025	76.5	82.6
1999	74.0	79.7
1998	73.8	79.5
1997	73.6	79.4
1996	73.1	79.1
1995	72.5	78.9
1994	72.4	79.0
1993	72.2	78.8
1992	72.3	79.1
1991	72.0	78.9
1990	71.8	78.8
1980	70.0	77.4
1970	67.1	74.7
1960	66.6	73.1
1950	65.6	71.1
Change		
1999–2050	5.5	5.2
1990–1999	2.2	0.9
1950–1990	6.2	7.7

Source: National Center for Health Statistics, Health, United States, 2000; *and* Projections of the Resident Population by Age, Sex, Race, and Hispanic Origin: 1999 to 2100, *Internet web site <http://www.census.gov/population/www/projections/natproj.html>; and* Deaths: Final Data for 1998, *National Vital Statistics Report, Vol. 48. No. 11, 2000; calculations by New Strategist*

Life Expectancy by Age and Sex, 1998

(years of life remaining at selected ages by sex, 1998)

	total	males	females
Aged 0	76.7	73.8	79.5
Aged 1	76.3	73.4	79.0
Aged 5	72.4	69.5	75.1
Aged 10	67.4	64.6	70.2
Aged 15	62.5	59.7	65.2
Aged 20	57.7	55.0	60.3
Aged 25	53.0	50.3	55.5
Aged 30	48.2	45.7	50.6
Aged 35	43.5	41.0	45.8
Aged 40	38.8	36.4	41.1
Aged 45	34.3	31.9	36.4
Aged 50	29.8	27.6	31.8
Aged 55	25.5	23.5	27.4
Aged 60	21.5	19.6	23.2
Aged 65	17.8	16.0	19.2
Aged 70	14.3	12.8	15.5
Aged 75	11.3	10.0	12.2
Aged 80	8.6	7.5	9.2
Aged 85	6.3	5.5	6.7
Aged 90	4.7	4.1	4.9
Aged 95	3.5	3.0	3.6
Aged 100	2.6	2.3	2.7

Source: National Center for Health Statistics, Deaths: Final Data for 1998, *National Vital Statistics Report, Vol. 48, No. 11, 2000; calculations by New Strategist*

Bibliography

Agency for Health Care Policy and Research, "Health Status and Limitations: A Comparison of Hispanics, Blacks, and Whites, 1996." *MEPS Research Findings* 10, AHCPR Pub. No. 00-0001, 1999. <www.ahcpr.gov>.

"Alternative Medicine Use Common among the Elderly." *The Back Letter* 14, no. 14 (May 1999): 50.

"AMA to Provide Online Initiatives for America's Physicians, Patients." *The Journal of the American Medical Association* 282, no. 20 (November 24, 1999): 51.

American Association of Colleges of Osteopathic Medicine. <www.aacom.org>.

American Association of Colleges of Pharmacy. <www.aacp.org>.

American Association of Colleges of Podiatric Medicine. <www.aacpm.org>.

American Dental Association. <www.ada.org>.

American Dietetic Association. *Americans' Food and Nutrition Attitudes and Behaviors — American Dietetic Association's Nutrition and You: Trends 2000,* January 3, 2000. <www.eatright.org>.

American Hospital Association. <www.aha.org>.

American Medical Association. *Journal of the American Medical Association.* <www.ama.assn.org>.

The American Society for Aesthetic Plastic Surgery. <www.surgery.org>.

Anders, George. *Health Against Wealth: HMOs and the Breakdown of Medical Trust.* New York: Houghton Mifflin, 1996.

"Anger Doubles Risk of Attack for Heart Disease Patients." *The New York Times* (March 19, 1994): 7.

"Are DTC Ads Losing Their Punch?" *Drug Topics* 144, no. 6 (March 20, 2000): 8.

Association of American Medical Colleges. <www.aame.org>.

Association of Schools and Colleges of Optometry. <www.opted.org>.

Astin, John A. "Why Patients Use Alternative Medicine." *Journal of the American Medical Association* 279, no. 19 (May 20, 1998): 1548–1554.

"Balance of Power Needed in Industry." *Health Management Technology* 19, no. 1 (December 1998): 8.

Baransky, Barbara; Jonas, Harry S.; and Etzel, Sylvia I. "Educational Programs in U.S. Medical Schools, 1998-1999." *Journal of the American Medical Association* 282, no. 9 (September 1, 1999): 840–846.

Barret, Joi; Detre, Thomas; Pincus, Harold Alan; et al. "Mental Health Benefits in the Era of Managed Care." *Patient Care* 31, no. 14 (September 15, 1997): 76–83.

Bender, J.P. "Medicare Home Health Care Plunges." *South Florida Business Journal* 20 (May 26, 2000): 1.

Beresford, Larry. "The Good Death: The People of Missoula, Montana, Open a Dialogue on Better Ways to Die." *Hospitals and Health Networks* 71, no. 12 (June 20, 1997): 60–63.

"Black Men Push for More Funding, Education for Prostate Cancer." *Jet* (February 2, 1998): 24–26.

"Black, Hispanic Gay Men Surpass Whites in US AIDS cases." *Medical Industry Today* (January 17, 2000).

Black, Paul Sheldon; and Shimberg, Elaine Fantle. *How to Get Out of the Hospital Alive.* New York: Macmillan, 1997.

"Body Wash and Logo Revamp Enliven Olay's Image." *Drug Store News* (March 6, 2000): 41.

Bower, Bruce. "Social Links May Counter Health Risks." *Science News* 152 (August 30, 1997): 135.

Bureau of the Census. <www.census.gov>.

—. "Americans with Disabilities: 1994–95." *Current Population Reports* P70–61, 1997.

—. *Historical Statistics of the United States: Colonial Times to 1970*, Part 1, 1975.

—. "Preliminary Estimates on Caregiving from Wave 7 of the 1996 Survey of Income and Program Participation." No. 231. The Survey of Income and Program Participation, 1999.

—. Projections of the Resident Population by Age, Sex, Race, and Hispanic Origin: 1999 to 2100. <www.census.gov/population/www/projections/natproj.html>.

—. Unpublished disability data from <www.census.gov/hhes/www/disable/cps/cps199.html> and <www.census.gov/hhes/www/disable/sipp/disable9495.html>.

—. Unpublished health insurance data from the 1998 Current Population Survey and from <www.census.gov/hhes/hlthins/historic/hihist2.html>.

Bureau of Labor Statistics. <www.bls.gov>.

—. *Employee Benefits in Medium and Large Private Establishments, 1997*, Bulletin 2517, 1999.

—. *Employee Benefits in Small Private Establishments, 1996*, Bulletin 2507, 1999.

—. Unpublished data from the 1998 Consumer Expenditure Survey.

Burke, Wylie; Thomson, Elizabeth; Choi, Muin J.; McDonnell, Sharon; Press, Nancy; Barton, James C.; and Beutler, Ernest. "Hereditary Hemochromotosis Gene Discovery and Its Implications for Population Based Screening." *Journal of the American Medical Association* 280, no. 2 (July 8, 1998): 172A.

"California County Women Say Cancer Is God's Punishment." *Cancer Weekly Plus* (January 6, 1997): 14.

Castro, Janice. *The American Way of Health: How Medicine Is Changing and What It Means to You*. Boston: Little, Brown, 1994.

"CDC Finds Low Breastfeeding Rates, More Children Overweight." *Public Health Reports* 3, no. 2 (May 1999): 209.

Centers for Disease Control and Prevention. <www.cdc.gov>.

—. "Media Dissemination of and Public Response to the Ultra Violet Index." *Mortality and Morbidity Weekly Report* 46, no. 17 (1997): 370–374.

—. "Selected Cigarette Smoking Initiation and Quitting Behaviors among High School Students— United States, 1997." *Mortality and Morbidity Weekly Report* 47, no. 19 (1998): 386–389.

—. "Surveillance for Foodborne Disease Outbreaks—United States, 1993–1997." *Mortality and Morbidity Weekly Report* 49, no. 10 (2000): 201–205.

—. "World No-Tobacco Day, May 31, 1999." *Mortality and Morbidity Weekly Report* 7, no. 19 (1998): 1.

Champion, Victoria. "Relationship of Age to Mammography Compliance." *Cancer* 74, no. 1 (July 1, 1994): 329–337.

Camarow, Avery. "The Best Hospitals Are the Best." *US News and World Report* 126, no. 5 (February 8, 1999): 67.

Chronic Disease Notes and Reports Newsletter 13, no. 1 (Winter 2000): 1.

Coe, Jenny. *Blockbuster Lifestyle Drugs*. Datamonitor, 2000.

Collins, Karen Scott; Hall, Allyson; and Neuhaus, Charlotte. *U.S. Minority Health: A Chartbook*. The Commonwealth Fund, 1999.

"Community Indicators of Health-Related Quality of Life—United States 1993–1997." *The Journal of the American Medical Association* 283, no. 6 (April 26, 2000): 2097.

"Computer Terminal Aids Hospital Patients." *Business First of Buffalo* (February 14, 2000): 3.

Conlan, Michael F. "Consumers Speak Out—Our Exclusive Survey Reveals How Consumers Rate Herbals, Internet Pharmacies, DTC Ads and Their Own Rx and More." *Drug Topics* 44, no. 6 (March 20, 2000): 71.

Consumer Healthcare Products Association. *OTC Retail Sales 1964–1999*. July 11, 2000. <www.nmdainfo.org>.

Contreras, Russell. "Texas Official's Remarks Stereotype Latinos." Knight Ridder/Tribune News Service (April 13, 2000): 1983.

Cooper, Laura. "Finding Non-Employment Based Health Insurance." *Inside MS* (Spring 1998): 42–44.

Cuellar, Israel, and Roberts, Robert E. "Relations of Depression, Acculturation, and Socioeconomic Status in a Latino Sample." *Hispanic Journal of Behavioral Sciences* 19, no. 2 (May 1997): 230–239.

David, Richard J., and Collins, James W. Jr. "Differing Birthweights among Infants of U.S. Born Blacks, African Born Blacks and U.S. Born Whites." *The New England Journal of Medicine* 337, no. 17 (October 23, 1997): 1209–1214.

Digman, James J. "Outcomes among African Americans and Caucasians in Colon Cancer Adjuvant Therapy Trials: Findings from the National Surgical Adjuvant Breast and Bowel Project." *Journal of the American Medical Association* 283, no. 5 (February 2, 2000): 583.

Dolliver, Mark. "100." *Adweek* eastern edition 40, no. 150 (December 13, 1999): 74.

Dreyfuss, Ira. "Health Club Targets Truckers." The Associated Press via America Online News (December 14, 1997).

"DTC Drug Ads Should Hit $1 Bil for 1998." *Advertising Age* (January 4, 1999): 1.

Eisenberg, David M.; Kessler, Ronald C.; Foster, Cindy; Norlock, Frances E.; Calkins, David R.; and Delbanco, Thomas L. "Unconventional Medicine in the United States—Prevalence, Cost and Patterns of Use." *The New England Journal of Medicine* 328, no. 4 (January 28, 1993): 246–252.

Elias, Marilyn. "Half of Kids' Ailments Tied to Adults' Smoking," *USA Today* (February 3, 1998). Report available at <www.pediatrics.org>.

—."Violent Home Is a War Zone for Kids." *USA Today* (February 4, 1998): 8B.

Elliot, Stuart. "A Seminar Examines the Plethora of Prescription Drug Pitches Since Regulations Were Loosened." *The New York Times* (June 15, 1998): C11.

Enge, Marilee. "San Carlos, California, Bar Owner's Smoking-Ban Protest Draws Fire." Knight-Ridder/Tribune News Service (January 4, 2000).

The Equifax/Harris Consumer Privacy Survey, 1996. <www.equifax.com>.

"Explosive Growth of Cyberchondriacs Continues." *The Harris Poll* 47 (August 5, 1999). <www.harrisinteractive.com>.

Federal Interagency Forum on Child and Family Statistics. *America's Children: Key National Indicators of Well-Being, 1999*. <http://childstat.gov>.

"Feds Eye Dueling Diets." Third Age News Service (June 1, 2000). <www.thirdage.com>.

Ferry, Jon."Virtual Doctors on the Horizon in Seattle." *The Lancet* 354, no. 9182 (September 11, 1999): 926.

Fleming, Harris Jr. "New Jersey Insurers to Cover Experimental Cancer Treatments." *Drug Topics* 144, no. 3 (February 7, 2000): 115.

"Following ER." Johns Hopkins School of Public Health (June 28, 2000). <http://er.jhsph.edu>.

Food Marketing Institute. *Shopping for Health 1997.*

—. *Trends in the United States—Consumer Attitudes and the Supermarket, 2000.*

"The Frankenfood Monster Stalks Capitol Hill." *Business Week* (December 13, 1999): 55.

Freudenheim, Milt. "Advice Is the Newest Prescription for Health Costs." *The New York Times Online* (April 9, 2000). <www.nytimes.com>.

Furfaro, Danielle. "New York Based Maker of Drug Testing Kits Markets Products to Schools." Knight Ridder Tribune Business News (August 25, 1999).

Gang, Jing; Madhavan, Shantha; and Alderman, Michael H. "The Association between Birthplace and Mortality from Cardiovascular Causes among Black and White Residents of New York City." *The New England Journal of Medicine* 335, no. 21 (November 21, 1996): 1545–1552.

Gellert, George A.; Higgins, Kathleen V.; Lowery, Rosann M.; and Maxwell, Roberta N. "A National Survey of Public Health Officer's Interactions with Media." *Journal of the American Medical Association* 271, no. 16 (April 27, 1994): 1285–1291.

"Generation XXL: Childhood Obesity Now Threatens One in Three Kids with Long Term Health Problems, and the Problem Is Growing." *Newsweek* (July 3, 2000): 40.

Geronimus, Arline T.; Bound, John; Waidmann, Timothy A.; Hillemeier, Marianne H.; and Burns, Patricia B. "Excess Mortality among Blacks and Whites in the United States." *The New England Journal of Medicine* 335, no. 21 (November 21, 1996): 1552–1559.

Ginzberg, Eli. "Managed Care and the Competitive Market: What They Can and Cannot Do." *Journal of the American Medical Association* 277, no. 22 (June 11, 1997): 1812–1814.

Goedert, Joseph. "Medical Societies Enter Web Portal Wars." *Health Data Management* (December 1999).

Goetzl, David. "Second Magazine Study Touts Value of DTC Drug Ads." *Advertising Age* (June 28, 1999): 22.

Golden, Frederic. "Good Eggs, Bad Eggs: The Growing Power of Prenatal Genetic Tests Is Raising Thorny New Questions about Ethics, Fairness and Privacy." *Time* 153, no. 1 (January 11, 1999): 56.

Goldman, Jane."Preventing Malpractice." *Hippocrates* 11, no. 10 (1997): 27–33.

Goldman, Janlori, J.D.; and Hudson, Zoe. "Promoting Health/Protecting Privacy: A Primer," Health Privacy Project, Georgetown University, written for the California HealthCare Foundation and Consumers Union, January 1999. <www.chcf.org>.

Goldman, Janlori, J.D.; Hudson, Zoe; and Smith, Richard M. "Report on the Privacy Policies and Practices of Health Web Sites." Health Privacy Project, Georgetown University, January 2000. <www.chcf.org>.

Gordon, Suzanne. "Nurse, Interrupted." *The American Prospect* (February 14, 2000): 26.

"Guaranteed: Lose 1 Pound in 90 Days." *US News and World Report* 126, no. 7 (February 22, 1999): 67.

Hager, Robert. "Weight-Loss Gurus Debate Fad Diets." MSNBC (February 24, 2000). <www.msnbc.com>.

"The Halt, the Blind and the Dyslexic: Has the Americans with Disabilities Act Gone Too Far, or Not Far Enough?" *The Economist* (April 18, 1998): 25–27.

Harris Interactive. "Harris Interactive Study Reveals a Lack of Information Technology Use in Medicine" (March 28, 2000). <www.harrisinteractive.com>.

Healthcare Financing Administration. <www.hefa.gov>.

Henry J. Kaiser Family Foundation. *Key Facts: Race, Ethnicity and Medical Care*, 1999.

—. *Sources of Financing and the Level of Health Spending for Native Americans*, 1999.

Hingley, Audrey T. "Alzheimers: Few Clues on the Mystery of Memory." *FDA Consumer* 32, no. 2 (May-June 1998): 26.

Industry Week Online Editor (January 7, 1998). <www.industryweek.com>.

International Food Information Council Foundation. <www.ific.org>.

—. "Diets: Look before You Leap," July 1, 2000.

—. *Food for Thought II—Reporting of Diet, Nutrition and Food Safety, Executive Summary*, February 1998.

—. *U.S. Attitudes toward Food Biotechnology*, 2000.

International Food Information Council Foundation and the Center for Media and Public Affairs. *Food for Thought III, A Quantitative and Qualitative Content Analysis of Diet, Nutrition and Food Safety Reporting*, February 2000.

"The Internet Goes Wireless." IDC (February 8, 2000). <www.idc.com>.

"Japanese Fearful Parents Seek Ways to Track Kids." *The Democrat and Chronicle* (June 18, 1998): 14A.

"Japanese Menopause is Different." *Menopause News* (November–December 1996): 1–3.

Joch, Alan. "Getting a Network Transplant." *eWeek* (June 26, 2000): 74.

Jubbel, F. Allan; Chavez, Leo R.; Mishra, Shirz I.; and Valedez, R. Burciaga. "Differing Beliefs about Breast Cancer Among Latinas and Anglo Women." *The Western Journal of Medicine* 164, no. 5. (May 1996): 405–410.

"The Judge Has Not Yet Ruled in a Suit Challenging FDA's Policy on Biotech Food." *Food Chemical News* 42, no. 9 (April 17, 2000): 38.

Kleber, Herbert. "Chapter Six: Abuse and Addiction." In *The Columbia University College of Physicians and Surgeons Complete Home Medical Guide*, 3rd ed. New York: Crown Publishers, 1995.

Kline and Company Inc. *Economic Benefits of Self-Medication—A Final Report to the Nonprescription Drug Manufacturers Association*. May 15, 1997.

Kolata, Gina. "Web Research Transforms Visit to the Doctor." *The New York Times Online* (March 6, 2000). <www.nytimes.com>.

Krueger, Alan; and Levy, Helen. "Accounting for the Slowdown in Employer Health Care Costs." National Bureau of Economic Research *Working Paper* 589, 1998.

Landmark Healthcare Inc. *The Landmark Report on Public Perceptions of Alternative Care*, January 1998.

Landwher, Joseph B.; Zador, Ivan E.; Wolfe, Honor M.; Dombroski, Mitchell P.; and Treadwell, Marjorie C. "Telemedicine and Fetal Ultrasonography: Assessment of Technical Performance and Clinical Feasibility." *American Journal of Obstetrics and Gynecology* 177, no. 3 (September 1997): 846–849.

Lang, Forest. "The Evolving Role of Patient and Physician." *Archives of Family Medicine 9*, no. 1 (January 2000).

Leo, John. "A New Medical Skill: Counting." *US News and World Report* (December 8, 1997): 20.

Little, Jan. " The Changing Images of Disability." *Accent on Living* (Winter 1995): 116–120.

Localio, A. Russell; Hamory, Bruce H.; Sharp, Tonya J.; Weaver, Susan L.; TenHave, Thomas R.; and Landis, J. Richard. "Comparing Hospital Mortality in Adult Patients with Pneumonia: A Case Study of Statistical Methods in a Managed Care Program." *Annals of Internal Medicine* 122, no. 2 (January 15, 1995): 125–133.

Lucas, Beverly D. "White House Focuses on America's Mental Health Needs." *Patient Care* 33, no. 13 (August 15, 1999): 20.

Lynn, Joanne. "An 88-Year-Old Woman Facing the End of Life." *Journal of the American Medical Association* 277, no. 20 (May 28, 1997): 1633–1641.

MacPherson, Peter. "Is This Where We Want to Go?" *The Hastings Center Report* 27, no. 6 (November-December 1997): 17–23.

Makosky, Patti. "HMOs." *Accent on Living* (Fall 1996): 34–38.

Malone, Fergal D.; Nores, Jose A.; Athanassiou, Achilles; Craigo, Sabrina D.; Simpson, Lynn L.; Carmel, Sara H.; and D'Alton, Mary E. "Validation of Fetal Telemedicine as a New Obstetric Technique." *American Journal of Obstetrics and Gynecology* 177, no. 3 (September 1997): 626–629.

Marcus, Bess H. "Exercise Behavior and Strategies for Intervention." *Research Quarterly for Exercise and Sport* 66, no. 4 (December 1995): 319–326.

Martin, Douglas. "Eager to Bite the Hands That Would Feed Them." *The New York Times* (June 1, 1997): D1.

Martin, Sean. "Drug Ads for Consumers Hurt Quality of Care, Article Says. Pharmaceutical Firms Say the Spots Empower Patients." *WebMD* (April 18, 2000). <www.webmd.com>.

Martinez, Yleana. "Sexual Silence: To Battle Aids, Hispanics Must Overcome Cultural Barriers." *Hispanic* (January-February 1997): 100-104.

McCann, Jean. "Friendly Computer Voice Gets People to Take Their Medicine." *Drug Topics* 140, no. 18 (September 16, 1996): 50–52.

McCarthy, Robert. "Rx Ads Hit Consumer Bull's Eye." *Drug Benefit Trends* 10, no. 1 (January 1998): 23.

McCombs, Janet. "Hormone Replacement Therapy." *Drug Store News* (September 22, 1997): 31–35.

McEntee, Christopher. "Florida to Receive $11.3 Billion from Tobacco Industry in Settlement." *The Bond Buyer* 321, no. 30217 (August 26, 1997): 2.

Media Metrix, November 1999. <www.mediametrix.com>

"Medical Monitoring: Web Shirts." *The Economist* 353, no. 8148 (December 4, 1999): 78.

Meier, Diane E.; Emmons, Carol-Ann; Wallenstein, Sylvan; Quill, Timothy; Morrison, R. Sean; and . Cassel, Christine K. "A National Survey of Physician-Assisted Suicide and Euthanasia in the United States." *The New England Journal of Medicine* 338, no. 17 (April 23, 1998): 1193–2000.

Messina, Judith. "Hospital Fights Surgery Sights." *Crain's New York Business* 16 (April 30, 2000): 3.

"Minority Health: Paucity of Docs in Ethnic Communities." *American Health Line* (June 9, 1999).

Natelson, Benjamin H. *Tomorrow's Doctors: The Path to Successful Practice in the 1990's*. New York: Plenum Press, 1990.

National Cancer Institute. "New Project Launched to Study Minority Populations." Press Release, March 26, 1999. <http://rex.nci.nih.gov>.

National Cancer Institute Office of Special Populations Research. "The Cancer Burden." January 28, 2000. <ospr.nci.nih.gov/burden.html>.

National Center for Health Statistics. <www.cdc.gov/nchs>.

—. 1998 Summary: National Hospital Discharge Survey. *Advance Data* 316, 2000.

—. Adoption, Adoption Seeking, and Relinquishment for Adoption in the United States. *Advance Data* 306, 1999.

—. Ambulatory Care Visits to Physician Offices, Hospital Outpatient Departments, and Emergency Departments: United States: 1997. *Vital and Health Statistics*, Series 13, No. 143 (1999).

—. Births: Final Data for 1998, *National Vital Statistics Report* 48, No. 3 (2000).

—. Characteristics of Elderly Home Health Care Users: Data from the 1996 National Home and Hospice Care Survey. *Advance Data* 309 (1999).

—. Characteristics of Elderly Nursing Home Current Residents and Discharges: Data from the 1997 National Nursing Home Survey. *Advance Data* 312 (2000).

—. Characteristics of Hospice Care Users: Data from the 1996 National Home and Hospice Care Survey. *Advance Data* 299 (1998).

—. Current Estimates from the National Health Interview Survey, 1996. *Vital and Health Statistics*, Series 10, No. 200 (1999).

—. Deaths: Final Data for 1998. *National Vital Statistics Report* 48, No. 11 (2000).

—. Fertility, Family Planning, and Women's Health: New Data from the 1995 National Survey of Family Growth. *Vital and Health Statistics*, Series 23, No. 19 (1997).

—. *Health, United States, 1999*. Washington, D.C.: Government Printing Office, 1999.

—. *Health, United States, 2000*. Washington, D.C.: Government Printing Office, 2000.

—. *Healthy People 2000 Review, 1998-99*. Washington, D.C.: 1999.

—. Highlights of Trends in Pregnancies and Pregnancy Rates by Outcome: Estimates for the United States, 1976–96. *National Vital Statistics Reports* 47, No. 29 (1999).

—. National Ambulatory Medical Care Survey: 1998 Summary. *Advance Data* 315 (2000).

—. National Health Interview Survey data from NCHS Health E-Stats.

—. National Hospital Ambulatory Medical Care Survey: 1998 Emergency Department Summary. *Advance Data* 313 (2000).

—. National Hospital Ambulatory Medical Care Survey: 1998 Outpatient Department Summary. *Advance Data* 317 (2000).

—. National Hospital Discharge Survey: Annual Summary: 1997. *Vital and Health Statistics*, Series 13, No. 144 (2000).

—. An Overview of Home Health and Hospice Care Patients: 1996 National Home and Hospice Care Survey. *Advance Data* 297 (1998).

—. "Prevalence of Sedentary Leisure-Time Behavior among Adults in the United States." NCHS Health E-Stats (July 2, 2000).

—. Prevalence of Selected Chronic Conditions: United States, 1990–92. *Vital and Health Statistics*, Series 10, No. 194 (1997).

—. "Trends and Differential Use of Assistive Technology Devices: United States, 1994." *Advance Data* 292 (1997).

—. Trends in Hospital Utilization: United States, 1988–92. *Vital and Health Statistics*, Series 13, No. 124 (1996).

—. Trends in Twin and Triplet Births: 1980–97. *National Vital Statistics Reports* 47, No. 24 (1999).

National Council on Disability. *National Disability Policy: A Progress Report, November 1, 1998–November 19, 1999*. Washington, D.C., 2000.

National Institute of Environmental Health Sciences. "Fact Sheet: The Report on Carcinogens—9th Edition." Press Release (May 15, 2000). <www.niehs.nih.gov>.

National Institute of Mental Health. <www.nimh.nih.gov>.

—. *Mental Illness in America*, June 4, 1998.

—. NIMH Expert Panel on Youth Violence Intervention Research, February 29, 2000.

—. NIMH Research on Treatment for Attention Deficit Hyperactivity Disorder (ADHD): The Multimodal Treatment Study—Questions and Answers, March 2000.

—. "Questions and Answers about St. John's Wort," March 10, 2000.

National Institute on Disability and Rehabilitation Research. "Computer and Internet Use Among People with Disabilities." *Disability Statistics Report 13* (2000).

National Institute on Drug Abuse. *Monitoring the Future National Results on Adolescent Drug Use, Overview of Key Findings, 1999*. 2000. <www.nida.nih.gov>.

National Institutes of Health. "NINDS Funds Five Specialized Neuroscience Programs at Minority Institutions." Press Release, January 18, 2000. <www.nih.gov>.

National League for Nursing. <www.nln.org>.

National Opinion Research Center. Unpublished data from the 1974, 1975, 1996, and 1998 General Social Surveys. <www.norc.uchicago.edu>.

"National Study Finds Most Pharmaceutical Advertising Ineffective with Consumers." *PR Newswire*, December 2, 1998.

Newman, Laura. "U.S. Panel Examines Mental-Health Policies in New York." *The Lancet* 355, no. 9201 (January 29, 2000): 386.

Nielsen//NetRatings. "Nielsen//NetRatings Reports on Internet Year 1999 in Review." (January 20, 2000). < www.nielsentnetratings.com>.

Nonprescription Drug Manufacturers Association. *Self-Medication in the '90's: Practices and Perceptions*. November 1992.

North American Menopause Society. "NAMS 1997 Menopause Survey." <www.menopause.org>.

Office of Minority Health Resource Center. "Why Minorities Are Under-Represented in Clinical Studies." *Closing the Gap* (December 1997/January 1998). <www.omhrc.gov>.

"Open Letter from the Ad Hoc Committee to Defend Health Care." *Journal of the American Medical Association 278*, no. 21 (December 3, 1997): 1733–1739.

"Panel Sees Sharp Upturn for Organics." *Food Processing* 60, no. 10 (October 1999): 16.

Paulin, G.D. and Weber, W.D. "The Effects of Health Insurance on Consumer Spending." *Family Economics and Nutrition Review 9* (Winter 1996): 42–47.

Pew Research Center for the People & the Press. "Investors Now Go Online for Quotes, Advice— Internet Sapping Broadcast News Audience." (June 11, 2000). <www.people-press.org>.

Podell, Richard N. *When Your Doctor Doesn't Know Best: Medical Mistakes that Even the Best Doctors Make and How to Protect Yourself.* New York: Simon and Schuster, 1995.

Pollock, Allyson M.; and Rice, Dorothy P. "Monitoring Health Care in the United States—A Challenging Task." *Public Health Reports* 112, no. 2 (March-April 1997): 108–114.

Poplin, Barry M.; Siega-Riz, Anna Maria; and Haines, Pamela S. "A Comparison of Dietary Trends among Racial and Socioeconomic Groups in the U.S." *The New England Journal of Medicine* 335, no. 21 (November 21, 1996): 716–721.

Pretzer, Michael. "Protecting Patients' Privacy Isn't Coming Easy." *Medical Economics* 77, no. 8 (April 24, 2000): 31.

Prevention Magazine and the American Pharmaceutical Association, *Navigating the Medication Marketplace.* 1997.

"Prevention Magazine Teams with National Colorectal Cancer Research Alliance on Colorectal Cancer Awareness Survey." *PR Newswire*, May 22, 2000.

Quick, Rebecca. "CybeRx: Getting Medical Advice and Moral Support on the Web." *The Wall Street Journal Interactive Edition* (April 30, 1998). <www.wsj.com>.

"Racial Disparities: Whites Get Better Primary Care." *American Health Line* (October 7, 1999).

"Racist Slights That Blacks Face Every Day Are Linked to Their Higher Illness Rates: Study." *Jet* (October 20, 1997): 24–26.

Radford, Tim. "Public Understanding and Biomedical Advance." *The Lancet* 349, no. 9070 (July 5, 1997): 55–57.

"Rating the Diets." *Consumer Reports* (June 1993): 353–355.

Redfearn, Suz. "Hospitals Look to Hotels for Business Tips." *Baltimore Business Journal* 16, no 47 (April 9, 1999): 20.

Rentmeester, Marlene. "Balancing Act." *Women's Sports and Fitness* 2, no. 4 (May 1999): 31.

"Report: Elderly Get Wrong Drugs." Associated Press report via America Online News (November 17, 1996). Attributed to *USA Today.*

Rimm, Eric B.; Willet, Walter C.; Hu, Frank B.; Sampson, Laura; Colditz, Graham A; Manson, JoAnn E. Hennekens, Charles; and Stampfer, Meir J. "Folate and Vitamin B6 From Diet and Supplements in Relation to Risk of Coronary Heart Disease Among Woman." *Journal of the American Medical Association* 279, no. 5 (February 4, 1998): c15.

Ritter, Jim., "Women Redefining Art of Being a Doctor; Gender a Factor in Patient Choices," Sunday News, *Chicago Sun-Times* (February 13, 2000): 6.

Rosa, Linda; Rosa, Emily; Sainer, Larry; and Barret, Stephen. "A Close Look at Therapeutic Touch." *Journal of the American Medical Association* 279, no. 13 (April 1, 1998) 1005–1011.

Rose, Joan R. "Who Else Is Treating Your Patients." *Medical Economics* 77, no. 7 (April 10, 2000): 33.

Rosenthal, Gary E.; Harper, Dwain L.; Quinn, Linda M.; and Cooper, Gregory S. "Severity-adjusted Mortality and Length of Stay in Teaching and Nonteaching Hospitals: Results of a Regional Study." *Journal of the American Medical Association* 278, no. 6 (August 13, 1997): 485–491.

Rothman, David J. *Strangers at the Bedside: A History of How Law and Bioethics Transformed Medical Decision Making*. New York: Basic Books, 1991.

Sanabria, Virna. "Dr. Scholl's in Step." *Global Cosmetic Industry* 166, no. 5 (May 2000): 64.

Saunders, Carol S. "The Surgeon General Advocates for Mental Health." *Patient Care* 34, no. 115 (March 15, 2000): 11.

Savitz, S. Alan. "Mental Health Plans Help Employees, Reduce Costs." *Best's Insurance Review, Life-Health Insurance Edition* 96, no. 3 (July 1995): 60–63.

Shapiro, Joseph P. *No Pity: People with Disabilities Forging a New Civil Rights Movement*. New York: Times Books, 1994.

Sheehy, Gail. "Beyond Virility, A New Vision: Men and Their Doctors Need to Understand That Impotence Is Just One Part of a Complicated Midlife Passage: Call it MANopause." *Newsweek* (November 17, 1997): 69.

Shelton, Deborah L. "Group Focuses on Closing Gap in Minority, White Health." *American Medical News* 42, no. 44 (November 22, 1999): 25.

—. "Home Tests Test Doctor's Role." *American Medical News* 42, no. 13 (April 5, 1999): 26.

Sherrow, Victoria. *The U.S. Health Care Crisis*. Brookfield, Connecticut: Millbrook Press, 1994.

Skolnick, Andrew A. "Hard to Reach Hispanics Get Health News Via Physician's Radio, TV Shows." *Journal of the American Medical Association* 278, no. 4 (July 23, 1997): 269–272.

—. "Lessons from U.S. History of Drug Abuse." *The Journal of the American Medical Association* 277, no. 24 (June 25, 1996): 1919–1921.

"Smoking Cessation in Recovering Alcoholics: Fiction Versus Fact." *American Family Physician* 61, no. 6 (March 15, 2000): 1883.

Sporting Goods Manufacturers Association. *Sports Participation Trends 1999, Statistical Highlights from the Superstudy of Sports Participation* (April 2000). <www.sgma.com>.

Stashenko, Joel. "New York State Gets First Tobacco Settlement Payment." *Marketing News* 34, no. 10 (May 8, 2000): 27.

Stephenson, Joan. "Genetic Test Information Fears Unfounded." *The Journal of the American Medical Association* 282, no. 23 (December 15, 1999): 2197.

Stolberg, Sheryl Gay. "FDA Considers Switching Some Prescription Drugs to Over-the-Counter Status." *New York Times* Online (June 28, 2000). <www.nytimes.com>.

"Study Suggests Poor Cardiac Care Given Blacks and Women is Fault of Doctors' Prejudices." *Jet* 95, no. 15 (March 15, 1999): 46.

"Success Is Working with the Community's Natural Support System." *The Addiction Letter* 12, no. 4 (April 1996): 1–3.

"Texas A&M Bonfire Suspended Two Years." United Press International, June 19, 2000.

Todd, Knox H. "Ethnicity and Analgesic Practice." *The Journal of the American Medical Association* 283, no. 11 (March 15, 2000): 1395.

"Tribe Will Use Casino Profits for Housing, Health Care." *Nation's Cities Weekly* 23, no. 13 (April 3, 2000): 12.

U.S. Department of Agriculture. ARS Food Surveys Research Group. <www.barc.usda.gov/bhnrc/foodsurvey/home.htm>.

—. *Data Tables: Results from USDA's 1994–96 Continuing Survey of Food Intakes by Individuals.*

—. *Diet and Health Knowledge Survey, 1994-95*, 1997.

—. *Diet and Health Knowledge Survey, 1994-96*, 1999.

—. *Food Consumption, Prices, and Expenditures, 1970–1997.* Economic Research Service, 1999.

—. *Supplementary Data Tables: USDA's 1994–96 Continuing Survey of Food Intakes by Individuals*, 1999.

U.S. Department of Justice. "Statement By Attorney General Janet Reno On Impending Television Advertisements For Hard Liquor," Press Release, April 1, 1997.

U.S. Department of Transportation. *Traffic Safety Facts 1998.* National Center for Statistics and Analysis, Washington D.C. <www.nhtsa.dot.gov>.

"U.S. Doctors under Pressure from DTC Ads." *Chemist and Druggist* (November 27, 1999): 11.

U.S. Food and Drug Administration and Nonprescription Drug Manufacturers Association. *Nonprescription Medicines: What's Right for You?* Publication 621-C. Pueblo, Colorado: Consumer Information Center.

U.S. Forest Service. 1994-95 National Survey of Recration and the Environment.

U.S. House of Representatives. Statement of Dr. Steven E. Hyman, Director of the National Institute of Mental Health to the Subcommittee on Labor-DHHS, Education and Related Agencies. Committee on Appropriations, March 4, 1999. <www.nimh.nih.gov>.

U.S. Substance Abuse and Mental Health Services Administrations.

—. *Drug Abuse Warning Network, Annual Examiner Data 1998*, 2000.

—. *Summary of Findings from the 1998 National Household Survey on Drug Abuse*, 1999. <www.samhsa.gov>.

Van Dan, Laura. "The Gene Doctor Is In." *Technology Review*, Massachusetts Institute of Technology (July 1997): 46–52.

Voelker, Rebecca. "Do Ask, Do Tell." *Journal of the American Medical Association* 283, no. 24 (June 28, 2000): 3189.

Wagner, Mary. "Rx Solution: Hispanic Households Most Attractive, Attentive Target with Proper In-Language Approach." *Advertising Age* (August 30, 2000): S16.

"Warning on Elderly Mental Health." *Science News* 156, no. 12 (September 18, 1999): 189.

Weber, Joseph; and Barrett, Amy. "The New Era of Lifestyle Drugs: Viagra and Other Blockbusters Are Transforming the $300 Billion Industry." *Business Week* (May 11, 1998): 98.

Wechsler, Henry; Lee, Jae Eun; Kuo, Meichun; and Lee, Hang. "College Binge Drinking in the 1990s: A Continuing Problem—Results of the Harvard School of Public Health 1999 College Alcohol Study." Harvard School of Public Health. Cambridge, Massachusetts: 2000. <www.hsph.harvard.edu/cas/rpt2000/CAS2000rpt2.html>.

Wells, Claudia. "Faith and Healing." *Time* (June 24, 1996): 58.

WeMedia.com. "People with Disabilities are the Next Consumer Niche." (December 15, 1999). <www.wemedia.com>.

What Do Families Say about Health Care for Children with Special Health Care Needs? The Family Partners Project Report to Families. Family Voices and Brandeis University, 1998. <www.familyvoices.org>.

"What It Would Really Take: Tipper Gore Has Brought a Welcome Focus on the Problem. But Millions of Mentally Ill Americans Aren't Getting the Treatment They Need. And There's No Easy Fix." *Time* 153, no. 22 (June 7, 1999): 54.

"Why Big Tobacco Can't Be Killed." *Business Week* (April 24, 2000): 68.

Wilhelm, Carolyn. "Leveling Demand for Dietary Supplements." *Chemical Market Reporter* 257, no. 22 (May 29, 2000): 8.

Williams, Mark E. *The American Geriatric Society's Complete Guide to Aging and Health.* New York: Harmony Books, 1995.

"Workouts at Work Can Sweeten Long Days, But Don't Cut Loose on the Boss." *US News and World Report* 128, no. 24 (June 19, 2000): 57.

Youngkhill, Lee; and Skalko, Thomas K. "Redefining Health for People with Chronic Disabilities." *The Journal of Physical Education, Recreation and Dance* 67, no. 9 (November-December 1996): 64–66.

Zaldivar, R.A. "Health Statistics Misleading among Members of Asian, Pacific Islander Groups." Knight Ridder Tribune News Service (July 21, 1998): 721k2570.

—. "Long Term Immigrants from Asian, Latin Countries, Gradually Lose Health Advantages." Knight Ridder/Tribune News Service (July 21 1998): 721k2558.

Zanca, Jane. "The Challenge of Multiculturality, or How Do You Say Cancer Care in America?" *Cancer News* 48, no. 1 (Spring 1994): 8–10.

Glossary

Abortion Includes legal abortions only; defined as a procedure performed by a licensed physician or someone acting under the supervision of a licensed physician to induce the termination of a pregnancy.

Acquired immunodeficiency syndrome (AIDS) All 50 states and the District of Columbia report AIDS cases to the Centers for Disease Control and Prevention (CDC) using a uniform case definition and case report form. The data are published semiannually by CDC in HIV/AIDS Surveillance Report. *See* Human immunodeficiency virus (HIV) infection.

Active physician *See* Physician.

Acute condition *See* Condition.

Addition An addition to a psychiatric organization is defined by the Center for Mental Health Services as a new admission, readmission, return from long-term leave, or transfer from another service of the same organization or another organization.

Admission The American Hospital Association defines admissions as patients, excluding newborns, accepted for inpatient services during the survey reporting period. *See* Days of care; Discharge; Patient.

Age of householder *See* Householder, age of.

AIDS *See* Acquired immunodeficiency syndrome.

Ambulatory care Medical care provided at a health care facility or provider's office to persons who are not currently admitted to the health care institution on the premises. *See* Ambulatory patient.

Ambulatory patient Person seeking care from a health care facility or provider's office who is not currently admitted to the health care institution on the premises. *See* Ambulatory care.

Asian In this book, the term Asian includes both Asians and Pacific Islanders. *See* Race.

Average length of stay In the National Health Interview Survey, average length of stay per discharged patient is computed by dividing the total number of hospital days for a specified group by the total number of discharges for that group. In the National Hospital Discharge Survey, average length of stay is computed by dividing the total number of days of care, counting the date of admission but not the date of discharge, by the number of patients discharged. The American Hospital Association computes average length of stay by dividing the number of inpatient days by the number of admissions. Because length of stay computations differ between the organizations, length of stay figures also differ. *See* Days of care; Discharge; Patient.

Baby-boom generation Americans born between 1946 and 1964.

Bed Any bed that is set up and staffed for use by inpatients. For the American Hospital Association, the number of hospital beds is the average number of beds, cribs, and pediatric bassinets during the reporting period. *See* Occupancy rate.

Birth rate *See* Rate: Birth and related rates.

Birthweight The first weight of the newborn obtained after birth. Low birthweight is defined as less than 2,500 grams, or 5 pounds 8 ounces.

Cause of death For the purpose of national mortality statistics, every death is attributed to one underlying condition based on information reported on the death certificate and using the international rules for selecting the underlying cause of death from the reported conditions.

Chronic condition *See* Condition.

Community hospital *See* Hospital.

Condition A health condition is a departure from a state of physical or mental well-being. An impairment is a health condition that includes chronic or permanent health defects resulting from disease, injury, or congenital malformations. Based on duration, there are two categories of conditions, acute and chronic. An acute condition is a condition that has lasted less than three months and has involved either a physician visit (medical attention) or restricted activity. A chronic condition is a condition lasting three months or more or one that is classified as chronic regardless of its time of onset (for example, diabetes, heart conditions, emphysema, and arthritis).

Consumer price index (CPI) The CPI is prepared by the U.S. Bureau of Labor Statistics. It is a monthly measure of the average change in prices paid by urban consumers for a fixed basket of goods and services. The medical care component of the CPI shows trends in medical care prices based on specific indicators of hospital, medical, dental, and drug prices. *See* Health expenditures, national; Gross domestic product.

Consumer unit (on selected spending tables only) The term consumer unit is used by the Bureau of Labor Statistics in the annual Consumer Expenditure Survey. For convenience, the terms consumer unit and household are used interchangeably in the spending tables of this book, although consumer units are somewhat different from households. A consumer unit comprises all related members of a household or a financially independent member of a household. Thus, a household may include more than one consumer unit. *See* Household.

Current smoker Before 1992 a current smoker was determined by the following questions: "Have you ever smoked 100 cigarettes in your lifetime?" and "Do you smoke now?" In 1992, the question was modified to "Do you smoke everyday, some days, or not at all?" Those who smoke everyday or some days are current smokers.

Days of care According to the American Hospital Association, days of care is the number of adult and pediatric days of care rendered during the entire reporting period. Days of care for newborns are excluded. In the National Health Interview Survey, days of care refers to the total number of hospital days of care occurring in the 12-month period before the interview week. A hospital day is defined as one night spent in the hospital by one person admitted as an inpatient. In the National Hospital Discharge Survey, days of care refers to the total number of patient days accumulated by patients at the time of discharge from nonfederal short-stay hospitals during a reporting period. All days from and including the date of admission but not including the date of discharge are counted. *See* Admission; Average length of stay; Discharge; Hospital; Patient.

Death rate *See* Rate: Death and related rates.

Diagnosis *See* First-listed diagnosis.

Discharge The National Health Interview Survey defines a hospital discharge as the completion of any continuous period of stay of one or more nights in a hospital by an inpatient, not including well newborn infants. According to the National Hospital Discharge Survey and American Hospital Association, discharge is the formal release of an inpatient (excluding newborn infants) by a hospital, that is, the termination of a period of hospitalization (including stays of zero   nights) by death or by disposition to a place of residence, nursing home, or another hospital. *See* Admission; Average length of stay; Days of care; Patient.

Emergency department An emergency department is a hospital facility staffed 24-hours a day for the provision of unscheduled outpatient services to patients whose conditions require immediate care. Off-site emergency departments open less than 24 hours are included if staffed by the hospital's emergency department. An emergency department visit is a direct personal exchange between a patient and a physician or other health care provider working under the physician's supervision for the purpose of seeking care and receiving personal health services. *See* Hospital; Outpatient department.

Expenditures *See* Health expenditures, consumer; Health expenditures, national.

Family All persons within a household related to each other by blood, marriage, or adoption. *See* Household; Unrelated individuals.

Family income Each member of a family is classified according to the total income of the family. Unrelated individuals are classified according to their own income. Income is the total income received by the members of a family or by an unrelated individual in the 12 months before the interview. Income includes wages, salaries, rents from property, interest, dividends, profits and fees from a business, pensions, and help from relatives.

Federal hospital *See* Hospital.

Federal physician *See* Physician.

Fertility rate *See* Rate: Birth and related rates.

First-listed diagnosis In the National Hospital Discharge Survey, this is the first recorded final diagnosis on the medical record face sheet.

General hospital *See* Hospital.

Geographic regions The four regions and nine census divisions of the United States are composed as follows:

Northeast:
—New England: Connecticut, Maine, Massachusetts, New Hampshire, Rhode Island, and Vermont
—Middle Atlantic: New Jersey, New York, and Pennsylvania

Midwest:
—East North Central: Illinois, Indiana, Michigan, Ohio, and Wisconsin
—West North Central: Iowa, Kansas, Minnesota, Missouri, Nebraska, North Dakota, and South Dakota

South:
—South Atlantic: Delaware, District of Columbia, Florida, Georgia, Maryland, North Carolina, South Carolina, Virginia, and West Virginia
—East South Central: Alabama, Kentucky, Mississippi, and Tennessee
—West South Central: Arkansas, Louisiana, Oklahoma, and Texas

West:
—Mountain: Arizona, Colorado, Idaho, Montana, Nevada, New Mexico, Utah, and Wyoming
—Pacific: Alaska, California, Hawaii, Oregon, and Washington

Generation X Americans born between 1965 and 1976.

Gestation The period of gestation is defined as beginning with the first day of the last normal menstrual period and ending with the day of birth or day of termination of pregnancy. *See* Abortion; Live birth.

Gross domestic product (GDP) GDP is the market value of the goods and services produced by labor and property located in the United States. The suppliers (that is, the workers and, for property, the owners) may be either U.S. residents or residents of the rest of the world.

Health expenditures, consumer Consumer spending statistics show the amounts spent out-of-pocket on health care products and services by individual consumer units during a 12-month period, including the amount spent on sales tax. The full cost of each purchase is recorded even though full payment may not have been made at the date of purchase. Average expenditure figures may be artificially low for infrequently purchased items such as eyeglasses because figures are calculated using all consumer units within a demographic segment rather than just purchasers. *See* Consumer unit.

Health expenditures, national These statistics show the total amount spent for all health services and supplies and health-related research and construction activities in the United States during one calendar year. Detailed estimates are available by source of expenditure (for example, out-of-pocket payments, private health insurance, and government programs) and by type of expenditure (for example, hospital care, physician services, and drugs). They are in current dollars for the year of report.

—*Personal health care expenditures* National outlays for goods and services relating directly to patient care. Expenditures in this category are total national health expenditures minus expenditures for research and construction, expenses for administering health insurance programs, and government public health activities.

—*Private expenditures* Outlays for services provided or paid for by nongovernmental sources— consumers, insurance companies, private industry, and philanthropic and other nonpatient care sources.

—*Public expenditures* Outlays for services provided or paid for by federal, state, and local government agencies or expenditures required by governmental mandate (such as workmen's compensation insurance payments).

Health maintenance organization (HMO) A prepaid health plan delivering comprehensive care to members through designated providers, having a fixed monthly payment for health care services, and requiring beneficiaries to be plan members for a specified period of time (usually one year). Pure HMO enrollees use only the prepaid capitated health services of the HMO's panel of medical care providers. Open-ended HMO enrollees use the prepaid HMO health services and in addition may receive medical care from providers who are not part of the HMO's panel. Usually a substantial deductible, co-payment, or coinsurance is associated with the use of nonpanel providers. The types of HMOs are:

—*Group* Delivers health services through a physician group that is controlled by the HMO unit or an HMO that contracts with one or more independent group practices to provide health services.

—*Individual practice association (IPA)* Contracts directly with physicians in independent practice and/or one or more associations of physicians in independent practice and/or one or more multispecialty group practices. The plan is predominantly organized around solo-single-specialty practices.

—*Mixed* Combines features of group and IPA. This category was introduced in mid-1990 because HMOs are continually changing and many now combine features of group and IPA plans in a single plan.

Hispanic origin Of Mexican, Puerto Rican, Cuban, Central and South American, and other or unknown Spanish origins. Persons of Hispanic origin may be of any race. In other words, there are black Hispanics, white Hispanics, and Asian Hispanics. *See* Race.

HIV *See* Human immunodeficiency virus infection.

Home health care Care provided to individuals and families in their place of residence for promoting, maintaining, or restoring health or for minimizing the effects of disability and illness including terminal illness.

Hospice care A program of palliative and supportive care services providing physical, psychological, social, and spiritual care for dying persons, their families, and other loved ones. Hospice care is available in home and inpatient settings.

Hospital According to the American Hospital Association, hospitals are licensed institutions with at least six beds whose primary function is to provide diagnostic and therapeutic patient services for medical conditions by an organized physician staff and which have continuous nursing services under the supervision of registered nurses. Hospitals may be classified by type of service, ownership, number of beds, and length of stay. In the National Hospital Ambulatory Medical Care Survey, hospitals include all those with an average length of stay for all patients of less than 30 days (short-stay) and hospitals whose specialty is general (medical or surgical) or children's general. Federal hospitals, hospital units of institutions, and hospitals with fewer than six beds staffed for patient use are excluded. *See* Average length of stay; Bed; Days of care; Emergency Department; Outpatient department; Patient.

—*Community hospital* A nonfederal short-stay hospital except facilities for the mentally retarded, hospital units of institutions, and alcoholism and chemical dependency facilities.

—*Federal hospital* Hospital operated by the federal government.

—*General hospital* Hospital providing diagnostic, treatment, and surgical services for patients with a variety of medical conditions. Excluded are hospitals, usually in rural areas, that provide a more limited range of care.

—*Nonprofit hospital* Hospital operated by a church or other nonprofit organization.

—*Proprietary hospital* Hospital operated for profit by an individual, partnership, or corporation.

—*Short-stay hospital* The National Hospital Discharge Survey defines short-stay hospitals as those in which the average length of stay is less than 30 days. The National Health Interview Survey defines short-stay hospitals as any hospital or hospital department in which the type of service provided is general; maternity; eye, ear, nose, and throat; children's; or osteopathic.

—*Specialty hospital* Hospital that provides a particular type of service to the majority of its patients, such as psychiatric, tuberculosis, chronic disease, rehabilitation, maternity, and alcoholic or narcotic and others.

Hospital-based physician *See* Physician.

Hospital days *See* Days of care.

Household All the persons who occupy a housing unit. A household includes the related family members and all the unrelated persons, if any, such as lodgers, foster children, wards, and employees who share the housing unit. A person living alone is counted as a household. A group of unrelated people who share a housing unit as roommates or unmarried partners is also counted as a household, but group quarters such as college dormitories, prisons, and nursing homes are not.

Householder, age of The age of the householder is used to categorize households into age groups. Married couples, for example, are classified according to the age of either husband or wife depending on which one identified him- or herself as the householder.

Human immunodeficiency virus (HIV) infection In 1987, the National Center for Health Statistics introduced a specific category for classifying HIV infection as a cause of death. Prior to that time, HIV deaths were classified under a variety of codes depending on the specific course taken by the disease. Therefore, beginning with 1987, death statistics for HIV infection are not strictly comparable with data for earlier years. *See* Acquired immunodeficiency syndrome; Cause of death.

Incidence The number of cases of disease having their onset during a prescribed period of time. It is often expressed as a rate, for example, the incidence of measles per 1,000 children aged 5 to 15 during a specified year. Incidence is a measure of morbidity or other events that occur within a specified period of time. *See* Prevalence.

Length of stay *See* Average length of stay.

Life expectancy The average number of years of life remaining to a person at a particular age and is based on a given set of age-specific death rates, generally the mortality conditions existing in the period mentioned. Life expectancy may be determined by race, sex, or other characteristics using age-specific death rates for the population with that characteristic. *See* Rate: Death and related rates.

Limitation of activity A long-term reduction in a person's capacity to perform the usual kind or amount of activities associated with his or her age group. Each person is classified according to the extent to which his or her activities are limited, as follows: unable to carry on major activity, limited in the amount or kind of major activity performed, not limited in major activity but otherwise limited, and not limited in activity. *See* Condition; Major activity.

Live birth The complete expulsion or extraction from its mother of a product of conception, irrespective of the duration of the pregnancy, which, after such separation, breathes or shows any other evidence of life such as heartbeat, umbilical cord pulsation, or definite movement of voluntary muscles, whether the umbilical cord has been cut or the placenta is attached. Each product of such a birth is considered live born. *See* Rate: Birth and related rates.

Live-birth order The total number of live births the mother has had, including the present birth, as recorded on the birth certificate. Fetal deaths are excluded. *See* Live birth.

Low birthweight *See* Birthweight.

Major (or usual) activity The principal activity of a person or of his or her age-sex group. For children aged 1 to 5, major activity refers to ordinary play with other children; for children aged 5 to 17, major activity refers to school attendance; for adults aged 18 to 69, major activity usually refers to a job, housework, or school attendance; for persons aged 70 or older, major activity refers to the capacity for independent living (bathing, shopping, dressing, and eating without needing the help of another person). *See* Limitation of activity.

Marital status The term married encompasses all married people including those separated from their spouses. Unmarried includes those who are single (never married), divorced, or widowed.

Medicaid This program provides health care services for certain low-income persons. It is state operated and administered but has federal financial participation. Within certain broad federally determined guidelines, states decide on eligibility; the amount, duration, and scope of services covered; rates of payment for providers; and methods of administering the program. Medicaid does not provide health services to all poor people in every state. It categorically covers participants in the Aid to Families with Dependent Children program and in the Supplemental Security Income program. In most states it also covers certain other people deemed to be medically needy. The program was authorized in 1965 by Title XIX of the Social Security Act. *See* Health expenditures, national; Health maintenance organization; Medicare.

Medical specialties *See* Physician specialty.

Medicare This nationwide health insurance program provides health insurance protection to people aged 65 or older, people entitled to Social Security disability payments for two or more years, and people with end-stage renal disease, regardless of income. The program was enacted July 30, 1965, as Title XVIII, Health Insurance for the Aged of the Social Security Act, and became effective on July 1, 1966. It consists of two separate but coordinated programs, hospital insurance (Part A) and supplementary medical insurance (Part B). *See* Health expenditures, national; Health maintenance organizations; Medicaid.

Mental health organization The Center for Mental Health Services defines a mental health organization as an administratively distinct public or private agency or institution whose primary concern is the provision of direct mental health services to the mentally ill or emotionally disturbed. Excluded are private office-based practices of psychiatrists, psychologists, and other mental health providers; psychiatric services of all types of hospitals and outpatient clinics operated by federal agencies other than the Department of Veterans Affairs; general hospitals that have no separate psychiatric services but admit psychiatric patients to nonpsychiatric units; and psychiatric services of schools, colleges, halfway houses, community residential organizations, local and county jails, state prisons, and other human service providers. The major types of mental health organizations are described below.

—*Freestanding psychiatric outpatient clinic* Provides only outpatient services on either a regular or an emergency basis. Medical responsibility for services is generally assumed by a psychiatrist.

—*General hospital providing separate psychiatric services* Nonfederal general hospital that provides psychiatric services either in a separate psychiatric inpatient or outpatient unit or through partial hospitalization service with assigned staff and space.

—*Multiservice mental health organization* Directly provides two or more of the program elements defined under mental health service type and is not classifiable as a psychiatric hospital, general hospital, or residential treatment center for emotionally disturbed children.

—*Partial care organization* Provides a program of ambulatory mental health services.

—*Private mental hospital* Operated by a sole proprietor, partnership, limited partnership, corporation, or nonprofit organization primarily for the care of persons with mental disorders.

—*Psychiatric hospital* Primarily concerned with providing inpatient care and treatment for the mentally ill. Psychiatric inpatient units of Department of Veterans Affairs general hospitals and Department of Veterans Affairs neuropsychiatric hospitals are combined into the category Department of Veterans Affairs psychiatric hospitals because of their similarity in size, operation, and length of stay.

—*Residential treatment center for emotionally disturbed children* Must meet all of the following criteria: (a) not licensed as a psychiatric hospital and primary purpose is to provide individually planned mental health treatment services in conjunction with residential care; (b) include a clinical program directed by a psychiatrist, psychologist, social worker, or psychiatric nurse with a graduate degree; (c) serve children and youths primarily under the age of 18; and (d) primary diagnosis for the majority of admissions is mental illness classified as other than mental retardation, developmental disability, and substance-related disorders.

—*State and county mental hospital* Under the auspices of a state or county government or operated jointly by state and county governments.

Mental health service type Refers to the following kinds of mental health services:

—*Inpatient care* The provision of 24-hour mental health care in a mental health hospital setting.

—*Outpatient care* The provision of ambulatory mental health services for less than three hours per single visit to an individual, group, or family, usually in a clinic or similar facility. Also includes emergency walk-in care, as well as care provided by mobile teams that visit patients outside these facilities. "Hotline" services are excluded.

—*Partial care treatment* A planned program of mental health treatment services generally provided in units of three or more hours to groups of patients. Includes treatment programs that emphasize intensive short-term therapy and rehabilitation; programs that focus on recreation and/or occupational activities, including sheltered workshops; and education and training programs, including special education classes, therapeutic nursery schools, and vocational training.

—*Residential treatment care* The provision of overnight mental health care in conjunction with an intensive treatment program in a setting other than a hospital. Facilities may offer care to emotionally disturbed children or mentally ill adults.

Metropolitan area A county or group of counties that includes at least one city having a population of 50,000 or more plus adjacent counties that are metropolitan in character and are economically and socially integrated with the central city. In New England, towns and cities rather than counties are the units used in defining metropolitan areas. There is no limit to the number of adjacent counties included in the metropolitan area as long as they are integrated with the central city. A metropolitan area's boundaries may cross state lines.

Nonfederal physician *See* Physician.

Nonprofit hospital *See* Hospital.

Non-Hispanic People who do not identify themselves as Hispanic. Non-Hispanics may be of any race. *See* Hispanic; Race.

Nonmetropolitan area Counties that are not classified as metropolitan. *See* Metropolitan area.

Nursing home An establishment with three or more beds that provides nursing or personal care services to the aged, infirm, or chronically ill.

Occupancy rate The American Hospital Association defines the hospital occupancy rate as the average daily census divided by the average number of hospital beds during a reporting period. Average daily census is defined as the average number of inpatients, excluding newborns, receiving care each day during a reporting period.

Office In the National Health Interview Survey, the term office refers to the office of any physician in private practice not located in a hospital. In the National Ambulatory Medical Care Survey, an office is any location for a physician's ambulatory practice other than a hospital, nursing home, other extended care facility, patient home, industrial clinic, college clinic, and family planning clinic. Private offices in hospitals, however, are included. *See* Office visit; Outpatient visit; Physician; Physician contact.

Office-based physician *See* Physician.

Office visit In the National Ambulatory Medical Care Survey, an office visit is any direct personal exchange between an ambulatory patient and a physician or member of his or her staff for the purposes of seeking care and rendering health services. *See* Ambulatory care; Ambulatory patient; Outpatient visit; Physician contact.

Operation *See* Procedure.

Outpatient department According to the National Hospital Ambulatory Medical Care Survey, an outpatient department is a hospital facility where nonurgent ambulatory medical care is provided, excluding ambulatory surgical centers, employee health services, and facilities providing chemotherapy, renal dialysis, methadone maintenance, and radiology. An outpatient department visit is a direct personal exchange between a patient and a physician or other health care provider working under the physician's supervision for the purpose of seeking care and receiving personal health services. *See* Ambulatory care; Ambulatory patient; Emergency department, Hospital.

Outpatient visit The American Hospital Association defines outpatient visits as visits for receipt of medical, dental, or other services by patients who are not lodged in the hospital. Each appearance by an outpatient to each unit of the hospital is counted individually as an outpatient visit. *See* Ambulatory care, Ambulatory patient, Office visit, Physician contact.

Patient A person who is formally admitted to the inpatient service of a hospital for observation, care, diagnosis, or treatment. *See* Admission; Ambulatory patient; Average length of stay; Days of care; Discharge; Hospital.

Percent change The change (either positive or negative) in a measure expressed as a proportion of the starting measure.

Percentage point change The change (either positive or negative) in a value which is already expressed as a percentage.

Personal health care expenditures *See* Health expenditures, national.

Physician Physicians are classified by the American Medical Association and others as licensed doctors of medicine or osteopathy, as follows:

—*Active (or professionally active) physician* Physician currently practicing medicine for a minimum of 20 hours per week. Excluded are physicians who are inactive, practicing medicine less than 20 hours per week, have unknown addresses, or practice specialties not classified (when specialty information is presented).

—*Federal physician* Physician employed by the federal government.

—*Hospital-based physician* Physician who spends plurality of time as salaried physician in a hospital.

—*Office-based physician* Physician who spends plurality of time working in a practice based in a private office. *See* Office; Physician contact; Physician specialty.

Physician contact In the National Health Interview Survey, a physician contact is defined as a consultation with a physician, in person or by telephone, for examination, diagnosis, treatment, or advice. The service may be provided by the physician or by another person working under the physician's supervision. Contacts involving services provided on a mass basis (for example, blood pressure screenings) and contacts for hospital inpatients are not included. In the National Health Interview Survey, physician contacts are based on a two-week recall period and are adjusted to produce average annual number of contacts. *See* Place of contact.

Physician specialty Any specific branch of medicine in which a physician may concentrate. Data are based on physician self-reports of their primary area of specialty. Physician data are broadly categorized into two general areas of practice: generalists and specialists.

—*Generalist physician* Synonymous with primary care generalist. Includes physicians practicing in the general fields of family and general practice, general internal medicine, and general pediatrics. Specifically excludes primary care specialists.

—*Primary care specialist* Physician practicing in the subspecialties of general and family practice, internal medicine, and pediatrics. The primary care subspecialties for family practice include such specialties as geriatric medicine and sports medicine. For internal medicine they include such specialties as infectious diseases, medical oncology, and rheumatology. For pediatrics they include such specialties as critical care pediatrics, and pediatric cardiology.

—*Specialist physician* Those practicing in primary care subspecialties and all other specialist fields not included in the generalist definition. Specialist fields include allergy and immunology, anesthesiology, child and adolescent psychiatry, dermatology, general surgery, obstetrics and gynecology, and psychiatry.

Place of contact The location at which patients receive the services of a physician. This could be an office, hospital outpatient clinic, emergency room, telephone call (advice given by a physician in a telephone call), at home (any place in which a person was staying at the time a physician was called there), or at a clinic, HMO, and other place located outside a hospital. *See* Physician contact.

Prevalence The number of cases of a disease, infected persons, or persons with some other problem during a particular interval of time. It is often expressed as a rate, for example, the prevalence of diabetes per 1,000 persons during one year. *See* Incidence.

Primary admission diagnosis In the National Home and Hospice Care Survey, the primary admission diagnosis is the first-listed diagnosis at admission on the patient's medical record as provided by the agency staff member most familiar with the care provided to the patient.

Primary care specialties *See* Physician specialty.

Private expenditures *See* Health expenditures, national.

Procedure The National Hospital Discharge Survey defines procedure as a surgical or nonsurgical operation, diagnostic procedure, or special treatment assigned by the physician and recorded on the medical record of patients discharged from the inpatient service of short-stay hospitals. A maximum of four operations or diagnostic procedures are permitted per discharge. Procedures are subdivided into diagnostic and other nonsurgical procedures and surgical operations.

—Diagnostic and other nonsurgical procedures Procedures generally not considered to be surgery, including diagnostic endoscopy, radiography, and other tests as well as physical medicine and rehabilitation.

—Surgical operations The American Hospital Association defines surgery as a major or minor surgical episode performed in the operating room. During a single episode, multiple surgical procedures may be performed, but the episode is considered as one surgical operation. In contrast to this definition, the National Hospital Discharge Survey codes up to four surgical procedures per surgical episode.

Proprietary hospital *See* Hospital.

Public expenditures *See* Health expenditures, national.

Race The racial groups are American Indian or Alaskan Native, Asian or Pacific Islander, black, and white. Newborns and children of mixed race are classified according to the race of the mother. *See* Asian; Hispanic.

Rate The measure of some event, disease, or condition in relation to a unit of population, along with some specification of time.

Birth and related rates:
—Birth rate: Calculated by dividing the number of live births in a population in one year by the midyear resident population. Birth rate is expressed as the number of live births per 1,000 population. The rate may be restricted to births to women of specific age, race, marital status, or geographic location.
—Fertility rate: The number of live births per 1,000 women of reproductive age, 15 to 44.

Death and related rates:
—Death rate: Calculated by dividing the number of deaths in a population in one year by the midyear resident population. Death rate is expressed as the number of deaths per 100,000 population. The rate may be restricted to deaths in specific age, race, sex, or geographic groups or from specific causes of death.
—Infant mortality rate: Calculated by dividing the number of infant deaths during one year by the number of live births reported in the same year.

Region *See* Geographic regions.

Short-stay hospital *See* Hospital.

Smoker *See* Current smoker.

Specialty hospital *See* Hospital.

Surgical operations *See* Procedure.

Unrelated individuals Persons who live alone or with others to whom they are not related by blood, marriage, or adoption. *See* Family; Household.

Index

Quality of Life's End Missoula Demonstration
Project, 401

Race. *See also* Asian, Black, Hispanic, Native, and
White Americans.
  factor in health status, 107–117, 123
Radford, Tim, author, 170
Real Med Corporation, 58
Recreational activities, 255, 262, 268–270
Restaurants, 258, 286–287
Riche, Martha Farnsworth, former Census Bureau
director, 396
Robert Wood Johnson Medical Center, 56
Robert's American Gourmet, 261
Robertson, Kai, researcher, 253
Rochester General Hospital, 116
Rolling Strong Gym, 260
Rosa, Emily, researcher, 198
Rothman, David J., author, 53

Saccharine, 253
Satcher, David, surgeon general, 359
Savitz, S. Alan, author, 358
Schizophrenia, 351–353
Scripps Health, 192
Self-care, 183–199
Shalala, Donna, secretary of Department of Health
and Human Services, 20
Shapiro, Joseph P., author, 335
Sheehy, Gail, author, 396
Skolnick, Andre A., researcher, 109–110, 372
Smoking. *See* Cigarette smoking.
Sobe, 261
Society of Human Resource Managers, 260
Sporting Goods Manufacturers Association, 255,
262
State Children's Health Insurance Program
(SCHIP), 22
Substance Abuse and Mental Health Services
Administrations, 371
Suicide, physician-assisted, 398, 401, 428
Supreme Court, 330–331, 339, 398
Surgery,
  centers, 191
  cosmetic, 391, 395, 420–421
  outpatient, 17, 191–192

Teenagers
  abortion rate, 407
  alcohol consumption, 377–378, 384–385
  births, 392–393, 412–416, 418
  cigarette smoking, 377–379, 382–383, 389
  contraceptive use, 404–405
  illegal drug use, 371, 377–379, 386–387
  physical activity of, 254
  risk behavior, 377–379
  surveillance of, 379
  targeted by tobacco advertising, 378
Telemedicine, 195–196
Texas A & M University, 378
Title IX, 253
Tobacco industry
  advertising directed at teenagers, 378
  regulation of, 372–374, 378
Tolbert, Al, bar owner, 373
Tropicana, 261
Tuskegee Syphilis Study, 108

Ultraviolet index, 166
United States Government
  regulation of alternative medicine, 197–198
  regulation of home health care, 195
  regulation of organic food industry, 197
  regulation of tobacco industry, 372–373, 378
Universal design, 338
University Medical Center, Las Vegas, 190
University of California at San Francisco, 189
University of Michigan Institute for Social
Research, 108
University of Pennsylvania Cancer Center, 189
University of Puerto Rico, 115

Virtual Cinic, 62
Vitamins
  media reporting on, 181
  spending on, 31, 33, 35, 37
  use by age and sex, 257, 275

Wake Forest University, 115
Walking for exercise, 255, 268
Wayne-Doppke, Jennifer, author, 170
Webb, Susan, company president, 336
Weber, W.D., author, 19–20
WebMD.com, 168, 179